Urology: A Clinician's Guide

Urology: A Clinician's Guide

Editor: Ezra Martin

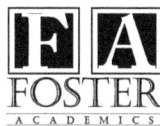

FA
FOSTER
ACADEMICS

www.fosteracademics.com

www.fosteracademics.com

FA FOSTER
ACADEMICS

Cataloging-in-Publication Data

Urology : a clinician's guide / edited by Ezra Martin.
      p. cm.
Includes bibliographical references and index.
ISBN 978-1-63242-966-7
1. Urology. 2. Genitourinary organs--Diseases. 3. Urinary organs--Diseases.
4. Urologists--Guidebooks. I. Martin, Ezra.

RC871 .U76 2020

616.6--dc23

Foster Academics,
118-35 Queens Blvd., Suite 400,
Forest Hills, NY 11375, USA

ISBN 978-1-63242-966-7 (Hardback)

Contents

Preface IX

Chapter 1 **Association between the hemodialysis adequacy and sexual dysfunction in chronic renal failure** 1
Jae Heon Kim, Seung Whan Doo, Won Jae Yang, Soon Hyo Kwon, Eun Seop Song, Hong Jun Lee, Ik Sung Lim, Hyun Hwang and Yun Seob Song

Chapter 2 **Survival and prognostic factors for adrenocortical carcinoma** 7
Zlatibor Loncar, Vladimir Djukic, Vladan Zivaljevic, Tatjana Pekmezovic, Aleksandar Diklic, Svetislav Tatic, Dusko Dundjerovic, Branislav Olujic, Nikola Slijepcevic and Ivan Paunovic

Chapter 3 **Modern extraction techniques and their impact on the pharmacological profile of *Serenoa repens* extracts for the treatment of lower urinary tract symptoms** 14
Celeste De Monte, Simone Carradori, Arianna Granese, Giovanni Battista Di Pierro, Costantino Leonardo and Cosimo De Nunzio

Chapter 4 **Early results of a novel technique for anterior vaginal wall prolapse repair: anterior vaginal wall darn** 25
Osman Köse, Hasan S Sağlam, Şükrü Kumsar, Salih Budak, Hüseyin Aydemir and Öztuğ Adsan

Chapter 5 **Vapoenucleation of the prostate using a high-power thulium laser** 31
Ching-Hsin Chang, Tzu-Ping Lin, Yen-Hwa Chang, William JS Huang, Alex TL Lin and Kuang-Kuo Chen

Chapter 6 **Prediction of open urinary tract in laparoscopic partial nephrectomy by virtual resection plane visualization** 38
Daiki Ueno, Kazuhide Makiyama, Hiroyuki Yamanaka, Takashi Ijiri, Hideo Yokota and Yoshinobu Kubota

Chapter 7 **Treatment by a nurse practitioner in primary care improves the severity and impact of urinary incontinence in women** 44
Doreth T. A. M Teunissen, Marjolein M. Stegeman, Hans H. Bor and Toine A. L. M Lagro-Janssen

Chapter 8 **Simultaneous retrograde intrarenal surgery for ipsilateral asymptomatic renal stones in patients with ureteroscopic symptomatic ureteral stone removal** 52
Dehui Lai, Meiling Chen, Yongzhong He and Xun Li

Chapter 9 **Does visualisation during urethrocystoscopy provide pain relief?** 58
J. Koenig, S. Sevinc, C. Frohme, H. Heers, R. Hofmann and A. Hegele

Chapter 10   **Protocol for a randomized, placebo-controlled, double-blind clinical trial investigating sacral neuromodulation for neurogenic lower urinary tract dysfunction** 64
Stephanie C Knüpfer, Martina D Liechti, Livio Mordasini, Dominik Abt,
Daniel S Engeler, Jens Wöllner, Jürgen Pannek, Bernhard Kiss,
Fiona C Burkhard, Marc P Schneider, Elena Miramontes, Alfons G Kessels,
Lucas M Bachmann and Thomas M Kessler

Chapter 11   **Wide-neck renal artery aneurysm: parenchymal sparing endovascular treatment with a new device**... 70
Michele Rossi, Gianluca Maria Varano, Gianluigi Orgera, Alberto Rebonato,
Florindo Laurino and Cosimo De Nunzio

Chapter 12   **Extravascular stent management for migration of left renal vein endovascular stent in nutcracker syndrome**... 75
Lu Tian, Shanwen Chen, Gaoyue Zhang, Hongkun Zhang,
Wei Jin and Ming Li

Chapter 13   **Pain and satisfaction during rigid cystoscopic ureteral stent removal**.. 79
Jae Heon Kim, Sun Young Park, Mun Gyu Kim, Hoon Choi, Dan Song,
Sung Woo Cho and Yun Seob Song

Chapter 14   **Disease-specific outcomes of Radical Prostatectomies in Northern Norway; a case for the impact of perineural infiltration and postoperative PSA-doubling time**.. 85
Sigve Andersen, Elin Richardsen, Yngve Nordby, Nora Ness,
Øystein Størkersen, Khalid Al-Shibli, Tom Donnem, Helena Bertilsson,
Lill-Tove Busund, Anders Angelsen and Roy M Bremnes

Chapter 15   **Treatment of genital lesions with diode laser vaporization** 96
Mário Maciel de Lima Jr, Mário Maciel de Lima and Fabiana Granja

Chapter 16   **Measuring the improvement in health-related quality of life using King's health questionnaire in non-obese and obese patients with lower urinary tract symptoms after alpha-adrenergic medication** 101
Jae Heon Kim, Hoon Choi, Hwa Yeon Sun, Seung Whan Doo, Jong Hyun Yoon,
Won Jae Yang, Byung Wook Yoo, Joyce Mary Kim, Soon-Sun Kwon,
Eun Seop Song, Hong Jun Lee, Ik Sung Lim and Yun Seob Song

Chapter 17   **The role of diagnostic ureteroscopy in the era of computed tomography urography**.. 109
Shay Golan, Andrei Nadu and David Lifshitz

Chapter 18   **Clinical relevance of aortic calcification in urolithiasis patients** 114
Toshikazu Tanaka, Shingo Hatakeyama, Hayato Yamamoto, Takuma Narita,
Itsuto Hamano, Teppei Matsumoto, Osamu Soma, Yuki Tobisawa,
Tohru Yoneyama, Takahiro Yoneyama, Yasuhiro Hashimoto, Takuya Koie,
Ippei Takahashi, Shigeyuki Nakaji, Yuriko Terayama, Tomihisa Funyu and
Chikara Ohyama

Chapter 19   Probiotics [LGG-BB12 or RC14-GR1] versus placebo as prophylaxis for urinary
tract infection in persons with spinal cord injury [ProSCIUTTU]...................................... 123
Bonsan Bonne Lee, Swee-Ling Toh, Suzanne Ryan, Judy M. Simpson, Kate Clezy,
Laetitia Bossa, Scott A. Rice, Obaydullah Marial, Gerard Weber, Jasbeer Kaur,
Claire Boswell-Ruys, Stephen Goodall, James Middleton, Mark Tudehope and
George Kotsiou

Chapter 20   Genomic copy number variation association study in Caucasian patients
with nonsyndromic cryptorchidism.. 131
Yanping Wang, Jin Li, Thomas F. Kolon, Alicia Olivant Fisher, T. Ernesto Figueroa,
Ahmad H. BaniHani, Jennifer A. Hagerty, Ricardo Gonzalez, Paul H. Noh,
Rosetta M. Chiavacci, Kisha R. Harden, Debra J. Abrams, Deborah Stabley,
Cecilia E. Kim, Katia Sol-Church, Hakon Hakonarson, Marcella Devoto and
Julia Spencer Barthold

Chapter 21   Developing a preoperative predictive model for ureteral length for ureteral
stent insertion.. 139
Takashi Kawahara, Kentaro Sakamaki, Hiroki Ito, Shinnosuke Kuroda,
Hideyuki Terao, Kazuhide Makiyama, Hiroji Uemura, Masahiro Yao,
Hiroshi Miyamoto and Junichi Matsuzaki

Chapter 22   Sacral neuromodulation for the treatment of neurogenic lower urinary tract
dysfunction caused by multiple sclerosis... 144
Daniel S. Engeler, Daniel Meyer, Dominik Abt, Stefanie Müller and
Hans-Peter Schmid

Chapter 23   Design of a single-arm clinical trial of regenerative therapy by periurethral
injection of adipose-derived regenerative cells for male stress urinary
incontinence in Japan: the ADRESU study protocol 150
Shinobu Shimizu, Tokunori Yamamoto, Shinobu Nakayama, Akihiro Hirakawa,
Yachiyo Kuwatsuka, Yasuhito Funahashi, Yoshihisa Matsukawa, Keisuke Takanari,
Kazuhiro Toriyama, Yuzuru Kamei, Kazutaka Narimoto, Tomonori Yamanishi,
Osamu Ishizuka, Masaaki Mizuno and Momokazu Gotoh

Chapter 24   Protocol for a prospective, randomized study on neurophysiological
assessment of lower urinary tract function in a healthy cohort 157
Stéphanie van der Lely, Martina Stefanovic, Melanie R. Schmidhalter,
Marta Pittavino, Reinhard Furrer, Martina D. Liechti, Martin Schubert,
Thomas M. Kessler and Ulrich Mehnert

Chapter 25   Sociodemographic correlates of urine culture test utilization in Calgary,
Alberta 164
Thomas P. Griener, Christopher Naugler, Wilson W. Chan and
Deirdre L. Church

Chapter 26   An observational study of the use of beclomethasone dipropionate
suppositories in the treatment of lower urinary tract inflammation in men 171
Giorgio Bozzini, Marco Provenzano, Nicolò Buffi, Mauro Seveso,
Giovanni Lughezzani, Giorgio Guazzoni, Alberto Mandressi and
Gianluigi Taverna

Chapter 27   **Role for intravesical prostatic protrusion in lower urinary tract symptom: a fluid structural interaction analysis study** 179
Junming Zheng, Jiangang Pan, Yi Qin, Jiale Huang, Yun Luo, Xin Gao and Xing Zhou

Chapter 28   **Wilms tumor with inferior vena cava duplication** 188
Feng Guo, Tianyou Li, Wei Liu, Gang Wang, Rui Ma and Rongde Wu

Chapter 29   **Spontaneous ureteric rupture, a reality or a faux pas?** 192
Gaurav Aggarwal and Samiran Das Adhikary

Chapter 30   **Bioelectrical activity of the pelvic floor muscles during synchronous whole-body vibration** 196
Magdalena Stania, Daria Chmielewska, Krystyna Kwaśna, Agnieszka Smykla, Jakub Taradaj and Grzegorz Juras

Chapter 31   **A rare diaphragmatic ureteral herniation case report: endoscopic and open reconstructive management** 206
Frank C. Lin, Jamie S. Lin, Samuel Kim and Jonathan R. Walker

Chapter 32   **Spontaneous renal allograft rupture complicated by urinary leakage** 210
Evaldo Favi, Samuele Iesari, Alessandro Cina and Franco Citterio

Chapter 33   **Congenital mid-ureteral stricture: a case report of two patients** 217
Hamdan Alhazmi and Abdullah Fouda Neel

Chapter 34   **Systemic analysis of urinary stones from the Northern, Eastern, Central, Southern and Southwest China** 221
Rui-hong Ma, Xiao-bing Luo, Qin Li and Hai-qiang Zhong

Permissions

List of Contributors

Index

Preface

Urology is a field of medical science which deals with the diseases of the male and female urinary tract. The disorders of the bladder, male reproductive organs, prostate and the urethra are treated in this medical discipline. This includes the management of bladder stones, congenital disorders, erectile dysfunction, incontinence, tumors and cancers, infertility, sterilization, etc. Various techniques of urologic imaging are used for the visualization of the urinary tract. These include antegrade pyelography, cystography, cystourethrography, intravenous pyelogram, radioisotope renography, etc. The treatment of many urologic disorders can be achieved with minimally invasive techniques such as key-hole surgery and endoscopic procedures. Some disorders may require open surgery, such as removal of kidney, bladder or prostate for treating cancer, bladder construction after removal, vasectomy, etc. This book is a valuable compilation of topics, ranging from the basic to the most complex advancements in the field of urology. From theories to research to practical applications, case studies related to all contemporary topics of relevance to this field have been included in this book. It will help new researchers by foregrounding their knowledge in this field.

The information shared in this book is based on empirical researches made by veterans in this field of study. The elaborative information provided in this book will help the readers further their scope of knowledge leading to advancements in this field.

Finally, I would like to thank my fellow researchers who gave constructive feedback and my family members who supported me at every step of my research.

Editor

Association between the hemodialysis adequacy and sexual dysfunction in chronic renal failure

Jae Heon Kim[1], Seung Whan Doo[1], Won Jae Yang[1], Soon Hyo Kwon[2], Eun Seop Song[3], Hong Jun Lee[4], Ik Sung Lim[5], Hyun Hwang[6] and Yun Seob Song[1*]

Abstract

Background: The core question of the study was whether adequately achieved HD affected the sexual dysfunction in women on hemodialysis (HD) with chronic renal failure (CRF).

Methods: Thirty-seven female patients on HD, including 18 women with adequate HD and 19 women with non-adequate HD, and 36 healthy controls were included in this study. Demographic and clinical variables, including the sexual hormones estradiol and testosterone, were recorded. Sexual function was assessed according to the Female Sexual Function Index (FSFI) and results were compared between groups. Adequate HD was defined as an average urea clearance of over 1.3 (Kt/V) over three consecutive months.

Results: All domains of the FSFI questionnaire, with the exception of satisfaction, were higher in the control group than in the HD group. In comparing the adequate and non-adequate HD groups, there was no difference in any of the six domains of the FSDI questionnaire. Among the clinical variables, the number of menopausal women was higher in the HD group than in the control group ($P = 0.023$). Estradiol and testosterone levels were higher in the control group than in the HD group ($P = 0.003$, 0.027, respectively). The number of menopausal women and estradiol and testosterone levels showed no differences between the adequate and non-adequate HD groups. Correlation analysis between Kt/V and FSFI showed no significant relationship, but estrogen did show a significant relationship with FSFI (correlation coefficient $= 0.399$, $P = 0.001$).

Conclusions: HD adequacy alone does not have a significant impact on sexual dysfunction. Other treatments options should be considered to treat sexual dysfunction in women with CRF.

Keywords: Hemodialysis, Hemodialysis adequacy, Urea clearance, Female, Sexual dysfunction

Background

Female sexual dysfunction is common in women experiencing chronic renal failure (CRF) and is estimated to occur at a rate of 60-70% despite the use of dialysis [1,2].

Hemodialysis (HD) is the most commonly used option for dialysis, and often patients on HD have no choice but to continue HD until they undergo a kidney transplant (KT). Although there have been many reports regarding the improvement of sexual dysfunction after KT [3,4], those outcomes are not consistent [5,6], and moreover, from the patients' perspective, the chance for a KT is not likely.

In HD patients, adequate HD is important because it enables the patient to live clinically asymptomatic and be reasonably active and to maintain correction of the altered metabolic and homeostatic components secondary to the loss of the kidney function [7]. Ultimately, adequacy of HD is related to reduced morbidity and mortality associated with CRF [7].

Urea clearance (Kt/V) is a fractional clearance and represents HD adequacy [8]. However, few studies have investigated whether HD adequacy can improve sexual function in women with CRF. The aim of this study was to assess the

* Correspondence: yssong@schmc.ac.kr
[1]Department of Urology, Soonchunhyang University Hospital, Soonchunhyang University College of Medicine, Seoul, Korea
Full list of author information is available at the end of the article

impact of HD adequacy on sexual dysfunction in women with CRF and on HD.

Methods
Study sample
From March 2008 to February 2011, a total of 37 consecutive married women with CRF who were on HD were eligible and willing to participate in the study. Healthy female volunteers ($n = 36$) from the health promotion center at Soonchunhyang University Hospital were included as controls.

Approval for this study was obtained from the Internal Review Board at Soonchunhyang University Hospital. The HD group was composed of patients receiving HD treatment three times a week for 4 hours at one dialysis procedure for at least 6 months at the HD center at Soonchunhyang University Hospital.

The eligibility criteria for inclusion were: between the ages of 18 and 60 years, female gender, married, sexually active, no psychiatric disease including depression in the previous 6 months, and the intellectual and mental capacity to understand and answer the questionnaire. Exclusion criteria were having undergone surgical menopause, having undergone pelvic surgery including hysterectomy, clinical depression or other major psychiatric disease and having used hormonal replacement therapy within the past 5 years. A total of 37 patients were included in this study (Figure 1).

Clinical investigation
All patients and controls provided informed consent and underwent detailed clinical examination including testing hemoglobin, testosterone and estradiol levels, and recording of urea clearance (Kt/V).

To limit the influence of fluctuations in plasma hormone levels, blood samples were always drawn at the same time of day (08:00 to 10:00 hours).

Methodology
This was a cross-sectional study. A single investigator conducted face-to-face interviews with all study participants using a structured questionnaire.

FSFI questionnaire
To obtain sexual function assessments, the patients were asked to answer the Female Sexual Function Index (FSFI) questionnaire after undergoing HD treatment. The FSFI is an instrument used for the assessment of sexual function and consists of 19 questions [9,10].

The FSFI has been validated based on the DSM IV diagnoses of desire disorder, arousal disorder, and orgasmic dysfunction, and is intended for patients that have been sexually active in the previous four weeks [9,10]. The FSFI been previously validated in the Korean language and in the Korean population [11]. The questions are grouped and scored for domains of desire (two questions), arousal (four questions), lubrication (four questions), orgasm

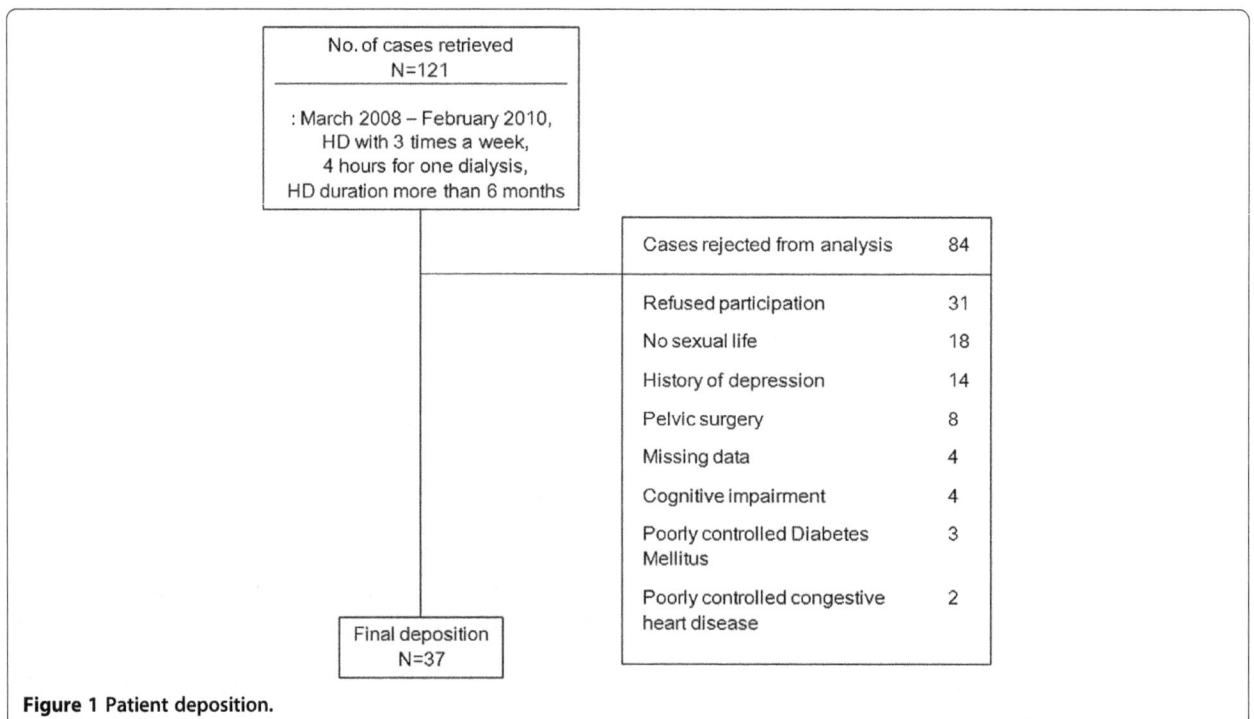

Figure 1 Patient deposition.

(three questions), satisfaction (three questions), and pain (three questions). Each domain is scored on a scale of 0 to 6, with higher scores indicating better function for each domain. A domain score of zero indicates that the women reported no sexual activity during the previous month and the full score ranges from 2 to 36. The individual domain scores are totaled and multiplied by a predetermined factor to weigh each domain equally.

Assessment of urea clearance (Kt/V)

Urea clearance (Kt/V) is a fractional clearance and is indicative of HD adequacy. [8] Kt/V is calculated using the following natural logarithm formula: Kt/V = – Ln (R - 0.008 × t) + (4 − 3.5 × R) × UF/W, where Ln is the natural logarithm, R is the ratio between post-dialysis blood urea nitrogen (BUN) and pre-dialysis BUN, t is the dialysis session length in hours, UF is the ultrafiltration volume in liters, and W is the patient's post-dialysis weight in kilograms.

Definition of adequate HD

Adequate HD was defined as over 1.3 (Kt/V) average urea clearance over three consecutive months. The Kidney Disease Outcomes Quality Initiative (KDOQI) guidelines (2006) recommend that the Kt/V dose targets are 1.4 with a 1.2 minimum, and the Renal Association Clinical Practice guidelines recommend a single pool Kt/V of greater than 1.3.

Statistical analyses

The Kolmogorov-Smirnov test was used to verify the normality of the distribution of continuous variables. Nonparametric comparison tests were used for variables evaluated as not normally distributed. Scores from the FSFI showed a nonparametric distribution; therefore, the mean value with standard deviation and the median value were used together as appropriate to describe statistics. Differences between groups were determined using the Kruskal-Wallis test and the Mann–Whitney test as appropriate. Spearmann's correlation test was used to investigate the association between Kt/V and sexual functional scores. All statistics were two-tailed and a P value < 0.05 was considered significant. All calculations were performed using SPSS version 18.0 (SPSS, Chicago, Ill., USA).

Results

Baseline analysis among the adequate HD, non-adequate HD, and normal control groups

There were no differences in age and height between the control and patient groups. Body weight and body mass index were significantly lower in the CRF patient group. The underlying etiologies of renal failure were chronic glomerulonephritis ($n = 6$), diabetic nephropathy ($n = 12$), hypertensive nephropathy ($n = 6$), adult polycystic kidney

($n = 1$) and other etiologies ($n = 11$). The mean duration of HD was 8.1 years.

Demographic variables did not differ, with the exception of body mass index, which was higher in the control groups. The rate of menopause was significantly higher in the HD groups, and testosterone and estradiol showed higher levels in the control groups. The average single–pool Kt/V in the adequate and non-adequate HD groups was 1.47 ± 0.11 and 1.14 ± 0.05, respectively (Table 1).

Comparative analysis of FSFI scores among the adequate HD, non-adequate HD, and normal control groups

When comparing the FSFI scores in the control and study groups, all domain scores except 'satisfaction', namely 'desire', 'arousal', 'lubrication', 'orgasm', 'pain' and 'total', were significantly lower in the HD groups than the scores of the control groups. The adequate and non-adequate groups did not differ in any of the domains or total FSFI (Table 2).

Correlation analysis between Kt/V and FSFI scores

Spearman's correlation test was performed to evaluate the associations among the FSFI questionnaire and Kt/V. The correlation analysis showed no significant relationship between FSFI and Kt/V (Table 3).

Correlation analysis between other factors and FSFI scores

Age, duration of dialysis, body mass index and testosterone showed no significant correlation with FSFI scores. Estrogen showed a significant correlation with all FSFI domains: 'desire' ($P < 0.001$), 'arousal' ($P < 0.001$), 'lubrication' ($P < 0.001$), 'orgasm' ($P < 0.001$), 'satisfaction' ($P = 0.047$), 'pain' ($P = 0.003$), and 'total FSFI' ($P = 0.001$).

Discussion

Female patients with CRF often suffer from sexual dysfunction [1,4]. Sexual dysfunction in women with CRF is largely due to loss of sexual interest, difficulties with arousal and reaching orgasm, reduced libido and lubrication, and pain during intercourse [1,12,13].

Considering that there are no other treatment options except KT, maintaining HD is an important treatment strategy for patients with CRF. HD adequacy is directly related to a patient's well–being, including physical activity, and is directly related to mortality and morbidity [7]. Considering there is no standard protocol for treating sexual dysfunction in women with CRF on HD, one important motivation for this study arose from the need to investigate the impact of HD adequacy on female sexual dysfunction.

Kt/V, urea fractional clearance, is a standard method to assess HD adequacy. This kinetic model is a clear was of determining adequacy [8]. There have been few reports regarding the role of Kt/V in female sexual dysfunction in

Table 1 Patient characteristics

	Controls ($n = 36$)	Adequate HD ($n = 18$)	Non-adequate HD ($n = 19$)	P value
Age (years)	48.19 ± 6.94	47.89 ± 6.82	47.53 ± 6.39	0.671
Height (cm)	155.65 ± 5.46	155.61 ± 4.07	155.741 ± 4.50	0.978
Weight [24]	58.84 ± 7.27	56.11 ± 9.46	54.18 ± 5.76	0.052
Body mass index (kg/m^2)	24.31 ± 3.02	23.08 ± 3.26[†]	22.37 ± 2.60[‡]	0.036[*]
Educational level				0.321
Middle school or less	8 (22.2%)	3 (16.6%)	3 (15.7%)	
High school	10 (27.7%)	10 (55.5%)	9 (47.3%)	
College or more	18 (50.0%)	5 (27.7%)	7 (36.8%)	
Monthly income (won)				0.072
<1 million	7 (19.4%)	6 (33.3%)	7 (36.8%)	
1-3 million	19 (52.7%)	7 (38.8%)	8 (42.1%)	
>3 million	10 (27.7%)	5 (27.7%)	4 (21.0%)	
Menopause (%)	10 (27.7%)	13 (66.5%)	12 (63.1%)	0.023[**]
Hematocrit (%)	29.8	28.1	28.3	0.057
Testosterone (ng/ml)	1.25 ± 2.25	0.45 ± 0.06[†]	0.26 ± 0.08[‡]	0.027[*]
Estradiol (pg/ml)	80.93 ± 77.24	27.55 ± 20.82[†]	34.68 ± 55.69[‡]	0.003[*]
Duration of HD (years)		7.4 ± 6.99	8.5 ± 3.99	0.781
Onset of CRF		10.5 ± 5.29	11.5 ± 6.72	0.574
Average single-pool Kt/V		1.47 ± 0.11	1.14 ± 0.05	0.021[***]

HD, hemodialysis, CRF, chronic renal failure. [*]analyzed by Kruskal-Wallis test; [**]analyzed by Fisher's exact test; [***]analyzed by Mann Whitney test. [†]Control versus adequate HD, [‡]Control versus non-adequate HD.

patients with CRF [14,15]. Previous studies reported that HD adequacy was not related to female sexual dysfunction. One of the limitations of those studies was the application of the Kt/V results. Recently, the recommended dose was increased to a target of 1.4. The KDOQI guidelines (2006) recommend a Kt/V dose target of 1.4 with a minimum of 1.2, and the Renal Association Clinical Practice guidelines recommend a single pool Kt/V of greater than 1.3. More importantly, HD adequacy cannot determined by a single Kt/V, but rather consecutive and consistent target doses of Kt/V are more important. In our study, adequate HD was defined as an average Kt/V of 1.3 over three consecutive months.

Although our study did not find an association between HD adequacy and female sexual dysfunction, this is the first study to assess the relation between sexual dysfunction and HD adequacy as measured using the consecutive method in women with CRF.

We reported in a previous study that the score of all domains of the FSFI questionnaire, 'desire', 'arousal', 'lubrication', 'orgasm', 'satisfaction' and 'pain', were significantly lower in the patient group than in the control group [16]. However, it is not clear that HD adequacy is related to sexual dysfunction. Our results show that HD adequacy alone does not restore sexual dysfunction in women with CRF. This is in agreement with a report

Table 2 Female sexual function index in patients with chronic renal failure who are on hemodiaysis

FSFI	Controls ($n = 36$)	Adequate HD ($n = 18$)	Non-adequate HD ($n = 19$)	P value[*]
Desire	2.4 ± 0.90, 2.4	1.43 ± 0.68[†], 1.2	2.08 ± 2.47[‡], 1.2	<0.001
Arousal	2.68 ± 1.90, 3.0	1.11 ± 1.71[†], 0	0.93 ± 1.87[‡], 0	0.001
Lubrication	3.30 ± 2.33, 3.9	1.66 ± 2.44[†], 0	1.16 ± 2.33[‡], 0	0.004
Orgasm	2.88 ± 2.11, 3.6	1.48 ± 2.23[†], 0	0.96 ± 1.93[‡], 0	0.004
Satisfaction	3.45 ± 1.66, 4.0	2.06 ± 1.70, 0.8	2.88 ± 1.79, 4.0	0.052
Pain	3.37 ± 2.27, 4.0	1.75 ± 2.59[†], 0	1.20 ± 2.40[‡], 0	0.011
Total	18.11 ± 10.24, 22.0	9.52 ± 10.64[†], 2	8.76 ± 9.52[‡], 5.2	0.003

Values are expressed as mean ± SD, median value.
HD, hemodialysis; FSFI, Female Sexual Function Index. [*]analyzed by Kruskal-Wallis test.
[†]Control versus adequate HD, [‡]Control versus non-adequate HD.

Table 3 Correlation coefficients between average single-pool Kt/V and female sexual function index score

FSFI	Correlation coefficients urea clearance	P value[*]
Desire	−0.156	0.355
Arousal	0.194	0.250
Lubrication	0.194	0.251
Orgasm	0.243	0.147
Satisfaction	−0.113	0.504
Pain	0.227	0.177
Total	−0.052	0.761

FSFI, Female Sexual Function Index. [*]analyzed by Spearman's correlation test.

that sexual dysfunctions does not improve with dialysis treatment [17].

As the genesis of sexual dysfunction is multifactorial in CRF patients, one aspect of HD adequacy alone was insufficient for explaining sexual dysfunction. It is believed that the lack of estradiol-stimulated cyclic LH secretion in women on dialysis leads to ovarian failure, which is presumed to be the primary cause of infertility [13,15,18,19]. Our results showed that levels of testosterone and estradiol were significantly decreased in the patient group. Moreover, estradiol showed a significant relationship with the scores in all domains of the FSFI. A previous study demonstrated that hormone replacement therapy allows sustained physiological serum estradiol concentrations in women with estrogen deficiency undergoing HD, with an associated improvement in sexual function [20]. It is suggested that adequate treatment of multiple factors, including emotional derangement and sex hormone change, is also necessary for improvement in sexual function in female CRF patients. Among them, hormonal replacement therapy (HRT) could be a promising treatment option. To date, only 17% of dialysis women had ever been treated with HRT and even less (6%) were currently on such therapy [21]. The benefits of HRT in premenopausal women on dialysis with estrogen deficiency treated with transdermal HRT have been reported to show a sustained increase in estrogen and recovery of menstruation [20].

This study had some limitations. First, our patient population was quite small. Generally, the participation rate in sex research is very low and the degree of conservatism in sexual attitudes was very high in those who refused participation. Second, the patients represented only a small geographic area, which limits the generalization of our findings. Third, we did not investigate the depression quantification by questionnaire. Although we excluded those patients with depression, concurrent and subclinical depression could be determined through a questionnaire. However, the diagnostic cut-off values of the Beck depression inventory, which is one of most commonly used questionnaires to assess depression, is not consistent between the DSM-IV criteria and Korean

validation form [22]. Therefore, the Beck depression inventory was not applied in our study. Fourth, we have not investigated other factors such as vascular abnormalities, medications, family interactions, and personal and social characteristics. Lastly, this study was not a prospective study. A prospective study of CRF patients is difficult as symptom onset is diverse, and indication and the method of dialysis differ according to each patient's medical condition. Further research, including a multi-center prospective study, is warranted for investigating sexual dysfunction in females with CRF who are undergoing HD.

Conclusion

In summary, sexual dysfunction was found in women with CRF who were on HD. HD adequacy alone does not have an impact on sexual dysfunction. Our results indicate that new strategies for the treatment of sexual dysfunction in women with CRF who are on HD are needed.

Abbreviations
CRF: Chronic renal failure; HD: Hemodialysis; FSFI: Female sexual function index; HRT: Hormonal replacement therapy.

Competing interest
The authors have no competing interest to disclose.

Authors' contributions
JHK and YSS contributed with the conception and design of the study and drafted the manuscript, SWD, SHK, ISL, and HH collected data and performed the analyses, WJY, ESS, and HJL assisted with conception and design of the study, conceived of the study and supervised the study and helped draft the manuscript. All authors read and approved the final manuscript.

Acknowledgement
This research was supported by Research Program through the National Research Foundation of Korea (NRF) funded by the Ministry of Education, Science and Technology (2010–0011678) and Soonchunhyang University Research Fund.

Author details
[1]Department of Urology, Soonchunhyang University Hospital, Soonchunhyang University College of Medicine, Seoul, Korea. [2]Department of Nephrology, Soonchunhyang University Hospital, Soonchunhyang University College of Medicine, Seoul, Korea. [3]Department of Obstetrics and Gynecology, Inha University School of Medicine, Incheon, Korea. [4]Medical Research Institute, Chung-Ang University College of Medicine, Seoul, Korea. [5]Department of Industrial Management and Engineering, Namseoul University College of Engineering, Cheonan, Korea. [6]North London Collegiate School, Jeju, Korea.

References
1. Toorians AW, Janssen E, Laan E, Gooren LJ, Giltay EJ, Oe PL, Donker AJ, Everaerd W: Chronic renal failure and sexual functioning: clinical status versus objectively assessed sexual response. *Nephrol Dial Transplant* 1997, 12(12):2654–2663.
2. Kettas E, Cayan F, Akbay E, Kiykim A, Cayan S: Sexual dysfunction and associated risk factors in women with end-stage renal disease. *J Sex Med* 2008, 5(4):872–877.
3. Tauchmanova L, Carrano R, Sabbatini M, De Rosa M, Orio F, Palomba S, Cascella T, Lombardi G, Federico S, Colao A: Hypothalamic-pituitary-gonadal axis function after successful kidney transplantation in men and women. *Hum Reprod* 2004, 19(4):867–873.

4. Basok EK, Atsu N, Rifaioglu MM, Kantarci G, Yildirim A, Tokuc R: Assessment of female sexual function and quality of life in predialysis, peritoneal dialysis, hemodialysis, and renal transplant patients. *Int Urol Nephrol* 2009, **41**(3):473–481.

5. Muehrer RJ, Keller ML, Powwattana A, Pornchaikate A: Sexuality among women recipients of a pancreas and kidney transplant. *West J Nurs Res* 2006, **28**(2):137–150. discussion 151–161.

6. Filocamo MT, Zanazzi M, Li Marzi V, Lombardi G, Del Popolo G, Mancini G, Salvadori M, Nicita G: Sexual dysfunction in women during dialysis and after renal transplantation. *J Sex Med* 2009, **6**(11):3125–3131.

7. Eknoyan G, Beck GJ, Cheung AK, Daugirdas JT, Greene T, Kusek JW, Allon M, Bailey J, Delmez JA, Depner TA, *et al*: Effect of dialysis dose and membrane flux in maintenance hemodialysis. *N Engl J Med* 2002, **347**(25):2010–2019.

8. Daugirdas JT: Second generation logarithmic estimates of single-pool variable volume Kt/V: an analysis of error. *J Am Soc Nephrol* 1993, **4**(5):1205–1213.

9. Meston CM: Validation of the female sexual function index (FSFI) in women with female orgasmic disorder and in women with hypoactive sexual desire disorder. *J Sex Marital Ther* 2003, **29**(1):39–46.

10. Rosen R, Brown C, Heiman J, Leiblum S, Meston C, Shabsigh R, Ferguson D, D'Agostino R Jr: The female sexual function index (FSFI): a multidimensional self-report instrument for the assessment of female sexual function. *J Sex Marital Ther* 2000, **26**(2):191–208.

11. Hy K, Hs S, Ks P, Jeong SJ, Lee JY, Ryu SB: Development of the Korean-version of female sexual function index (FSFI). *Korean J Androl* 2002, **20**(1):50–56.

12. Diemont WL, Vruggink PA, Meuleman EJ, Doesburg WH, Lemmens WA, Berden JH: Sexual dysfunction after renal replacement therapy. *Am J Kidney Dis* 2000, **35**(5):845–851.

13. Zingraff J, Jungers P, Pelissier C, Nahoul K, Feinstein MC, Scholler R: Pituitary and ovarian dysfunctions in women on haemodialysis. *Nephron* 1982, **30**(2):149–153.

14. Neto AF, de Freitas Rodrigues MA, Saraiva Fittipaldi JA, Moreira ED Jr: The epidemiology of erectile dysfunction and its correlates in men with chronic renal failure on hemodialysis in Londrina, southern Brazil. *Int J Impot Res* 2002, **14**(2):S19–26.

15. Peng YS, Chiang CK, Kao TW, Hung KY, Lu CS, Chiang SS, Yang CS, Huang YC, Wu KD, Wu MS, *et al*: Sexual dysfunction in female hemodialysis patients: a multicenter study. *Kidney Int* 2005, **68**(2):760–765.

16. Song YS, Yang HJ, Song ES, Han DC, Moon C, Ku JH: Sexual function and quality of life in Korean women with chronic renal failure on hemodialysis: case–control study. *Urology* 2008, **71**(2):243–246.

17. Soykan A, Boztas H, Kutlay S, Ince E, Nergizoglu G, Dilekoz AY, Berksun O: Do sexual dysfunctions get better during dialysis? Results of a six-month prospective follow-up study from Turkey. *Int J Impot Res* 2005, **17**(4):359–363.

18. Mastrogiacomo I, De Besi L, Serafini E, Zussa S, Zucchetta P, Romagnoli GF, Saporiti E, Dean P, Ronco C, Adami A: Hyperprolactinemia and sexual disturbances among uremic women on hemodialysis. *Nephron* 1984, **37**(3):195–199.

19. Oksuz E, Malhan S: Prevalence and risk factors for female sexual dysfunction in Turkish women. *J Urol* 2006, **175**(2):654–658. discussion 658.

20. Matuszkiewicz-Rowinska J, Skorzewska K, Radowicki S, Sokalski A, Przedlacki J, Niemczyk S, Wlodarczyk D, Puka J, Switalski M: The benefits of hormone replacement therapy in pre-menopausal women with oestrogen deficiency on haemodialysis. *Nephrol Dial Transplant* 1999, **14**(5):1238–1243.

21. Kramer HM, Curhan GC, Singh A: Permanent cessation of menses and postmenopausal hormone use in dialysis-dependent women: the HELP study. *Am J Kidney Dis* 2003, **41**(3):643–650.

22. Koo JR, Yoon JW, Kim SG, Lee YK, Oh KH, Kim GH, Kim HJ, Chae DW, Noh JW, Lee SK, *et al*: Association of depression with malnutrition in chronic hemodialysis patients. *Am J Kidney Dis* 2003, **41**(5):1037–1042.

Survival and prognostic factors for adrenocortical carcinoma

Zlatibor Loncar[1*], Vladimir Djukic[1], Vladan Zivaljevic[2], Tatjana Pekmezovic[3], Aleksandar Diklic[2], Svetislav Tatic[4], Dusko Dundjerovic[4], Branislav Olujic[1], Nikola Slijepcevic[2] and Ivan Paunovic[2]

Abstract

Background: Adrenocortical carcinoma (ACC) is aggressive, but rare tumours that have not been sufficiently studied. The aim of our study was to present the demographic and clinical characteristics of patients with ACC, to determine the overall survival rates, analyse the effect of prognostic factors on survival, as well as to identify favorable and unfavourable predictors of survival.

Method: The study included 72 patients (42 women and 30 men) with ACC. We analysed the prognostic value of the demographic and clinical characteristics of the patients, tumour characteristics, therapy administered and survival rates. Kaplan-Meier survival curves and the log-rank test were used to estimate the overall and specific survival probabilities and the Cox regression model was used to identify independent prognostic factors for survival.

Results: The patients had mean age of 50 years. The 1-, 5-, and 10-year probabilities of survival in patients with ACC were 52.5 %, 41.1 %, and 16.4 %, respectively. The median survival time was 36 months. The results of multivariate Cox regression analysis showed that the presence of lymphatic metastases (HR = 7.37, 95 % CI = 2.31-23.48, p = 0.001) and therapy with mitotane (HR = 0.11, 95 % CI = 0.04-0.27, p = 0.001) were independent prognostic factors for survival.

Conclusion: The presence of lymphatic metastasis is an unfavourable prognostic factor, while postoperative therapy with mitotane is a favorable prognostic factor for survival in patients with ACC.

Keywords: Adrenal gland, Cortex, Carcinoma, Surgery, Survival, Mitotane

Background

The more frequent clinical use of ultrasound and computerized tomography have increased the detection of adrenal tumours. Such adrenal incidentalomas are usually benign adenomas. Adrenocortical carcinoma (ACC) is rare, but aggressive malignant endocrine tumour. An ACC is the second most aggressive endocrine tumour, after anaplastic thyroid cancer. In addition, an ACC is the second rarest cancer of the endocrine system, following parathyroid cancer. The annual incidence of ACC is one per million population and ACC is responsible for 0.2 % of all cancer-related mortality [1, 2]. Even though a multimodal approach is used in the treatment of these patients, in which surgery has the most important role, the prognosis for

these patients is poor. Most ACC occur as sporadic tumours, but ACC can be part of the rare hereditary Li-Fraumeni syndrome. The pathogenesis of ACC is not well-known. In agreement with the characteristics of benign tumours, ACC can be hormonally-active (functional) or hormonally-inactive (non-functional). Approximately 70 % of all ACC are hormonally active, and present in greater than one-half of cases with Cushing's syndrome [3, 4]. The most common first sign of a hormonally-inactive ACC is abdominal pain [4]. Because ACC is very rare tumour there are not many institutions that have had much experience with these tumours, and therefore clinical characteristics, optimal treatment approaches, prognosis, and prognostic factors are still in need of research.

The aims of our study were as follows: present the demographic and clinical characteristics of patients with ACC; determine the overall survival rates; analyse the role of prognostic factors on survival, and identify favourable and unfavourable predictors of survival.

---
* Correspondence: loncarz2014@gmail.com
[1]Emergency Centre, Clinical Centre of Serbia, Faculty of Medicine, University of Belgrade, Pasterova 2, 11000 Belgrade, Serbia
Full list of author information is available at the end of the article

Methods

This cohort study included 72 consecutive patients who were diagnosed with ACC based on definitive histopathologic findings and who underwent operative treatment at the Clinical Centre of Serbia between 1996 to 2014. The following data were collected from patient records, a specialized database, and other medical documentation: basic demographic characteristics of the patients (gender and age); clinical characteristics (stage of the disease, size and weight of the tumour, presence of lymphatic and distant metastases, tumour localization [i.e., left vs. right side and local tumour infiltration of surrounding tissues]; operative treatment (type of operation, surgeon who performed the surgery [i.e., as a prognostic factor based on experience], re-operation for local recurrence of the disease, and operative treatment of distant metastases); other modes of therapy (radiotherapy and chemotherapy); hormonal activity of the tumour (functional, or nonfunctional); and type of hypersecretion of functional tumours.

ACC was classified into one of four stages. The first stage included patients with a tumour sized ≤ 5 cm in diameter and without local or distant metastases. The second stage included patients with a tumour ≥ 5 cm in diameter and without infiltration of surrounding tissues, or local or distant metastases. The third stage included patients with a tumour of any size but with infiltration of surrounding tissue or local lymphatic metastasis. The fourth stage included patients with tumours of any size, but with infiltration of surrounding tissues and local lymphatic metastases or distant metastases only. Continuous variables (age, tumour weight, and tumour size) were transformed into dichotomous variables based on distribution. Other variables (stage of disease, surgical approach, and type of operation) were transformed into dichotomous variables. Surgical approaches were categorized as extraperitoneal or transperitoneal.

After analysing the stages of disease individually, we grouped stages I and II together and stages III and IV together. For the type of operation, we formed two groups also. The first group included patients with incomplete resection of the tumour (i.e., a sub-adrenalectomy). The second group included patients who had an adrenalectomy with or without resection of surrounding tissues.

Mitotane was the only form of chemotherapy, and when used, the dosage was 4 g/d. Hormonal activity was measured for all patients pre-operatively. All surgical procedures were performed by surgeons in highly specialized tertiary referral centres. Information on whether or not the patient was alive, and if not, the date of death, were retrieved through contact with the patients themselves, members of their families, and patient's general practitioner. Only patients with a cancer-specific cause of death were included in the probability of survival calculation. Median follow-up was 48 months.

The study was approved by the Ethical Committee of the Faculty of Medicine of the University of Belgrade and carried out in compliance with the Helsinki declaration. Participants signed an informed consent prior to enrolment in the study.

Statistical analysis

Kaplan-Meier survival curves and the log-rank test were used for determining overall survival and the specific probability of survival for each of the observed variables, respectively. We then performed univariate Cox regression analysis to determine which variables were significantly associated with length of survival. The variables which were significantly associated with length of survival at a $p < 0.05$ level of significance, were included in the multivariate regression analysis model to determine independent prognostic factors of survival.

Results

As shown in Table 1, ACC occurred in women nearly 50 % more often than men.

The highest number of ACC occurred in patients in their sixth decade of life; the youngest patient with an ACC was 17 years of age, while the oldest patient was 72 years of age, and the mean age was 50.4 years. Nearly one-half of the patients had stage II disease; patients with stage I disease were extremely rare. Approximately 70 % of patients had a tumour ≤ 10 cm in diameter weighing ≤ 300 gram. At time of diagnosis, ACC lymphatic metastases were present in 12 % of patients, while distant metastases were present in six patients (lung, n = 3; liver, n = 2; contralateral adrenal gland, n = 1. Local tumour invasion was present in ≥ 40 % of patients, which demonstrates the aggressive nature of the tumours. One patient presented with an IVC thrombus. Two-thirds of patients were operated through a subcostal laparotomy approach and 22 % through a transdorsal approach; other approaches were rarely used. An endoscopic approach was not used for this group of patients. There was a similar rate of tumour occurrence on the right and left sides. Most patients (88 %) underwent potentially radical surgery, while tumour reduction or biopsy was performed in one of nine patients. All operations were performed by one of seven specialist surgeons, and ≥ 70 % of the operations were performed by a surgeon with 10 years of experience. Transcutaneous radiotherapy was administered to only one patient, while two-thirds of the patients received chemotherapy with mitotane. Following primary surgery, over a period of 1–6 years, 6 patients underwent re-operation for local tumour recurrence. In addition, two patients underwent surgery for distant metastases to the lungs during this time period. Most of the tumours

Table 1 Basic demographics and clinical characteristics of patients with ACC

Variable	Number	Percent
Gender		
Females	42	58.3
Males	30	41.7
Age		
<20	2	2.8
21–30	4	5.6
31–40	7	9.7
41–50	24	33.3
51–60	19	26.4
61–70	16	22.2
70+		
Stage of disease		
I	2	3.1
II	31	48.4
III	20	31.3
IV	11	17.2
Tumour size		
<100	43	71.7
101+	17	28.3
Tumour weight		
<300	39	69.6
301+	17	30.4
Lymphatic metastasis		
Yes	8	12.1
No	58	87.9
Distant metastases		
Yes	6	8.8
No	62	91.2
Local infiltration		
Yes	29	42.6
No	39	57.4
Surgical approach		
Subcostal laparotomy	48	66.7
Transdorsal lumbotomy sec.Young	16	22.2
Median laparotomy	1	1.4
Bilateral subcostal laparotomy	3	4.2
Lumbotomy sec. Kifer	3	4.2
Transrectal laparotomy	1	1.4
Tumour localization		
Left side	34	47.2
Right side	37	51.4
Bilateral	1	1.4

Table 1 Basic demographics and clinical characteristics of patients with ACC *(Continued)*

Type of operation		
Biopsy	5	7.1
Tumour reduction	3	4.3
Adrenalectomy	50	71.4
Extended adrenalectomy	12	17.1
Surgeons experience		
Specialist up to 10 years	21	29.2
Specialist over 10 years	51	70.8
Mitotane		
Yes	30	63.8
No	17	36.2
Hormonal activity		
Functional	19	26.4
Afunctional	53	73.6
Clinical presentation		
Asymptomatic	28	38.9
Symptomatic	44	61.1

(73.6 %) were not hormonally-active. Of the 19 patients with functional tumours, 16 had Cushing's syndrome (hypersecretion of cortisol) one had hypersecretion of sex hormones, and two had mixed hypersecretion of cortisol and sex hormones. Most patients had clear symptoms at diagnosis, while nearly 40 % of patients were asymptomatic with general symptoms such as weight loss, anaemia or fatigue. Of the 44 symptomatic patients, pain was the predominant symptom in 25, while 19 had clinical manifestations of hypersecretion of cortisol (hypertension, hirsutism, amenorrhea).

Figure 1 shows the overall probability of survival for patients with ACC. The 6-month, 1-year, 3-year, 5-year, 10-year probabilities of survival were 69.8 %, 52.5 %, 48.2 %, 41.1 %, and 16.4 %, respectively. The median survival time was 36 months (95 % CI = 13.4–58.5) and the mean survival time was 61.5 months (95 % CI = 42.7–80.1).

The results of univariate Cox regression analysis are presented in Table 2. The variables significantly associated with patient survival include gender, age, disease stage, tumour weight, lymphatic and distant metastases, local tumour invasion, surgical approach, and therapy with mitotane.

The results of multivariate Cox regression analysis, which included all variables that were associated with patient survival at a $p < 0.05$ level of significance, are shown in Table 3. The independent prognostic factors of patient survival include lymphatic metastases (hazard ratio [HR] = 7.37, 95 % CI = 2.31–23.48) as an unfavourable prognostic factor, and therapy with mitotane

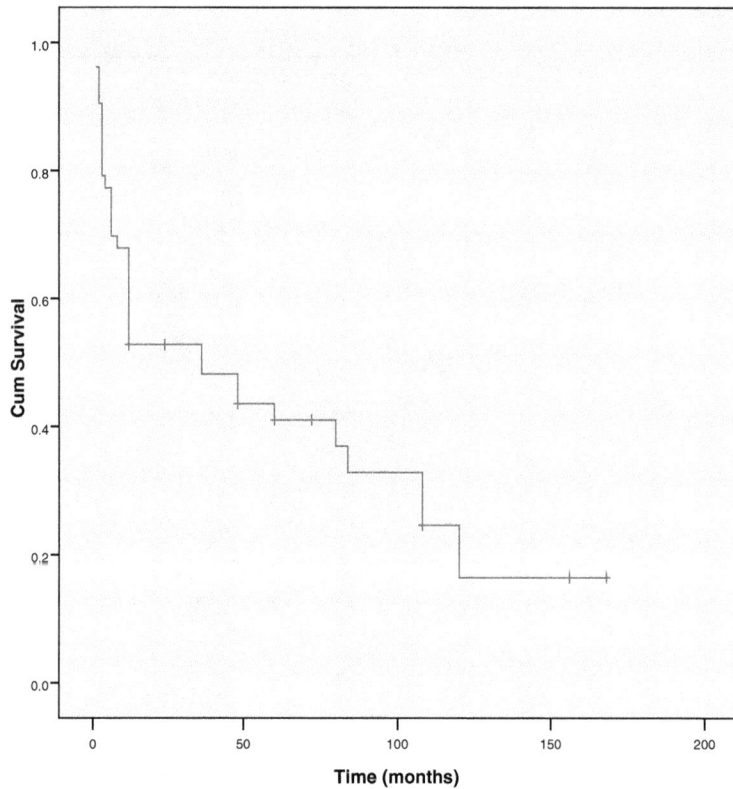

Fig. 1 Kaplan-Meier survival curve for ACC

Table 2 Results of univariate Cox regression analyses

Variable	P	HR	95 % CI
Gender (male vs. female)	0.028	2.17	1.09–4.32
Age (years) (50+ vs. <50)	0.015	2.40	1.18–4.86
Stage of disease (III–IV vs. I–II)	0.005	2.94	1.39–6.21
Tumour size (mm) (100+ vs. <100)	0.437	1.36	0.62–2.99
Tumour weight (gram) (300+ vs. <300)	0.047	2.26	1.01–5.05
Lymphatic metastasis (present vs. absent)	0.001	4.86	1.88–12.54
Distant metastases (present vs. absent)	0.001	4.31	1.45–12.83
Local infiltration (present vs. absent)	0.001	3.20	1.57–6.52
Surgical approach (extraperitoneal vs. transperitoneal)	0.022	0.29	0.10–0.84
Localization (right vs. left)	0.251	1.50	0.75–3.01
Type of surgery (biopsy and tumor reduction vs. adrenalectomy and extended adrenalectomy)	0.191	0.52	0.20–1.38
Reoperation (yes vs. no)	0.550	0.75	0.29–1.95
Surgeons experience (10+ vs. <10)	0.704	0.86	0.40–1.85
Mitotane (used vs. not used)	0.001	0.13	0.06–0.31
Hormonal activity (non-functional vs. functional)	0.544	1.28	0.57–2.86
Symptomatic presentation (yes vs. no)	0.536	0.81	0.41–1.60

HR–Hazard ratio; 95 % CI - Confidence interval

(HR = 0.11, 95 % CI = 0.04–0.27), as a favourable prognostic factor.

Discussion

Data on the incidence of ACC are limited, but there has been no increase in incidence, even though there has been an increase in the number of diagnosed adrenal tumours and the number of adrenal operations. This increase in the early diagnosis and operative treatment of adrenal tumours could in fact be the reason for the

Table 3 The prognostic factors for survival in patients with ACC (multivariate Cox regression analysis)

Variable	p	HR	95 % CI
Gender (male vs. female)	0.918	1.05	0.43–2.58
Age (years) (50+ vs. <50)	0.593	1.31	0.49–3.54
Stage of disease (III–IV vs. I–II)	0.879	1.15	0.20–6.71
Tumour weight (g) (300+ vs. <300)	0.665	1.35	0.34–5.36
Lymphatic metastasis (present vs. absent)	0.001	7.37	2.31–23.48
Distant metastases (present vs. absent)	0.491	1.82	0.33–10.09
Local infiltration (present vs. absent)	0.306	1.64	0.64–4.23
Surgical approach (extraperitoneal vs. transperitoneal)	0.381	0.55	0.15–2.09
Mitotane (used vs. not used)	0.001	0.11	0.05–0.27

HR–Hazard ratio; 95 % CI - Confidence interval

slight decrease in the incidence of ACC in Holland over the past 20 years; the incidence has declined from 1.3 to 1.0 per million inhabitants [2].

The gender prevalence in our study corresponds to data from the literature. Women are affected by ACC more often than men, with a ratio of 1.2–1.5:1 [1–4]. Even though most patients are in their fifth or sixth decade of life at the time of diagnosis, with a mean age of 43–56 years, ACC occurs in all age groups, including children [1–4]. The population-based age-standardized incidence rate for patients <20 years of age is 0.2 per million person-years [5].

ACC is rarely diagnosed as stage I. Indeed, in the current study study only 3 % of patients were diagnosed in stage I, compered to 6 % according to the literature [3, 6, 7]. Most patients (approximately 50 %) are diagnosed with stage II ACC, as was the case in the current study and published data [3, 4, 7]. ACC tumours are usually large in size. The mean size of ACC tumours according to published data is ≥ 10 cm [1, 6]. In the current study, the size of ACC tumours ranged from 3.5 to 23 cm (mean, 9.8 cm; standard deviation [SD], 4.0 cm), and the weight ranged from 15 to 2450 g (mean, 323 g; SD, 481 g). Lymphatic metastases are present in 20 % of patients with ACC at the time of diagnosis, while distant metastases occur in nearly 30 % of patients with ACC [1].

The most common sites for distant metastases are in lungs and liver [8]. Even though, lymphatic metastases are often present, locoregional lymph node dissection is not routinely performed, although Reibetanz et al. suggested that locoregional lymph node dessection improves oncologic outcome [9].

The optimal treatment plan for ACC has not been well-defined. The best results have been achieved with surgical treatment, which has the most important role in the treatment of ACC, while additional treatment options are still a matter of discussion [10]. Surgical treatment is relatively safe, considering that the perioperative mortality is approximately 5 % [3]. A subcostal laparotomy is the most common approach to ACC; a laparoscopic approach was not used at our institution, even though we perform laparoscopic surgery for other indications. Ferreira et al. also reported that a subcostal extended incision is the best approach for ACC and that it can be used even for ACC tumours ≥ 15 cm in size [11]. Laparoscopic adrenalectomy for ACC is associated with higher recurrence rates, particularly peritoneal recurrences. For this reason, open adrenalectomy is a better choice because of the oncologic benefit that surpasses the short-term benefits of minimally invasive surgery [12]. Miller et al. reported the mean size of laparoscopically-removed tumours to be 7 cm, whereas the size of tumours removed through open adrenalectomy

was 12 cm. In the same study, positive margins of resection were present in 50 % of laparoscopic operations and ≤ 20 % in open adrenalectomies. Furthermore, there was a shorter interval before recurrence after laparoscopic surgery compared to open surgery (9 months vs. 19 months). For all of these reasons, Miller et al. concluded that laparoscopic surgery should not be attempted for ACC [13].

Open adrenalectomy is superior to laparoscopic adrenalectomy because of a more complete resection of the tumour [14]. Brix et al. after analyzing 35 laparoscopic and 117 open adrenalectomies, concluded that for localized ACC tumours ≤ 10 cm in diameter, laparoscopic adrenalectomy performed by an experienced surgeon is not inferior to open adrenalectomy [15].

ACC is considered a radioresistant tumour, thus radiotherapy is rarely used; except as adjuvant radiotherapy to the tumour bed in patients with incomplete tumour resection or ACC metastases as a palliative measure [16]. Data on the results of the application of adjuvant radiotherapy to the tumour bed in patients with complete resection of the tumour are limited; and the results of the effect of such adjuvant radiotherapy on reducing high rates of local recurrence of ACC are controversial [17, 18].

In the current study, the 1-, 3-, 5-, and 10-year survivals in patients with ACC were 52.5 %, 48.2 %, 41.1 %, and 16.4 %, respectively; the median survival was 36 months and the mean survival was 61.5 months. Bilimoria et al. reported a median survival of 32 months and a 5-year survival of 38 % in patients with ACC, with no evident change in survival rates between 1985 and 2000 [1]. Tritos et al. reported a median survival of 17 months in patients with ACC [19]. Tauchmanova et al. found an overall survival of 41 months in patients with ACC [4]. Schulick et al. showed a median survival of 38 months and a 5-year survival of 37 % for patients with ACC [20]. According to Keskin et al. the median survival for patients with ACC was 18 months, while the 1-year survival was 73 % and the 5-year survival was 48 % [6]. In the current study, the presence of lymphatic metastasis was a negative prognostic factor, while postoperative therapy with mitotane was a positive prognostic factor of survival for patients with ACC. Keskin et al. reported that the absence of lymphatic metastasis was a favourable prognostic factor for patients with ACC [6]. Also, Keskin et al. showed that the absence of distant metastases and an early stage of the disease were favourable prognostic factors. Additionally, Keskin et al. found gender to be a favourable prognostic factor, because survival length was five times longer in men than women (58 months vs. 12 months). Based on a multivariate analysis, Bilimoria et al. demonstrated a high risk of death with an increase in age, involved margins, and nodal or distant metastasis [1]. The presence of lymphatic metastases in patients with ACC is stage III disease. The higher the stage of disease, the worse the survival rates. Kerkhofs et al. reported, a mean survival in patients with ACC of 159 months for stage I and II disease, 26 months for stage III disease, and 5 months for stage IV disease [2]. Gomez Rivera et al. reported a mean survival in patients with ACC of 67 months for stage II disease, 13 months for stage III disease, and 3 months for stage IV disease [21]. Furthermore, Gomez Rivera at al. concluded that prognostic factors that worsen survival are older age, distant metastases, non-surgical treatment and a locally invasive tumour that involves large veins. Even in stage IV disease, better survival is expected if an ACC is resected in toto (R0), but the question that arises is whether or not there are really negative resection margins in stage IV disease [8, 22]. Dong et al. do not recommend surgical treatment for stage IV ACCbecause the prognosis is not affected; in contrast, surgical treatment in stage I and II ACC are most effective, but surgery is also recommended for stage III ACC [7].

The worst prognosis is expected when the tumour invades large veins (inferior vena cava and renal veins), which shorten disease-free interval and survival six-fold compared to patients in whom invasion of veins is not present [23]. Peri-operative mortality is 13 % when the inferior vena cava is infiltrated, but experienced surgeons should aim for a radical operation even in these cases [24]. We did not show that the extent of surgery influenced the survival outcome, even though this is considered the most important factor with respect to survival of patients with ACC. Because most of our patients had complete resection of the tumour, it was not possible to statistically prove that surgery influenced survival outcome. Based on the results of regression analysis, Tritos et al. showed that the absence of metastases at the time of diagnosis, patients ≤ 54 years of age, and complete surgical resection are independent prognostic factors for improved survival in patients with ACC [19]. Resection for cure is reported in 50–75 % of patients with ACC [3, 7]. The outcome of ACC patients is influenced by the expertise of the surgeons and number of patients at the institution where the patients undergo surgery. For this reason, Hermsen et al. emphasize the relevance of national cooperation and centralized surgery for ACC [25]. Furthermore, Lombardi et al. classified institutions into high and low-volume centres [26]. High-volume centres annually perform more than ten adrenalectomies for ACC, and the outcomes are better in such centres. The survival benefit is not only the consequence of expert surgical treatment, but also the result of a multidisciplinary approach to ACC which is practiced in these specialized centres [27]. We could not statistically analyse this parameter, because all patients underwent surgery at the same centre, which is in fact the centre where most patients with ACC are surgically treated in our country.

The use of mitotane is still under debate, although mitotane is used in greater than one-half of patients with ACC [3]. Mitotane is usually used as monotherapy, at a high-dose, which is favourable [28]. Terzolo et al. reported that the application of mitotane extends the recurrence-free interval in radically-resected ACC patients [29]. Icard et al. concluded that mitotane is only beneficial for ACC patients who undergo complete resection of the tumour [3]. In contrast, Grubbs et al. reported that the recurrence-free interval is nearly the same for patients with ACC who underwent surgery and received mitotane and patients who did not receive mitotane [30]. The hormonal activity of the tumour also influences the outcome of patients with ACC. According to Berruti et al. hypercortisolism is a prognostic factor in completely resected ACC with respect to overall survival and recurrence-free survival [31]. Icard et al. reported that precursor-secreting tumours influenced outcome [3].

ACC has a high recurrence rate. Analysing 101 re-operations for ACC, Erdogan et al. reported prolonged survival for R0 resection, even if > 1 year elapsed between the primary operation and recurrence of the disease [32].

The reported responses to conventional treatment of ACC have not been favourable. Additionally, an alternative approach, such as a wide array of chromosomal, genetic, molecular, and immunohistochemical markers, has been tested in ACC to identify reliable diagnostic and prognostic factors [33–35]. Therefore, certain molecular markers, such as the IGF system, the Wnt pathway, and p53, may be considered as potential targets for treatment and available therapeutic options [33].

There were several limitations to the present study. It would be useful if this study could be conducted as a multicentric study with a higher number of patients, because it would allow better analysis of variables with low occurrences. Additionally, there were missing data for some variables. In our study histopathological and immunochemical parameters were not included, and which will be presented in forthcoming publication.

Conclusion

In conclusion, the presence of lymphatic metastasis at the time of diagnosis was a negative prognostic factor for survival, while postoperative therapy with mitotane was a favourable prognostic factor for survival in patients with ACC.

Abbreviations

ACC: Adrenocortical carcinomas; CI: Confidence interval; HR: Hazard ratio; SD: Standard deviation.

Competing interests

The authors declare that they have no competing interests.

Authors' contributions

ZL made substantial contributions to conception of the study, wrote the paper and has been involved in all steps of the study. VD, VZ and TP made substantial contributions to design of the study, and have been involved in critically revising the manuscript for important intellectual content. AD, ST, DD, BO, NS and IP have been involved in acquisition of data. All authors read and approved the final manuscript.

Author details

[1]Emergency Centre, Clinical Centre of Serbia, Faculty of Medicine, University of Belgrade, Pasterova 2, 11000 Belgrade, Serbia. [2]Centre for Endocrine Surgery, Clinical Centre of Serbia, Faculty of Medicine, University of Belgrade, Pasterova 2, 11000 Belgrade, Serbia. [3]Institute of Epidemiology, Faculty of Medicine, University of Belgrade, Visegradska 26A, Belgrade 11000, Serbia. [4]Institute of Pathology, Faculty of Medicine, University of Belgrade, Dr Subotica 1, 11000 Belgrade, Serbia.

References

1. Bilimoria KY, Shen WT, Elaraj D, Bentrem DJ, Winchester DJ, Kebebew E, Sturgeon C. Adrenocortical carcinoma in the United States: treatment utilization and prognostic factors. Cancer. 2008;113:3130-3136.
2. Kerkhofs TM, Verhoeven RH, Van der Zwan JM, Dieleman J, Kerstens MN, Links TP, et al. Adrenocortical carcinoma: a population-based study on incidence and survival in the Netherlands since 1993. Eur J Cancer. 2013;49:2579–86.
3. Icard P, Goudet P, Charpenay C, Andreassian B, Carnaille B, Chapuis Y, et al. Adrenocortical carcinomas: surgical trends and results of a 253 patient series from the French Association of Endocrine Surgeons study group. World J Surg. 2001;25:891–7.
4. Tauchmanovà L, Colao A, Marzano LA, Sparano L, Camera L, Rossi A, et al. Adrenocortical carcinomas: twelve-year prospective experience. World J Surg. 2004;28:896–903.
5. Kerkhofs TM, Ettaieb MH, Verhoeven RH, Kaspers GJ, Tissing WJ, Loeffen J, et al. Adrenocortical carcinoma in children: First population based clinicopathological study with long-term follow-up. Oncol Rep. 2014;32:2836–44.
6. Keskin S, Tas F, Vatansever S. Adrenocortical carcinoma: clinicopathological features, prognostic factors and outcome. Urol Int. 2013;90:435-438.
7. Dong D, Li H, Yan W, Ji Z, Mao Q. Surgical management and clinical prognosis of adrenocortical carcinoma. Urol Int. 2012;88:400-404.
8. Dy BM, Strajina V, Cayo AK, Richards ML, Farley DR, Grant CS, et al. Surgical Resection of Synchronously Metastatic Adrenocortical Cancer. Ann Surg Oncol. 2015;22:146–51.
9. Reibetanz J, Jurowich C, Erdogan I, Nies C, Rayes N, Dralle H, et al. Impact of lymphadenectomy on the oncologic outcome of patients with adrenocortical carcinoma. Ann Surg. 2012;255:363–9.
10. Ng L, Libertino JM. Adrenocortical carcinoma: diagnosis, evaluation and treatment. J Urol. 2003;169:5-11.
11. Ferreira U, Nardi Pedro R, Matheus WE, Prudente A, Mendonça Borges G, Rodrigues Netto Jr N. Open surgical treatment of right-sided adrenal carcinomas >15 cm. Urol Int. 2007;78:46–9.
12. Cooper AB, Habra MA, Grubbs EG, Bednarski BK, Ying AK, Perrier ND, et al. Does laparoscopic adrenalectomy jeopardize oncologic outcomes for patients with adrenocortical carcinoma? Surg Endosc. 2013;27:4026–32.
13. Miller BS, Ammori JB, Gauger PG, Broome JT, Hammer GD, Doherty GM. Laparoscopic resection is inappropriate in patients with known or suspected adrenocortical carcinoma. World J Surg. 2010;34:1380–5.
14. Miller BS, Gauger PG, Hammer GD, Doherty GM. Resection of adrenocortical carcinoma is less complete and local recurrence occurs sooner and more often after laparoscopic adrenalectomy than after open adrenalectomy. Surgery. 2012;152:1150–7.
15. Brix D, Allolio B, Fenske W, Agha A, Dralle H, Jurowich C, et al. German Adrenocortical Carcinoma Registry Group. Laparoscopic versus open adrenalectomy for adrenocortical carcinoma: surgical and oncologic outcome in 152 patients. Eur Urol. 2010;58:609–15.
16. Polat B, Fassnacht M, Pfreundner L, Guckenberger M, Bratengeier K, Johanssen S, et al. Radiotherapy in adrenocortical carcinoma. Cancer. 2009;115:2816–23.
17. Fassnacht M, Hahner S, Polat B, Koschker AC, Kenn W, Flentje M, et al. Efficacy of adjuvant radiotherapy of the tumor bed on local recurrence of adrenocortical carcinoma. J Clin Endocrinol Metab. 2006;91:4501–4.
18. Habra MA, Ejaz S, Feng L, Das P, Deniz F, Grubbs EG, et al. A retrospective cohort analysis of the efficacy of adjuvant radiotherapy after primary surgical resection in patients with adrenocortical carcinoma. J Clin Endocrinol Metab. 2013;98:192–7.
19. Tritos NA, Cushing GW, Heatley G, Libertino JA. Clinical features and prognostic factors associated with adrenocortical carcinoma: Lahey Clinic Medical Center experience. Am Surg. 2000;66:73-79.
20. Schulick RD, Brennan MF. Long-term survival after complete resection and repeat resection in patients with adrenocortical carcinoma. Ann Surg Oncol. 1999;6:719–26.
21. Gomez-Rivera F, Medina-Franco H, Arch-Ferrer JE, Heslin MJ. Adrenocortical carcinoma: a single institution experience. Am Surg. 2005;71:90-94.
22. Ohwada S, Izumi M, Kawate S, Hamada K, Toya H, Togo N, et al. Surgical outcome of stage III and IV adrenocortical carcinoma. Jpn J Clin Oncol. 2007;37:108–13.
23. Turbendian HK, Strong VE, Hsu M, Ghossein RA, Fahey TJ 3rd. Adrenocortical carcinoma: the influence of large vessel extension. Surgery. 2010;148:1057-1064.
24. Mihai R, Iacobone M, Makay O, Moreno P, Frilling A, Kraimps JL, et al. Outcome of operation in patients with adrenocortical cancer invading the inferior vena cava–a European Society of Endocrine Surgeons (ESES) survey. Langenbecks Arch Surg. 2012;397:225–31.
25. Hermsen IG, Kerkhofs TM, den Butter G, Kievit J, van Eijck CH, van Dijkum EJ N, et al. Surgery in adrenocortical carcinoma: Importance of national cooperation and centralized surgery. Surgery. 2012;152:50–6.
26. Lombardi CP, Raffaelli M, Boniardi M, De Toma G, Marzano LA, Miccoli P, et al. Adrenocortical carcinoma: effect of hospital volume on patient outcome. Langenbecks Arch Surg. 2012;397:201–7.
27. Kerkhofs TM, Verhoeven RH, Bonjer HJ, van Dijkum EJ, Vriens MR, De Vries J, et al. Surgery for adrenocortical carcinoma in The Netherlands: analysis of the national cancer registry data. Eur J Endocrinol. 2013;16:83–9.
28. Kerkhofs TM, Baudin E, Terzolo M, Allolio B, Chadarevian R, Mueller HH, et al. Comparison of two mitotane starting dose regimens in patients with advanced adrenocortical carcinoma. J Clin Endocrinol Metab. 2013;98:4759–67.
29. Terzolo M, Angeli A, Fassnacht M, Daffara F, Tauchmanova L, Conton PA, et al. Adjuvant mitotane treatment for adrenocortical carcinoma. N Engl J Med. 2007;356:2372–80.
30. Grubbs EG, Callender GG, Xing Y, Perrier ND, Evans DB, Phan AT, et al. Recurrence of adrenal cortical carcinoma following resection: surgery alone can achieve results equal to surgery plus mitotane. Ann Surg Oncol. 2010;17:263–70.
31. Berruti A, Fassnacht M, Haak H, Else T, Baudin E, Sperone P, et al. Prognostic role of overt hypercortisolism in completely operated patients with adrenocortical cancer. Eur Urol. 2014;65:832–8.
32. Erdogan I, Deutschbein T, Jurowich C, Kroiss M, Ronchi C, Quinkler M, et al. The role of surgery in the management of recurrent adrenocortical carcinoma. J Clin Endocrinol Metab. 2013;98:181–91.
33. Hubalewska-Dydejczyk A, Jabrocka-Hybel A, Pach D, Gilis-Januszewska A, Sokolowski G. Current and future medical therapy, and the molecular features of adrenocortical cancer. Recent Pat Anticancer Drug Discov. 2012;7:132–45.
34. Tacon LJ, Prichard RS, Soon PS, Robinson BG, Clifton-Bligh RJ, Sidhu SB. Current and emerging therapies for advanced adrenocortical carcinoma. Oncologist. 2011;16:36–48.
35. Volante M, Buttigliero C, Greco E, Berruti A, Papotti M. Pathological and molecular features of adrenocortical carcinoma: an update. J Clin Pathol. 2008;61:787–93.

Modern extraction techniques and their impact on the pharmacological profile of *Serenoa repens* extracts for the treatment of lower urinary tract symptoms

Celeste De Monte[1], Simone Carradori[1], Arianna Granese[1], Giovanni Battista Di Pierro[2*], Costantino Leonardo[2] and Cosimo De Nunzio[3]

Abstract

Background: Bioactive compounds from plants (*i.e.*, *Serenoa repens*) are often used in medicine in the treatment of several pathologies, among which benign prostatic hyperplasia (BPH) associated to lower urinary tract symptoms (LUTS).

Discussion: There are different techniques of extraction, also used in combination, with the aim of enhancing the amount of the target molecules, gaining time and reducing waste of solvents. However, the qualitative and quantitative composition of the bioactives depends on the extractive process, and so the brands of the recovered products from the same plant are different in terms of clinical efficacy (no product interchangeability among different commercial brands).

Summary: In this review, we report on several and recent extraction techniques and their impact on the composition/biological activity of *S. repens*-based available products.

Keywords: Benign prostatic hyperplasia, *Serenoa repens*, Extraction techniques, Supercritical fluid extraction, Lipidosterolic composition, Content standardization

Background

Benign prostatic hyperplasia (BPH) is a significant health concern and increases in prevalence as the population ages. Symptomatic BPH represents the most common urologic disease among elderly males, affecting about one-quarter of men in their '50s, one-third of men in their '60s, and about half of octogenarians. BPH is considered a chronic disease with early initiation and slow progression. BPH starts as a simple micro nodular hyperplasia and evolves into a macroscopic nodular enlargement that may result in bladder prostatic obstruction (BPO), causing lower urinary tract symptoms (LUTS) [1,2]. When considering options for managing LUTS, which may suggest BPO, the short term goal is to improve the individual's quality of life by relieving symptoms, however, the aim should be to prevent or reduce the worsening of symptoms over longer term and limiting BPH progression [3]. Medical treatment options of LUTS/BPO include α1-adrenoceptor antagonists, 5α-reductase inhibitors, anti-cholinergic agents, phosphodiesterase 5 inhibitors and plant extracts. Although the European Association of Urology is unable to make specific recommendations about plant extracts treatment in patients with LUTS/BPH because of the heterogeneity of the marketed products and the methodological problems associated with meta-analysis, their use in clinical practice is rising with an increased global prescription index, particularly in some European countries (Belgium, Hungary, Poland, France) [2,4,5]. Furthermore, the treatment of BPH with α-blockers and 5α-reductase inhibitors could play an important role in the alteration of sexual functions leading to ejaculatory and erectile disorders [6]. To avoid

* Correspondence: gb.dipierro@libero.it
[2]Department of Obstetrics, Gynecology and Urology, Sapienza University of Rome, Viale del Policlinico 155, Rome 00161, Italy
Full list of author information is available at the end of the article

this issue, natural products derived from plants have been using for treating BPH, especially extracts of *Serenoa repens* (saw palmetto) obtained from the American dwarf palm [7-9].

Nowadays, a lot of extractive strategies with differences in terms of methodology, time, temperature, pressure and solvents have been developed, also used in combination with other techniques in order to improve the recovery and, consequently, the pharmacological profile of their extracts. However, as a consequence of the differences among the extractive processes used by several companies, there is a discrepancy in the qualitative and quantitative composition of the extracts obtained from the same plant. Hence, each brand is different in quality and efficacy for the content of the bioactive compounds with repercussions on the beneficial effects for patients in response to clinical trials and treatments [10].

Discussion

The aim of this review is the evaluation of the available evidence on plant extraction and its possible clinical implications on *S. repens* therapeutic efficacy.

Serenoa repens as a standard reference material (SRM)

The knowledge of the exhaustive quali-quantitative composition of *S. repens* extracts is warranted not only due to the multiple variables associated to different extraction techniques, but also due to the not yet fully understood pharmacological profile of each active principle.

For this reason, the validation of appropriate analytical methods, to develop standard reference materials for selected dietary supplements, have been regulated by the National Institute of Health's Office of Dietary Supplements and the Food and Drug Administration's Center for Drug Evaluation and Research in collaboration with the National Institute of Standards and Technology (NIST) [11].

NIST, as a non-regulatory federal agency of USA, supports accurate and compatible measurements by certifying and providing over 1300 Standard Reference Materials® (SRMs) with well-characterized composition or properties. Each NIST Standard Reference Material® is supplied with a Certificate of Analysis and/or a Materials Safety Data Sheet. In addition, NIST has published many articles and practice guides that describe the development, analysis, traceability and use of SRMs. Certified concentration values are usually determined by two or more independent methods, which could be combined with data from other laboratories.

In the case of saw palmetto, two reference materials have been reported, SRM 3250 *S. repens* ground fruit and SRM 3251 *S. repens* extract. SRM 3250 has certified concentration values for specific phytosterols, and fatty acids (free or as triglycerides). On the other hand, the extract SRM 3251 has certified concentration values for phytosterols, fatty acids (free or as triglycerides), β-carotene and its isomers, and γ- and δ-tocopherol.

For SRM 3250 three extraction procedures and conditions for each procedure were evaluated including PFE (pressurized fluid extraction), Soxhlet extraction (with dichloromethane), and sonication. PFE and Soxhlet extraction gave the highest amounts of extracted fatty acids from the ground fruit. In the case of PFE (conditions: solvent mixture of 4:1 (v/v) of hexane/acetone with a four static cycle extraction at 125°C and 10.4 MPa), the choice of solvent, temperature of extraction, and pressure of extraction did not have significant effects on the composition of the extracted fractions. The solvent choice also did not have a deep impact on the efficiency of the Soxhlet extraction, although the duration of the extraction time was critical (at least 40 h). Conversely, SRM 3251 has been obtained as a supercritical CO_2 extract and analyzed with respect to the corresponding extracts obtained for SRM 3250.

As reported in Table 1, the concentrations of the fatty acids as triglycerides were 6–25 times higher in SRM 3251 compared with SRM 3250. In general, the concentration of each fatty acid as a triglyceride was higher than the corresponding free fatty acid for both extracts. The concentration of linoleic and α-linoleic acid in SRM 3250 was approximately six times lower than in SRM 3251. Linoleic and α-linolenic acids were also lower in concentration as free fatty acids in both SRM 3250 and SRM 3251 as compared with the corresponding fatty acids as triglycerides.

These SRMs could also furnish appropriate reference materials to make comparisons among dietary supplements. In fact, SRM 3251 has the second highest concentration of linoleic acid, as regards the triglycerides, compared with the other available SRMs (*i.e.*, fish oil and tissues), and the highest concentration of α-linolenic acid. As regards the phytosterols content, in both SRMs, campesterol, β-sitosterol and stigmasterol have certified concentration values (higher in SRM 3251 than SRM 3250). Furthermore, β-carotene (46.8 μg/g), γ-tocopherol (280 μg/g) and δ-tocopherol (35.3 μg/g) were also quantified.

Extraction techniques

Many plants possess bioactive metabolites that can be used as therapeutic agents for the treatment of human pathologies like BHP associated to LUTS. Because of the very low concentrations of therapeutic compounds in plants, their exhaustive recovery becomes a crucial issue in order to obtain high yields of the products with the use of an extractive method that should be reproducible, time saving and eco-friendly. Furthermore, in the choice of the extractive method, it is important to keep in mind

Table 1 Composition of *Serenoa repens* extracts as standard reference materials

Extract	Fatty acids content (as triglycerides)	Free fatty acids content on a dry mass basis
	2.96% (dodecanoic acid)	
	3.24% (oleic acid)	
	1.10% (myristic acid)	
	0.869% (palmitic acid)	
	0.824% (linoleic acid)	
	0.194% (linolenic acid)	
	0.179% (stearic acid)	
	0.117% (capric acid)	
	0.107% (caprylic acid)	
SRM 3250 (ground fruit)	0.0173% (gondoic acid)	From 0.0121 mg/g (pentadecanoic acid) to 33.7 mg/g (oleic acid)
	0.0158% (palmitoleic acid)	
	0.0107% (tetracosanoic acid)	
	0.0097% (arachidic acid)	
	0.0076% (tridecanoic acid)	
	0.0066% (docosanoic acid)	
	0.0061% (heptadecanoic acid)	
	0.0547% (vaccenic acid)	
	0.0047% (pentadecanoic acid)	
	34.73% (oleic acid)	
	26.34% (dodecanoic acid)	
	10.62% (myristic acid)	
	8.51% (palmitic acid)	
	5.99% (linoleic acid)	
	2.67% (capric acid)	
	2.65% (caprylic acid)	
	2.25% (hexanoic acid)	
	1.24% (linolenic acid)	
	0.830% (vaccenic acid)	
SRM 3251 (supercritical CO$_2$ extract)	0.271% (palmitoleic acid)	From 0.119 mg/g (pentadecanoic acid) to 221 mg/g (oleic acid)
	0.1931% (gondoic acid)	
	0.175% (stearic acid)	
	0.0932% (arachidic acid)	
	0.0926% (tetracosanoic acid)	
	0.069% (tridecanoic acid)	
	0.0644% (docosanoic acid)	
	0.0637% (heptadecanoic acid)	
	0.0515% (pentadecanoic acid)	
	0.0313% (undecanoic acid)	

the thermolability of the active molecules, hence the temperature and the other parameters should be optimized. For having an efficient process, three important factors must be mainly considered: the sample matrix, the type and the localization of bioactive compounds within the matrix. In fact, the target compound firstly must be removed from the site in which it is placed and then it must diffuse towards the extraction phase to be finally collected.

We briefly report on classical and innovative extraction techniques which have been or could be applied to obtain *S. repens* extracts enriched by specific active principles.

Solvent extraction

According to the solubility of the bioactive compounds there are a large number of inorganic, organic, polar and non-polar solvents to perform a good extraction, also in combination among them. If the substance of our interest is lipophilic, the organic solvents of choice will be non-polar, ranging from those with a very low polarity such as hexane, to those that are less non-polar like chloroform and dichloromethane. For example, the apolar solvents cyclohexane, hexane, toluene, benzene, ether, chloroform and ethyl acetate are currently used to extract alkaloids, coumarins, fatty acids (FAs), flavonoids and terpenoids. On the contrary, for hydrophilic compounds the choice will fall on a polar solvent which may be non-protic such as acetone, or protic such as ethanol, methanol or even water. In fact acetone, acetonitrile, butanol, propanol and ethanol are the solvents for the extraction of flavonols, lectins, alkaloids, quassinoids, flavones, polyphenols, tannins and saponins. One of the major pros of this procedure is the use of simple equipment and its limited cost.

Microwave-assisted extraction

Microwave-assisted extraction (MAE) is an extractive method based on the utilization of microwave energy that is produced when the perpendicular oscillation between the electric and the magnetic fields generates electromagnetic radiations with a frequency ranging from 0.3 to 300 GHz. If the microwave goes through and interacts with a substance there is a production of heat whose intensity depends on the absorption of the energy by the material and the dissipation of the resulting heat [12].

MAE techniques can be classified according to the pressure through which they operate: higher than the atmospheric pressure (closed MAE system) and lower than the atmospheric pressure (open MAE system). As regards closed systems, the temperature is set over the boiling point of the solvent and the pressure is under control to avoid an excessive development. Among the closed systems we can enumerate high pressure microwave-assisted extraction (HPMAE) which uses high pressure and temperature in order to enhance the capacity of the solvent to incorporate the energy from radiation and to avoid large amount of solvent for the extraction. In case of thermolabile molecules, soft conditions are needed and so the choice will fall on an open system or the vacuum microwave assisted extraction (VMAE) that allows the reduction of the boiling point of the solvent. For compounds that are susceptible of oxidation it has been developed the nitrogen-protected microwave-assisted extraction operating under pressurized inert gas. When the bioactive compounds are susceptible of hydrolysis such as the essential oils, solvent-free microwave-assisted extraction (SFME) is used to avoid the loss/degradation of these products. Moreover, MAE can be associated to ultrasonic energy (ultrasonic/microwave-assisted extraction UMAE) to reduce extraction times and the amounts of solvent leading to an improvement of the yield. Another way to gain time is coupling the extraction step with the analytical one in the dynamic microwave-assisted extraction (DMAE) which operates continuously and automatically. The choice of the solvent is influenced by its ability to absorb the microwave radiation: ethanol, methanol, water and the more selective room temperature ionic liquids are good solvents for MAE. The ratio of solvent to solid is important for improving MAE: if the amount of solvent is too much it absorbs all the energy with a resulting inefficient matrix heating, whereas if the ratio is too low the amount of solvent is not enough to allow the diffusion of the compounds out of the matrix. Also the vessel size is a critical factor because in a little vessel the internal pressure tends to augment and this could mean a degradation of the more delicate molecules.

Another parameter to consider in MAE is the power of extraction: an increased power boosts the temperature reducing the solvent viscosity and leading to a better efficiency, except in case of thermolabile molecules. Microwave-assisted extraction gives several advantages with respect to classical extractive processes such as Soxhlet: MAE allows a gain of time, higher quality and yields [13]. It is also cheaper than supercritical fluid extraction (SFE) and faster than ultrasonic-assisted extraction (UAE). On the other hand, MAE shows some drawbacks: it is more expensive than UAE, less eco-friendly than SFE due to the use of organic solvents, not suitable for thermolabile compounds because the irradiation could promote chemical reactions with the loss of the desirable products, and not efficient when the target molecules and/or the solvent of extraction are non-polar because they do not absorb energy from the source [14]. This technique has never been applied to *S. repens* extraction.

Ultrasound-assisted extraction

In recent times, ultrasound-assisted extraction has received a great interest to overcome the disadvantages of classical solvent extractions such as little yields and waste of time. UAE is based on the production of ultrasound waves and their transmission throughout the solvent with a resulting cavitation. When the cavitation bubbles collapse, there is a generation of liquid circulation currents and turbulence that improve the mass transfer rate. The fractures formed in the cell wall enhance its permeability and so a bigger amount of solvent can enter into the plant tissues to extract the bioactive metabolites. In order to perform an extraction based on sonochemistry, the choice of solvent becomes an important parameter because its physical properties like polarity, viscosity, vapour pressure and surface tension influence the cavitation phenomena. Ethanol, methanol and hexane are very used in UAE, and sometimes water could be added to ethanol, even if its amount must not be too much in order to avoid a decrease in extraction efficiency, probably due to the generation of radicals from the ultrasonic dissociation of water [15]. Other parameters to be considered are the frequency and the power: often the former ranges from 20 to 100 kHz and the latter from 100 to 800 W. Also the power dissipation is a critical factor, because the generation of physical effects like turbulence is directly proportioned to the power dissipated as heat. For the future, the design of reactors based on multiple transducers is needed in order to operate at multiple frequencies and improve the efficacy of UAE. Another problem that currently limits the use of UAE at large scales is the erosion of transducers and their continuous replacement to avoid a decrease in the transmitted energy. Nonetheless, UAE is less expensive than the traditional extractive techniques; it can give high quantities of products without spending time and without using large amounts of solvent. For a better performance, UAE can be also used in combination with other techniques like supercritical fluid process. This technique has never been applied to *S. repens* extraction.

Supercritical fluid extraction

Supercritical fluid extraction is a novel technique especially used for the recovery of essential oil from plants. SFE is based on the use of carbon dioxide in supercritical phase, which is at low pressure and temperature (74 bar and 32°C): in this state CO_2 possesses a polarity similar to pentane and so it is a good candidate for the extraction of lipophilic compounds. Furthermore supercritical CO_2 is non toxic, non-flammable, not expensive, and easy to remove in the end of the process (eco-friendly). Operating at low temperature it is possible to obtain in high yield thermolabile compounds like terpenes and terpenoids that normally have their boiling point over 150°C and so it is important to work at lower temperatures for preventing their degradation [16]. If the components to extract are polar, a cosolvent like water or ethanol in little percentage (5-10%) is needed to increase the extraction quality. When in the plant matrix there are bioactive compounds of different solubility, a method to improve the recovery of all the phytotherapeutics without any loss is the fractionation of the extract [17]. Two strategies could be applied: the multi-step fractionation and the on-line fractionation.

When the multi-step fractionation is performed, there are different successive steps of separation with different conditions in terms of density of CO_2: in the first step we will obtain the fraction of the more soluble compounds such as essential oils, whereas in the second step, increasing CO_2 density we will have the recovery of the less soluble components like antioxidants. Moreover, thanks to this strategy we can obtain in the first step the products extracted by the only use of supercritical CO_2, while in a second time we can add a cosolvent such as ethanol for the other compounds. The on-line fractionation works, instead, in a cascade depressurization system in order to obtain the precipitation of the several fractions according to their saturation conditions. The particular properties of the supercritical fluid characterized by a low viscosity and a high diffusion make this technique an excellent alternative to the others for the recovery of therapeutic products from plants.

Ionic liquids

The use of ionic liquid (IL) for analytical purposes has been developed in modern times with advantages in terms of quality and efficacy of extraction. In particular, an ionic liquid consists of a liquid organic salt that selectively interacts with specific polar and non-polar compounds thanks to ion-exchanges, π-stacking interactions, hydrophobic interactions or hydrogen bonds, improving the selectivity of the extractive method [18]. For example, the interaction of 1-butyl-3-methylimidazolium hexafluorophosphate ([BMIM][PF$_6$]) with hydrophilic amino acids enhances the extraction efficiency with respect to a traditional organic solvent extraction. Being ILs applied in several extractive processes such as MAE and UAE, they should be stable enough to resist to the high temperatures through which the technique works. About this matter, tetraalkylammonium cations and imidazolium ions like tetrafluoroborate $[BF_4]^-$, bis(trifluoromethylsulfonyl) imide $[NTf_2]^-$, trifluoromethanesulfonate $[CF_3SO_3]^-$, and hexafluorophosphate $[PF_6]^-$, possess a great thermal stability; moreover, the organic anions have shown to be more stable than the inorganic ones when operating at elevated temperatures. In conclusion, extraction based on ILs represents a good choice to recover in high yields organic and inorganic and metal ions as bioactive components of plants and herbs. This technique has never been applied to *S. repens* extraction.

Enzyme-assisted extraction

An alternative approach to classical solvent extraction techniques is the enzyme-assisted extraction: this method is innovative and convenient thanks to the fact that the enzymes catalyze reactions in a specific way without operating under strong conditions that could lead to the degradation of the desired products. In addition, proteins like cellulases, hemicellulases and pectinases disrupt cell wall with the hydrolysis of its components leading to a major permeability and allowing an easier release of the metabolites from plants [19]. The application of enzymes such as lipases, proteases, phospholipases, permits to reduce the use of the solvent for the extraction. For oil extraction from plants, cellulase, α-amylase and pectinase are the most used enzymes. These proteins can be obtained from fungi, bacteria, animals, and vegetables or from genetic engineering methods and, thanks to their selective catalysis, they can be used to recover a specific bioactive compound in high yields and in a "green" approach, without wasting too much energy. Nevertheless, there are some limitations due to the cost of the enzymatic approach, the incomplete disruption of the cell wall and the complicated application in a commercial scale because of the different behaviour of the enzymes according to the environmental circumstances such as the amount of oxygen, the variety of nutrients and the operating temperature. This technique has never been applied to *S. repens* extraction.

Pressurized liquid/fluid extraction

Pressurized liquid extraction (PLE or PFE in case of a general fluid) is a novel and eco-friendly approach for the recovery of bioactives from plants. This method often requires water as the solvent and so it can keep away from the environmental and health risks due to the use of organic solvents. Operating at high temperature (till 200°C) and pressure (from 35 to 200 bar), PLE improves the quality of the extraction that can be carried out in a dynamic mode in which the solvent is incessantly pumped through the vessel, or in a static mode in which there are more cycles with a continuous replacement of the solvent [20]. At elevated temperatures there is a reduction of the viscosity of the solvent that can better penetrate the matrix extracting the analytes of interest, even if this approach cannot be used for the thermally unstable compounds and it could lead to a co-extraction of other compounds because of the decreased selectivity of extraction at higher temperatures. The elevated pressure permits maintaining the solvent in the liquid phase and the disruption of plant cells wall exerting pressure on the matrix. In place of organic solvents, it is possible to use additives like non-ionic surfactants, antioxidants like ascorbic acid, CO_2 to drop aqueous pH or drying agents. Furthermore, PLE apparatus protects light sensitive and oxygen sensitive products from degradation, and it could be hyphenated with other modern extractive techniques like UAE to improve its efficacy.

Serenoa repens extracts: therapeutic properties and implication for the treatment of BPH

Natural products recovered from plants and herbs have been using for centuries for the treatment of several pathologies including benign prostatic hyperplasia. Among the phytotherapeutics used for BHP, bioactives extracted from the fruit of the American dwarf palm *S. repens* is the most widespread thanks to its safety, tolerability profile, and clinical benefits. The composition of free fatty acids, methyl and ethyl esters, long chain esters and glycerides found in *S. repens* extracts (SrE) is different from a brand to another according to the extractive strategy used [21].

Although the specific mechanism of action of SrE has not been completely understood yet, it has been reported that the therapeutic agents could exert an inhibitory activity towards 5α-reductase, in addition to pro-apoptotic, anti-estrogenic and anti-inflammatory properties [22].

In the past, two reviews compared a large number of different brands of marketed *S. repens* extracts on the basis of the quali-quantitative composition in free fatty acids and their esterified forms [23] and on their corresponding inhibitory activity against the two isoforms of 5α-reductase [24,25]. Results were contrasting among these natural products (and above all among the batches of the same product) and, consequently, their clinical efficacy could be recognized different as well.

The database (Pubmed, Scifinder) investigation has been directed towards the most recent and relevant studies regarding the biological properties and therapeutic applications of *S. repens* extracts and the comparison among these commercial products. We chose "*Serenoa repens*" and "*Serenoa repens* extraction" terms for the bibliographic research. As a matter of this, we collected in Table 2 studies on different extracts and active principles of *S. repens* to demonstrate how, despite the pharmacological interest in this plant for the treatment of lower urinary tract symptoms, little is known about its phytochemical/pharmacological complexity and a better standardization could improve the interchangeability among these brand products.

From this synoptic summary it is possible to extrapolate that:

- As regards Sabalselect® by Indena (supercritical carbon dioxide extract, SFE), despite the high content in free fatty acids, the quantitative composition in its single components depends on the natural source variability. The major findings of this study are that lauric acid, oleic acid, myristic acid and linoleic acid, the major constituents of SFE, as well as SFE itself, actively bound to pharmacologically relevant (α1-adrenergic, muscarinic and 1,4-DHP) receptors in rat brain, and significantly inhibited 5α-reductase activity in rat liver. In addition, these components and the whole extract were shown to inhibit specific binding of [³H]prazosin in rat brain. Based on their IC_{50} values, the affinity for α1-adrenergic, 1,4-DHP, and muscarinic receptors displayed by linoleic acid, oleic acid, and myristic acid was 1.3-4.5 times greater than that of SFE. Conversely, the receptor binding activity of lauric acid and palmitic acid was similar to that of SFE. In general, the receptor binding activity of unsaturated fatty acids tended to be greater than that of saturated fatty acids (correlation of the pharmacological activity with the degree of

Table 2 Different extracts of different brands of *Serenoa repens* discussed and compared in this review

Extract (composition)	Extraction technique	Isolated active compound (%)	Ref.
Sabal Select (>90% free fatty acids or their esterified forms, 0.01-0.15% fatty alcohols, 0.25-0.50% total sterols, 0.15-0.35% β-sitosterol)	Supercritical CO_2	Oleic acid (15%)	[26]
		Lauric acid (15%)	
Sabal Select (>90% free fatty acids or their esterified forms, 0.01-0.15% fatty alcohols, 0.25-0.50% total sterols, 0.15-0.35% β-sitosterol)	Supercritical CO_2	Lauric acid (30.2%)	[27,28]
		Oleic acid (28.5%)	
		Myristic acid (12.1%)	
		Palmitic acid (9.1%)	
		Linoleic acid (4.6%)	
		free fatty acids/mixed triglycerides ratio: ~55/45	
Permixon		Oleic acid (36.0%),	
		Lauric acid (27.5%),	
Free saturated and unsaturated fatty acids (>90%)	Solvent (hexane) extraction	Myristic acid (12.0%)	[29-33]
		Palmitic acid (9.7%).	
		Esterified FAs represent 7%, while the rest is composed of phytosterols, flavonoids, alcohols and polyprenic compounds	
Prostasan (95% total content of free fatty acids)	Solvent (96% ethanol) extraction	Not reported	[34]
Prostasan (86% total content of free fatty acids)	Solvent (96% ethanol) extraction	Not reported	[35]
Saw Palmetto Berry Powder (SPBE) (Madis Botanical, Inc., New Jersey) (90% free fatty acids, alcohols and sterols)	Solvent (20% ethanol) extraction of (phyto)sterols	β-sitosterol, Stigmasterol, Cholesterol	[36]
PC-SPES	Solvent (70% ethanol) extraction	Not reported	[37]
Talso, Talso uno	Supercritical CO_2	acid lipophilic compounds, fatty alcohols and sterols as main components	[38]
Prostamol Uno	Not reported	Saturated and unsaturated fatty acids and phytosteroids	[39,40]
ProstateEZE Max	Not reported	*Serenoa repens* standardized to fatty acids, *Pygeum africanum* standardized to β-sitosterol, *Epilobium parviflorum*, *Cucurbita pepo* seed oil, lycopene	[41]
Profluss	Oily extract	*Serenoa repens* extract 85%, lycopene 6%, selenium	[42]
SeR	Solvent (ethanol) extraction	Not reported	[43]

unsaturation and bond length). SFE, lauric acid, oleic acid, myristic acid and linoleic acid inhibited 5α-reductase activity in a concentration-dependent manner. The inhibitory effect of each fatty acid was similar or slightly more potent than that of SPE. Consistent with these results, Raynaud *et al.* reported that palmitic acid was inactive in the inhibition of 5α-reductase [25]. The inhibitory effect on 5α-reductase activity by each fatty acid was roughly similar to their affinity for pharmacologically relevant receptors [26,27]. In a recent research, the effect on rat prostate gland contractility of this extract was evaluated after fractioning. The inhibition of prostatic smooth muscle contractions

was preferentially induced by the ethyl acetate fraction (enriched in fatty acids) *via* a non-specific mechanism (not involving the inhibition of protein kinase C, myosin light chain kinase and Rho kinase) [28].

- Permixon® is the most studied extract in the literature both regarding its anti-proliferative activity and its anti-inflammatory ability. The former activity has been demonstrated, for the hexanic extract, against a large number of prostate carcinoma cell lines (PC3 and LNCaP) where it caused growth arrest and apoptosis at 50–80 μg/mL for 24–48 h (but not in MCF7 breast cancer cells). Treatment of cells with 100 μg/mL for 4 h resulted in morphological changes with massive vacuolization and swelling (derangement of the ultrastructure with major changes in membrane composition and function). Apoptosis seemed to depend on the intrinsic pathway, which appears to be triggered by opening of the mitochondrial PTP, a high-conductance channel that is involved in many forms of cell death, and complete release of mitochondrial TMRM (early mitochondrial depolarization and loss of membrane potential). Cell-cycle analysis showed the presence of a sub-G1 peak, a decreased G0/G1 peak and an accumulation of cells in G2/M phase after 48 h of treatment [29,30].

With respect to the latter mechanism of action, different research groups highlighted the anti-inflammatory property of this plant. Multiple inflammation functional systems, such as Cytokines family, Glucocorticoid/PPAR signalling, MAPK signalling, TNF superfamily, and COX/LOX pathways, seemed to be modulated by LSESr treatment. Recently, Latil *et al.* [31] have studied how this biological property could be ascribed only to the hexanic extract of this plant and not to the supercritical CO_2 extract. Both of the tested extracts belonged to six different batches of the same plant at Pierre Fabre Plantes et Industrie. Results showed that the hexanic extract was responsible of a strong attenuation of a large number of inflammation mediators and markers. Moreover, inhibition of MCP-1/CCL2 mRNA expression in a concentration-dependent manner has been registered only for the hexanic extract, whereas the supercritical CO_2 extract was not endowed with this inhibitory effect. This is the only one example in the literature of a direct comparison of the different pharmacological profile associated to two extraction techniques showing the impact of this procedures on the quality/efficacy of phytotherapeutic products [31-33];

- Prostasan® has been also studied both for its anti-proliferative and anti-inflammatory activities (as an ethanolic extract). Comparison of the obtained results with respect to Permixon® led to similar results in terms of low cytotoxicity against normal cells, dose-dependent reduction of cellular growth (especially in AR-positive prostate and ER-positive breast cancer cells), apoptosis induction, inhibition of IL-12, MCP-1 and GM-CSF secretion and, consequently, decreased inflammatory processes and production of cytokine pro-inflammatory from macrophages. The content in free fatty acids is almost comparable to that of Permixon®. Moreover, inhibitory effects on the epithermal growth factor (EGF) and the Gram-negative bacteria cell wall component LPS-induced proliferation of prostatic cells PC-3 were observed with this extract. In the case of EGF, the mechanism involves competition for the EGF receptor. LPS exerts a milder but still significant induction on proliferation of prostate cells, supporting the role of bacterial infection in the origin of BPH. The mechanism behind *S. repens* extract effecting LPS actions on prostatic cells remains to be elucidated since it does not apparently affect Toll-like receptor 4 intracellular signalling [34,35];

- Saw Palmetto Berry Powder (SPBE) biological activity has been investigated with respect to its phytosterols content. With increasing concentration, the authors observed a reduction in cell growth compared to control cells in the following order of substance effectiveness: SPBE > β-sitosterol > stigmasterol, and an increase in cell growth with rising cholesterol concentration on prostate cancer cells (DU145). Analysis of cell cycle regulating proteins (p53, p27, p21) and 2D traction microscopy were also performed. p53 increased after treatment with this extract, whereas p27 and p21 decreased. This report justifies the administration of the entire phytocomplex to ensure a proper pharmacological efficacy not limiting the interest only to free fatty acids [36];

- PC-SPES is a combination of herbs containing flavonoids, alkaloids, polysaccharides, amino acids, and trace minerals. The 8 herbs used were chrysanthemum, isatis, licorice, *Ganoderma lucidum*, *Panax pseudo-ginseng*, *Rabdosia rubescens*, saw palmetto, and skullcap. PC-SPES mediated an anti-proliferative effect on prostate cancer cells (LNCaP, DU145, and PC3) *in vivo* and *in vitro*, induced apoptosis of LNCaP cells in a dose- and time-dependent manner and reduced prostate specific antigen (PSA) or AR levels in LNCaP cells and in more than 80% of individuals with prostate cancer. In addition in the same cell line, saw palmetto might inhibit cell growth down-regulating basal and DHT- or IL-6-induced PSA expression in cytoplasmic protein and AR expression in nuclear proteins. Previous studies have demonstrated that STAT3 signalling has a critical role in the tumour formation of prostate cancer and IL-6 treatment results in the activation of STAT3 in prostate cancer cells. This extract down-regulated the IL-6-induced level of the phosphorylated form of STAT3 in LNCaP cells blocking this pathway and markedly inhibiting the growth of LNCaP cells [37];

- The SG 291 extract (Talso, Talso uno) was analyzed by gas chromatography and investigated for its dual inhibitory influence on cyclooxygenase (COX, IC_{50} = 28.1 μg/mL) and 5-lipoxygenase (5-LOX, IC_{50} = 18 μg/mL). After alkaline hydrolysis, ether extraction and preparative TLC the SG 291 extract was separated in three fractions containing acid lipophilic compounds (A), fatty alcohols (B) and sterols (C). Only fraction A inhibited COX and 5-LOX as the native SG 291 extract, whereas the fractions B, C and β-sitosterol showed no inhibitory effect on both enzymes [38].

- Prostamol Uno (Berlin-Chemie AG/Menarini Group) was shown to possess anti-inflammatory and antiedematous effects reducing the proliferation of prostatic epithelium. Moreover, its pharmacological activity in rats with BPH was compared to that of a complex of peptides isolated from the cattle prostate. The results showed that both treatments reduced the acinar epithelial area in this experimental model, but the response to S. repens extract was characterized by an enhanced stromal/epithelial proportion [39]. In addition, the safety and tolerability of this extract have been evaluated in two dosage regimes in experimental animals [40].

- ProstateEZE Max (Caruso's Natural Health) is an orally dosed herbal preparation containing S. repens (660 mg/day), among other prostatotropic agents of natural origin (Cucurbita pepo, Epilobium parviflorum, lycopene and Pygeum africanum). It has been studied in a short-term phase II randomized double-blind placebo controlled clinical trial to evaluate its efficacy and safety [41]. This combination of herbal extracts behaved as an effective treatment in the management of symptoms of BPH.

- Profluss® by Konpharma: to evaluate its efficacy on prostatic chronic inflammation, 168 subjects affected by LUTS due to bladder outlet obstruction were enrolled and subjected to Profluss with or without α-blockers treatment ("Flogosis And Profluss in Prostatic and Genital Disease" (FLOG) study). At follow-up there were statistical significant reductions of extension and grading of flogosis (mean values of CD20, CD3, CD68, and PSA). This product may have an anti-inflammatory activity that could be of interest in the treatment of PCI in BPH [42].

- SeR alcoholic extract, provided by Bernett, has been recently studied (alone and in association with selenium and lycopene) for the impact on the bax/bcl-2 ratio, caspase-3 activity, IAPs and survivin expression, and cytokines production in prostatic specimens from BPH patients. These analyses suggested that the impairment in the extrinsic pathway does not contribute to the cell death program in BPH, that the administration of SeR, either alone or in association, markedly mitigated survivin expression. Moreover, the expression of IL-6 was reduced preventing the histological features of BPH and inhibiting growth by 43.3% [43].

Review and conclusions

Benign prostate hyperplasia is one of the most common diseases in male population. In addition to pharmacological therapy with α-blockers or 5α-reductase inhibitors, also bioactive compounds derived from plants play an important role in the treatment of BPH associated to LUTS. Despite the benefits obtained from SrE, the variety of the extractive techniques and strategies makes one extract different from another in terms of bioactives composition and this could affect the quality and the clinical effects of natural therapies of different brands even if derived from the same plant. Thus, the clinical and biological activities of one preparation cannot be extrapolated to other preparations of the same plant source. Moreover, standardization of the composition through alternative and more reproducible techniques is warranted due to the complex pharmacological profile of the whole phytocomplex of S. repens. Results from different clinical trials must be compared strictly according to the same validated extraction technique and/or content in active principles.

At this time, few studies made a comparison among these different extracts. The solvent (hexane) extraction of lipidosterolic composition from S. repens is the most investigated in clinical and experimental trials although further large comparative trials should explore the possible clinical influence of the different extractions processes.

Competing interests

We disclose any conflict of interest such as consultancies, stock ownership or other equity interests, patents received and/or pending, or any commercial relationship which might be in any way considered related to the submitted article.

Authors' contributions

CDM conception and design, general supervision. SC conception and design, analysis and interpretation of data drafting of the manuscript. AG collection of data, drafting of the manuscript. GBDP conception and design, critical revision for intellectual content. CL general supervision, collection of data, CDN conception and design, general supervision, critical revision for intellectual content. All authors have made a significant contribution to the paper, and have read and approved the final draft. The work has not already been published and has not been submitted simultaneously to any other journal.

Acknowledgment

We thank Pierre Fabre for supporting and funding the study.

Author details

[1]Department of Drug Chemistry and Technologies, Sapienza University of Rome, P.le A. Moro 5, Rome 00185, Italy. [2]Department of Obstetrics, Gynecology and Urology, Sapienza University of Rome, Viale del Policlinico 155, Rome 00161, Italy. [3]Department of Urology, Ospedale Sant'Andrea, Sapienza University of Rome, Via di Grottarossa 1035/1039, Rome 00189, Italy.

References

1. De Nunzio C, Aronson W, Freedland S, Giovannucci E, Parsons JK: The correlation between metabolic syndrome and prostatic diseases. *Eur Urol* 2012, **61**:560–571.

2. Oelke M, Bachmann A, Descazeaud A, Emberton M, Gravas S, Michel MC, N'dow J, Nordling J, de la Rosette JJ: EAU guidelines on the treatment and follow-up of non-neurogenic male lower urinary tract symptoms including benign prostatic obstruction. *Eur Urol* 2013, **64**:118–140.

3. Miano R, De Nunzio C, Asimakopoulos T, Germani S, Tubaro A: Treatment options for benign prostatic hyperplasia in elderly men. *Med Sci Monit* 2008, **14**:94–102.

4. Cornu JN, Cussenot O, Haab F, Lukacs B: A widespread population study of actual medical management of lower urinary tract symptoms related to benign prostatic hyperplasia across Europe and beyond official clinical guidelines. *Eur Urol* 2010, **58**:450–456.

5. Fourcade RO, Théret N, Taïeb C: Profile and management of patients treated for the first time for lower urinary tract symptoms/benign prostatic hyperplasia in four European countries. *BJU Int* 2008, **101**:1111–1118.

6. Suter A, Saller R, Riedi E, Heinrich M: Improving BPH symptoms and sexual dysfunctions with a saw palmetto preparation? Results from a pilot trial. *Phytother Res* 2013, **27**:218–226.

7. MacDonald R, Tacklind JW, Rutks I, Wilt TJ: Serenoa repens monotherapy for benign prostatic hyperplasia (BPH): an updated Cochrane systematic review. *BJU Int* 2012, **109**:1756–1761.

8. Azimi H, Khakshur AA, Aghdasi I, Fallah-Tafti M, Abdollahi M: A review of animal and human studies for management of benign prostatic hyperplasia with natural products: perspective of new pharmacological agents. *Inflamm Allergy Drug Targets* 2012, **11**:207–221.

9. Tacklind J, Macdonald R, Rutks I, Stanke JU, Wilt TJ: *Serenoa repens* for benign prostatic hyperplasia. *Cochrane Database Syst Rev* 2012, **12**:CD001423.

10. Lowe FC: Phytotherapy in the management of benign prostatic hyperplasia. *Urology* 2001, **58**:71–77.

11. Schantz MM, Bedner M, Long SE, Molloy JL, Murphy KE, Porter BJ, Putzbach K, Rimmer CA, Sander LC, Sharpless KE, Thomas JB, Wise SA, Wood LJ, Yen JH, Yarita T, NguyenPho A, Sorenson WR, Betz JM: Development of saw palmetto (*Serenoa repens*) fruit and extract standard reference materials. *Anal Bioanal Chem* 2008, **392**:427–438.

12. Chan CH, Yusoff R, Ngoh GC, Kung FWL: Microwave-assisted extractions of active ingredients from plants. *J Chromatogr A* 2011, **1218**:6213–6225.

13. Capitani D, Sobolev AP, Delfini M, Vista S, Antiochia R, Proietti N, Bubici S, Ferrante G, Carradori S, De Salvador FR, Mannina L: NMR methodologies in the analysis of blueberries. *Electrophoresis* 2014. doi:10.1002/elps.201300629.

14. Zhang HF, Yang XH, Wang Y: Microwave-assisted extraction of secondary metabolites from plants: current status and future directions. *Trends Food Sci Tech* 2011, **22**:672–688.

15. Shirsath SR, Sonawane SH, Gogate PR: Intensification of extraction of natural products using ultrasonic irradiations - a review of current status. *Chem Eng Process* 2012, **53**:10–23.

16. Fornari T, Vicente G, Vàzquez E, Garcìa-Risco MR, Reglero G: Isolation of essential oil from different plants and herbs by supercritical fluid extraction. *J Chromatogr A* 2012, **1250**:34–48.

17. Akanda MJ, Sarker MZ, Ferdosh S, Manap MY, Ab Rahman NN, Ab Kadir MO: Applications of supercritical fluid extraction (SFE) of palm oil and oil from natural sources. *Molecules* 2012, **17**:1764–1794.

18. Tang B, Bi W, Tian M, Row KH: Application of ionic liquid for extraction and separation of bioactive compounds from plants. *J Chromatogr B* 2012, **904**:1–21.

19. Puri M, Sharma D, Barrow CJ: Enzyme-assisted extraction of bioactives from plants. *Trends Biotechnol* 2012, **30**:37–44.

20. Mustafa A, Turner C: Pressurized liquid extraction as a green approach in food and herbal plants extraction: A review. *Anal Chim Acta* 2011, **703**:8–18.

21. Geavlete P, Multescu R, Geavlete B: *Serenoa repens* extract in the treatment of benign prostatic hyperplasia. *Ther Adv Urol* 2011, **3**:193–198.

22. Buck AC: Is there a scientific basis for the therapeutic effects of *Serenoa repens* in benign prostatic hyperplasia? mechanisms of action. *J Urol* 2004, **172**:1792–1799.

23. Habib FK, Wyllie MG: Not all brands are created equal: a comparison of selected components of different brands of *Serenoa repens* extract. *Prostate Cancer Prostatic Dis* 2004, **7**:195–200.

24. Scaglione F, Lucini V, Pannacci M, Caronno A, Leone C: Comparison of the potency of different brands of *Serenoa repens* extract on 5α-reductase types I and II in prostatic co-cultured epithelial and fibroblast cells. *Pharmacology* 2008, **82**:270–275.

25. Raynaud JP, Cousse H, Martin PM: Inhibition of type 1 and type 2 5alpha-reductase activity by free fatty acids, active ingredients of Permixon. *J Steroid Biochem Mol Biol* 2002, **82**:233–239.

26. Abe M, Ito Y, Suzuki A, Onoue S, Noguchi H, Yamada S: Isolation and pharmacological characterization of fatty acids from saw palmetto extract. *Anal Sci* 2009, **25**:553–557.

27. Abe M, Ito Y, Oyunzul L, Oki-Fujino T, Yamada S: Pharmacologically relevant receptor binding characteristics and 5α-reductase inhibitory activity of free fatty acids contained in Saw Palmetto extract. *Biol Pharm Bull* 2009, **32**:646–650.

28. Chua T, Eise NT, Simpson JS, Ventura S: Pharmacological characterization and chemical fractionation of a liposterolic extract of saw palmetto (*Serenoa repens*): effects on rat prostate contractility. *J Ethnopharmacol* 2014, **152**:283–291.

29. Baron M, Mancini E, Caldwell A, Cabrelle P, Bernardi F, Pagano F: *Serenoa repens* extract targets mitochondria and activates the intrinsic apoptotic pathway in human prostate cancer cells. *BJUI* 2009, **103**:1275–1283.

30. Petrangeli E, Lenti L, Buchetti B, Chinzari P, Sale P, Salvatori L, Ravenna L, Lococo E, Morgante E, Russo A, Frati L, Di Silverio F, Russo MA: Lipido-sterolic extract of *Serenoa repens* (LSESr, Permixon®) treatment affects human prostate cancer cell membrane organization. *J Cell Physiol* 2009, **219**:69–76.

31. Latil A, Libon C, Templier M, Junquero D, Lantoine-Adam F, Nguyen T: Hexanic lipidosterolic extract of *Serenoa repens* inhibits the expression of two key inflammatory mediators, MCP-1/CCL2 and VCAM-1, *in vitro*. *BJUI* 2012, **110**:E301–E303.

32. Silvestri I, Cattarino S, Aglianò AM, Nicolazzo C, Scarpa S, Salciccia S, Frati L, Gentile V, Sciarra A: Effect of *Serenoa repens* (Permixon®) on the expression of inflammation-related genes: analysis in primary cell cultures of human prostate carcinoma. *J Inflammation* 2013, **10**:11–19.

33. Sirab N, Robert G, Fasolo V, Descazeaud A, Vacherot F, de la Taille A, Terry S: Lipidosterolic extract of *Serenoa repens* modulates the expression of inflammation related-genes in benign prostatic hyperplasia epithelial and stromal cells. *Int J Mol Sci* 2013, **14**:14301–14320.

34. Hostanska K, Suter A, Melzer J, Saller R: Evaluation of cell death caused by an ethanolic extract of *Serenoae repentis* fructus (Prostasan®) on human carcinoma cell lines. *Anticancer Res* 2007, **27**:873–882.

35. Iglesias-Gato D, Carsten T, Vesterlund M, Pousette A, Schoop R, Norstedt G: Androgen-independent effects of *Serenoa repens* extract (Prostasan) on prostatic epithelial cell proliferation and inflammation. *Phytother Res* 2012, **26**:259–264.

36. Scholtysek C, Krukiewicz AA, Alonso JL, Sharma KP, Sharma PC, Goldmann WH: Characterizing components of the Saw Palmetto Berry Extract (SPBE) on prostate cancer cell growth and traction. *Biochem Biophys Res Commun* 2009, **379**:795–798.

37. Yang Y, Ikezoe T, Zheng Z, Taguchi H, Koeffler HP, Zhu WG: Saw Palmetto induces growth arrest and apoptosis of androgen-dependent prostate cancer LNCaP cells via inactivation of STAT 3 and androgen receptor signaling. *Int J Oncol* 2007, **31**:593–600.

38. Breu W, Hagenlocher M, Redl K, Tittel G, Stadler F, Wagner H: Anti-inflammatory activity of sabal fruit extracts prepared with supercritical carbon dioxide. *In vitro* antagonists of cyclooxygenase and 5-lipoxygenase metabolism. *Arzneimittelforschung* 1992, **42**:547–551.

39. Duborija-Kovacevic N, Jakovljevic V, Sabo A, Tomic Z, Pajovic B, Perovic D: Tolerability and toxicity of lipidosterolic extract of American dwarf palm *Serenoa repens* in Wistar rats: well-known extract, new insight. *Eur Rev Med Pharmacol Sci* 2011, **15**:1311–1317.

40. Borovskaya TG, Fomina TI, Ermolaeva LA, Vychuzhanina AV, Pakhomova AV, Poluektova ME, Shchemerova YA: Comparative evaluation of the efficiency of prostatotropic agents of natural origin in experimental benign prostatic hyperplasia. *Bull Exp Biol Med* 2013, **155**:67–70.

41. Coulson S, Rao A, Beck SL, Steels E, Gramotnev H, Vitetta L: A phase II randomised double-blind placebo-controlled clinical trial investigating the efficacy and safety of ProstateEZE max: a herbal medicine

preparation for the management of symptoms of benign prostatic hypertrophy. *Compl Ther Med* 2013, **21**:172–179.

42. Morgia G, Cimino S, Favilla V, Russo GI, Squadrito F, Mucciardi G, Masieri L, Minutoli L, Grosso G, Castelli T: **Effects of** *Serenoa repens*, **selenium and lycopene (Profluss®) on chronic inflammation associated with benign prostatic hyperplasia: results of "FLOG" (flogosis and Profluss in prostatic and genital disease), a multicentre italian study.** *Int Braz J Urol* 2013, **39**:214–221.

43. Minutoli L, Altavilla D, Marini H, Rinaldi M, Irrera N, Pizzino G, Bitto A, Arena S, Cimino S, Squadrito F, Russo GI, Morgia G: **Inhibitors of apoptosis proteins in experimental benign prostatic hyperplasia: effects of** *Serenoa repens*, **selenium and lycopene.** *J Biomedical Sci* 2014, **21**:19.

Early results of a novel technique for anterior vaginal wall prolapse repair: anterior vaginal wall darn

Osman Köse[1,2*], Hasan S Sağlam[1], Şükrü Kumsar[1], Salih Budak[1], Hüseyin Aydemir[1] and Öztuğ Adsan[1]

Abstract

Background: The aim of this study was to describe the results of a 1-year patient follow-up after anterior vaginal wall darn, a novel technique for the repair of anterior vaginal wall prolapse.

Methods: Fifty-five patients with anterior vaginal wall prolapse underwent anterior vaginal wall darn. The anterior vaginal wall was detached using sharp and blunt dissection via an incision beginning 1 cm proximal to the external meatus and extending to the vaginal apex. The space between the tissues that attach the lateral vaginal walls to the arcus tendineus fasciae pelvis was then darned. Cough Stress Test, Pelvic Organ Prolapse Quantification, seven-item Incontinence Impact Questionnaire, and six-item Urogenital Distress Inventory scores were performed 1-year postoperatively to evaluate recovery.

Results: One-year postoperatively, all patients were satisfied with the results of the procedure. No patient had vaginal mucosal erosion or any other complication.

Conclusions: One-year postoperative findings for patients in this series indicate that patients with stage II–III anterior vaginal wall prolapse were successfully treated with the anterior vaginal wall darn technique.

Keywords: Anterior vaginal wall prolapse, Darn, Pelvic organ prolapse, Stress urinary incontinence, Surgical technique

Background

Pelvic organ prolapse (POP), a condition characterized by a downward descent of the pelvic organs, causing the vagina to protrude, afflicts millions of women worldwide and is increasingly recognized as a global burden on women's health [1]. The social, psychological, and economical cost of POP can be high [2,3]. During their lifetimes, nearly 10% of women will require surgery for POP, urinary incontinence, or both. Of these, 30% will undergo two or more surgical procedures, presenting a challenge to gynaecologist and urologist [4]. The anterior vaginal wall is the segment of the vagina that most commonly prolapses and is most likely to fail long term after surgical correction [5]. Central defects have trad-

itionally been treated with anterior colporrhaphy, which entails central plication of the fibromuscular layer of the anterior vaginal wall [6]. Paravaginal defects have been repaired with vaginal paravaginal repair. Combination vaginal repair of these defects has been performed with these two operations [7]. Recurrent anterior vaginal wall prolapse following conventional repair has been reported in more than 30% of cases [8].

In an effort to improve outcomes of transvaginal prolapse repair, a number of graft materials have been introduced to complement, reinforce, or replace native tissue in reconstructive surgical procedures. Although abdominal sacrocolpopexy and suburethral sling procedures, the standard of care, have been shown to be effective, there is considerable debate over the use of permanent mesh and biologic grafts for transvaginal POP repair [9,10].

The use of synthetic graft material for the repair of anterior vaginal wall prolapse has been limited by potential complications related to the mesh, including mesh erosion and contraction, dyspareunia, pelvic pain and infection. A

* Correspondence: koseonk@yahoo.com.tr
[1]Department of Urology, Faculty of Medicine, Sakarya University and Training and Research Hospital, 54100 Sakarya, Turkey
[2]Beyaz Kent Sitesi, Beşköprü M. Girne C., 54100 Sakarya, Turkey

lack of comparative data and an anticipated incidence of graft-related complications such as graft erosion and infection have caused debate among surgeons regarding the use of synthetic grafts [11].

For this reason, we introduce a new technique, anterior vaginal wall darn (AVWD) which is carried out without mesh. Unlike colporrhaphy, this technique does not cause tissue tension and is easy to perform, and in contrast to the use of mesh, it does not corrupt the anatomical structures.

Methods

Fifty-five patients who had been experiencing POP symptoms for the previous 9 months and stage II–III prolapse of the anterior vaginal wall were enrolled between September 2011 and July 2012. Patients provided written informed consent to participate, and the study protocol had been approved by the Ethics Committee of Sakarya University Medical Faculty.

Preoperative evaluation consisted of complete medical history, gynaecological examination, cough stress test (CST), voiding diary, daily pad use, Q-tip test, and seven-item Incontinence Impact Questionnaire (IIQ-7) and six-item Urogenital Distress Inventory (UDI-6) scores. Patients' symptoms were also evaluated via standard questions asked by the examining physician. The severity of prolapse was assessed using the POP Quantification (POPQ) system adopted by the International Continence Society. Daily pad weight was used to quantify patients' subjective complaints.

Exclusion criteria were a history of pelvic or vaginal surgery, predominant urge incontinence, pelvic or systemic infection, inguinal or vulvar abscess, pregnancy, urinary tract obstruction or renal insufficiency, pelvic pain unrelated to prolapse, vaginal bleeding of unknown aetiology, blood coagulation disorders, pelvic malignancy or previous irradiation of the pelvic region, vaginal erosion or severe vaginal atrophy, vaginal or urethral fistula, and known allergy to the suture material. Patients requiring concomitant vaginal vault suspension, such as sacrospinous ligament fixation; sacrocolpopexy for vaginal prolapse or uterine procidentia; or laparotomy or laparoscopy for any reason, were also excluded.

All AVWD procedures were performed by the same surgeon as follows: after insertion of an 18-Fr indwelling urethral catheter, an adequate volume of normal saline was injected under the vaginal mucosa to provide comfortable dissection in an accurate plane with limited haemorrhage. A midline incision was made beginning 1 cm proximal to the external urethral meatus and extending to the vaginal apex. The anterior vaginal wall was detached from the urinary bladder beyond the anterior vaginal sulcus using sharp and blunt dissection until the arcus tendinous fasciae pelvis (ATFP) was

exposed. Using a continuous locking 2–0 polypropylene suture, bites were taken on alternate sides from distal to proximal in the ATFP and the tissues that attach the lateral walls of the vagina to the ATFP (Figure 1). After 6 cm, at the point where the ATFP exits the anterior vaginal wall, the sutures were placed medial to the perivesical fascia for 2–3 cm. The running sutures were turned back from the cardinal ligaments without being tied and were extended continuously to the distal aspect to form a darn. The suture ends were tied together (Figures 2 and 3). The traumatized vaginal mucosa was trimmed and closed with a continuous absorbable sutures, and a vaginal pack soaked in antibiotic solution was inserted.

Postoperative evaluation, including POPQ measurement, UDI-6, and IIQ-7 scores, was performed for each patient, 1 year after the AVWD procedure. A Q-tip test was performed to evaluate urethral hypermobility. Pre- and postoperative questionnaire scores and POPQ measurements were analyzed using Wilcoxon signed rank test. SPSS for Windows, Version 12.0 (SPSS, Inc., Chicago, IL, USA) was used for data analysis. The level of statistical significance was set at $P < 0.05$.

Results

Fifty-five patients with anterior POP stage II–III were eligible to participate in the study. The patients age range was 35–67 years (median age 51 years). Baseline demographic and clinical parameters are shown in Table 1. Median surgical duration was 40 minutes (range: 30–45 min), mean duration of hospitalization was 1.7 days (range: 1–2

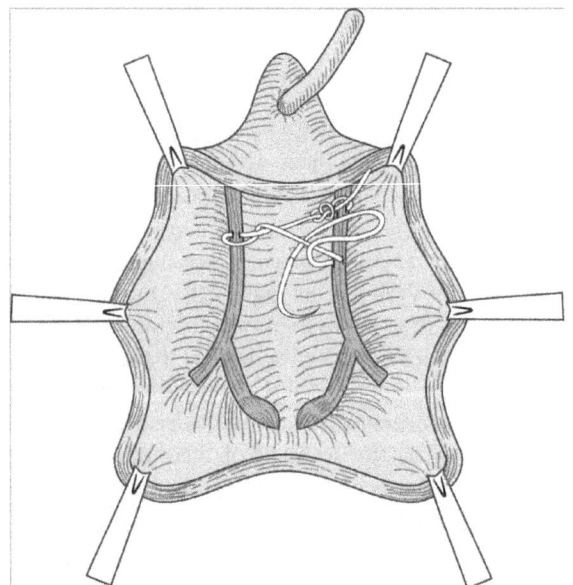

Figure 1 Bites were taken from alternate sides of the arcus tendineus fasciae pelvis using continuous locking 2–0 polypropylene suture, and the tissue edges were slightly approximated.

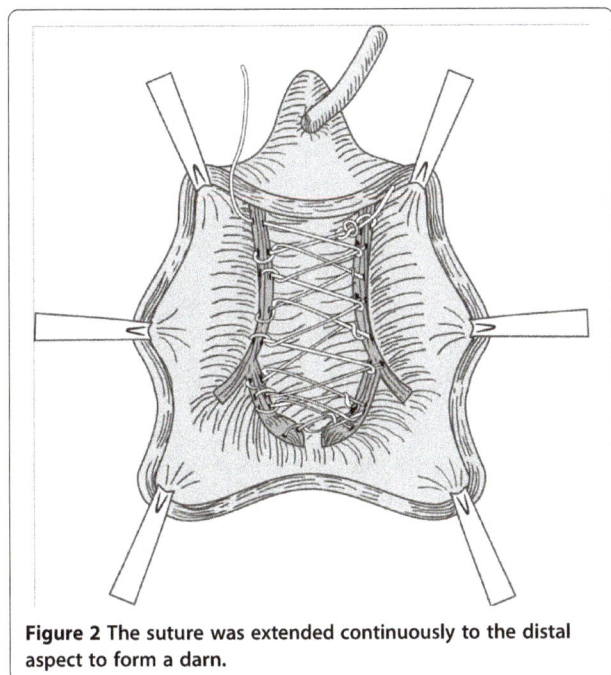

Figure 2 The suture was extended continuously to the distal aspect to form a darn.

Table 1 Patient characteristics at baseline

Characteristic	n = 55 (%)
Age	51 ± 16.3
Body mass index, kg/m²	
<30	36 (65.45)
30-40	12 (21.81)
>40	7 (12.72)
Parity	3 (0–6)
Topical oestrogen	13 (23.6)
Hypertension	15 (37.2)
Smoking status	
Current	10 (18.1)
Former	13 (23.6)

days), and the average time to void was 1.4 days (range: 1–2 days). Pre- and postoperative POPQ measurements, shown in Table 2, reveal significant improvements at points Aa and Ba. Similarly, UDI-6 and IIQ-7 scores were significantly lower postoperatively (P < 0.001) (Table 2). Similarly, UDI-6 and IIQ-7 scores were significantly lower postoperatively (p < 0.001) (Table 2).

Moderate groin discomfort was the most common complaint immediately postoperatively but disappeared within 10 days of analgesic therapy. One-year postoperatively, all patients underwent a complete evaluation. Symptom relief 12 months post-surgery is shown at Table 3. Upon examination, CST was negative in 90.9% of patients and vaginal examination were appeared normal in all patients. Bladder ultrasonography demonstrated no significant post-void residual urine volume.

Discussion

The goal of treatment of POP is to improve patient quality of life rather than prolong survival; therefore, when choosing a surgical method for anterior vaginal wall prolapse, it is important to consider all possible complications as well as treatment outcome [12]. Although conservative treatment is a reasonable initial approach for urinary incontinence, surgical management is usually required for symptomatic grade II-III vaginal prolapse. Many surgical methods are currently known, but unfortunately none can solve the problems caused by POP.

There is a lack of consensus concerning when, where, and how to perform surgery, preferably as a single procedure, to provide the best outcome in patients with POP. When selecting a surgical procedure for POP, pertinent factors, including history of anti-incontinence surgery, sexual activity, coital incontinence, obesity, chronic increases in intra-abdominal pressure, mixed incontinence and concurrent overactive bladder must be considered.

In an effort to improve the outcomes of transvaginal prolapse repair, a number of biologic and synthetic graft

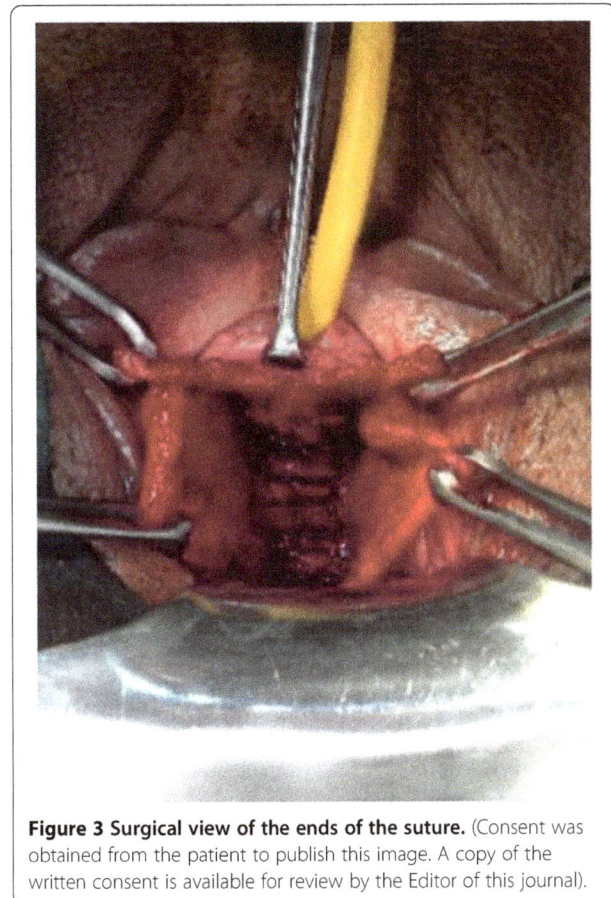

Figure 3 Surgical view of the ends of the suture. (Consent was obtained from the patient to publish this image. A copy of the written consent is available for review by the Editor of this journal).

Table 2 POPQ and incontinence-related quality values

	Before operation	After operation	P value
POPQ measurements Aa (cm)	1.6 ± 1.0	−2.1 ± 0.7	<0.001
POPQ measurements Ba (cm)	2.3 ± 1.5	−2.0 ± 0.8	<0.001
POPQ measurements Ap (cm)	−2.2 ± 0.6	−2 ± 0.7	0.17
POPQ measurements Bp (cm)	−2.78 ± 0.4	−2.61 ± 0.52	0.18
POPQ measurements TVL (cm)	7.62-0.51-	7.13-0.62	0.53
POPQ measurements C (cm)	−5.5 ± 1.4	−6.3 ± 1.2	0.046
UDI-6	8.9 ± 3.7	1.6 ± 1.2	<0.001
IIQ-7	10.5 ± 5.3	0.9 ± 0.8	<0.001
Q-TT	28.7 ± 6.2	15.3 ± 10.4	<0.018
Pad count (d)	4.3 ± 1.6	0.4 ± 0.9	<0.001
Residual urine volume (ml)	58.1 ± 13.2	32.2 ± 10.6	0.024

IIQ-7, seven-item Incontinence Impact Questionnaire; POPQ, Pelvic Organ Prolapse Quantification; Q-TT, Q-Tip test; UDI-6, six-item Urogenital Distress Inventory.

materials have been introduced since 1996 for use during reconstructive surgical procedures to reinforce or replace native tissue [13]. Results have been favourable, with anatomical success rates in the range of 59% to 94%; however, the use of mesh in vaginal repair procedures remains controversial [9,14-16]. Recently, significant problems associated with mesh use in vaginal prolapse surgery (dyspareunia, vaginal pain, mesh shrinkage, bladder erosion, fistula, mesh exposure and infection) have been reported [17-21]. Vaginal mesh erosion is one of the most common complications of introducing synthetic material via the vaginal route. Differences in mesh types, follow-up periods, and definitions of success and failure have contributed to inconsistent reported erosion rates. No generally accepted *"safety time zone"* for mesh exposure or erosion has been accepted, and the complication can occur many years after mesh placement. Young age and sexual activity are additional risk factors for mesh exposure [22].

Although there is increasing industry pressure on surgeons to adopt mesh-augmented repairs into their practice and many surgeons are employing the therapy liberally, health organizations such as the US Food and Drug Administration warn urogynaecologists and patients about the dangers of using mesh materials for the

Table 3 Postoperative symptom relief

	Preoperative	Postoperative
Pelvic pressure	33	4
Sensation of a mass bulging into the vagina	43	1
Stress urinary incontinence	16	2
Coital incontinence	11	1
Difficulties in emptying the bladder	10	1
Mixed urinary incontinence	13	3
Dyspareunia	12	3

treatment of POP [23,24]. The committee for POP at the 3rd International Consultation on Incontinence concluded that there were insufficient data to reach a definitive conclusion regarding the role of biologic or synthetic prosthetic materials in surgical procedures for primary or recurrent prolapse [25].

The available data concerning the results of prolapse surgery remain mixed. Success rate varies substantially depending on the technique used. Despite high anatomical recurrence rates, traditional anterior colporrhaphy, and paravaginal repair have been used for years for the treatment of combined anterior vaginal wall prolapse [26,27]. However, although pubocervical fascia is used to place plication sutures during anterior colporrhaphy, histologic examination of the anterior vaginal wall has failed to show a separate layer of fascia between the vagina and bladder [28], and paravaginal repair has been used only for paravaginal defects.

The tissue into which darn suture is placed during the novel AVWD procedure described herein is the ATFP, or *white line*, a fibrous thickening that consists of parietal fascia from the surrounding pubococcygeus and iliococcygeus portions of the levator ani and the obturator internus muscles [6]. The ATFP is important in providing support to pelvic structures. Cadaveric studies have shown that the anterior segment of the ATFP is attached to the lower posterior side of the body of the pubic bone, approximately 1 cm from the pubic symphysis; that the first 6 cm is attached anteriorly to the anterolateral vagina, creating the anteriorlateral vaginal sulci; and that it is also attached to the ischial spines and gets some fibres from adjacent fascias [29]. Detachment of this lateral support is the primary cause of paravaginal defects and can lead to prolapse of the anterior vaginal wall [30]. Although it may be injured during pregnancy, the ATFP is a point of attachment for many gynaecologic procedures.

However, as in hernia repair, tissue repairs are associated with a high risk of recurrence. Failed tissue repair is most often due to the apposition and suturing together under tension of structures in positions other than normal anatomic, as occurs in traditional anterior colporrhaphy. The principle behind AVWD for the repair of prolapse is similar to that of the nylon darn method, which was commonly used for the treatment of inguinal hernia before the advent of mesh and is still used by some general surgeons instead of mesh repair [31]. The rational for the darn procedure is that it forms a meshwork of non-absorbable sutures that is well tolerated by the tissues and fills the interstices with fibrous connective tissue, providing a buttress across the weakened area of the anterior vaginal wall. This technique is therefore a compensatory repair that facilitates the repair of anterior vaginal wall prolapse without distorting the normal anatomy and without creating suture-line tension, which can be used for central, lateral and combined defects. The procedure is in harmony with the anatomical structures and creates a hammock that reinforces the native support tissue, does not cause tension and confers very a low risk of vaginal mucosal erosion and urinary bladder injury.

The AVWD procedure also creates support under the bladder neck, and can therefore help to alleviate urethral hypermobility. Our postoperative 1-year Q-tip test results showed that average urethral angle dropped from 28.7 ± 6.2 degrees to 15.3 ± 10.4 degrees ($p < 0.018$). CST was negative in 90.9% of patients. We attribute this results to darn sutures passing under the bladder neck.

Conclusions

In the present initial series, early postoperative findings indicate that stage II-III anterior POP was successfully treated with the AVWD technique and that the complication rate was low; however, based on the early postoperative appearance of the anatomic site, AVWD does not appear to be as good as the mesh technique. Nevertheless, AVWD can be easily performed in patients who are concerned about serious adverse effects seen with mesh, such as erosion, mesh shrinkage, bladder erosion, fistula, mesh exposure and infection.

Abbreviations
ATFP: Arcus tendineus fasciae pelvis; AVWD: Anterior vaginal wall darn; CST: Cough stress test; IIQ-7: Seven-item incontinence impact questionnaire; POP: Pelvic organ prolapse; POPQ: POP Quantification; UDI-6: Six-item urogenital distress inventory.

Competing interests
The authors declare that they have no competing interests.

Authors' contributions
The project was developed by OK and ÖA. The clinical database of the patients was acquired by OK, HSS, SB, HA. The manuscript was written by OK, HSS, and ÖA. ŞK performed the statistical analyses. The operative procedures were performed by OK. All authors read and approved the final manuscript.

Acknowledgements
This work has not been funded by any commercial company or grant.

References
1. Kenton K, Mueller ER: **The global burden of female pelvic floor disorders.** *BJU Int* 2006, **98:**1–5.
2. Subak LL, Wactjen LE, van den Ecden S, Thom DH, Vittinghoff E, Brown JS: **Cost of pelvic organ prolapse surgery in the United States.** *Obstet Gynecol* 2001, **98:**646–651.
3. Melville JL, Fan M, Rau H, Nygaard IE, Katon WJ: **Major depression and urinary incontinence in women: temporal associations in an epidemiologic sample.** *Am J Obstet Gynecol* 2009, **201**(490):e1–e7.
4. Olsen AL, Smith VJ, Bergstrom JO, Colling JC, Clark AL: **Epidemiology of surgically managed pelvic organ prolapse and urinary incontinence.** *Obstet Gynecol* 1997, **89:**501–506.
5. Jelovsek JE, Maher C, Barber MD: **Pelvic organ prolapse.** *Lancet* 2007, **369:**1027–1038.
6. Weber AM, Walters MD: **Anterior vaginal prolapse: review of anatomy and techniques of surgical repair.** *Obstet Gynecol* 1997, **89:**311–318.
7. Mallipeddi PK, Steele AC, Kohli N, Karram MM: **Anatomic and functional outcome of vaginal paravaginal repair in the correction of anterior vaginal wall prolapse.** *Int Urogynecol J* 2001, **12:**83–88.
8. Maher C, Baessler K, Glazener CMA, Adams EJ, Hagen S: **Surgical management of pelvic organ prolapse in women.** *Cochrane Database Syst Rev* 2007, **18**(3):CD004014.
9. Maher C, Feiner B, Baessler K, Adams EJ, Hagen S, Glazener CM: **Surgical management of pelvic organ prolapse in women.** *Cochrane Database Syst Rev* 2010, **14**(4):CD004014.
10. Ogah J, Cody JD, Rogerson L: **Minimally invasive synthetic suburethral sling operations for stress urinary incontinence in women.** *Cochrane Database Syst Rev* 2009, **7**(4):CD006375.
11. Lee U, Raz S: **Emerging concepts for pelvic organ prolapse surgery: what is cure?** *Curr Urol Rep* 2011, **12:**62–67.
12. Bai SW, Sohn WH, Chung DJ, Park JH, Kim SK: **Comparison of the efficacy of Burch colposuspension, pubovaginal sling and tension-free vaginal tape for stress urinary incontinence.** *Int J Gynecol Obstet* 2005, **91:**245–246.
13. Julian TM: **The efficacy of Marlex mesh in the repair of severe, recurrent vaginal prolapse of the anterior midvaginal wall.** *Am J Obstet Gynecol* 1996, **175:**1472–1475.
14. Clemons JL, Myers DL, Aguilar VC, Arya LA: **Vaginal paravaginal repair with an Alloderm graft.** *Am J Obstet Gynecol* 2003, **189:**1612–1619.
15. Marcus-Braun N, von Theobald P: **Mesh removal following transvaginal mesh placement: a case series of 104 operations.** *Int Urogynecol J* 2010, **4:**423–430.
16. Milani R, Salvatore S, Soligo M, Pifarotti P, Meschia M, Cortese M: **Functional anatomical outcome of anterior and posterior vaginal prolapsed repair with prolene mesh.** *BJOG* 2005, **112:**107–111.
17. Deffieux X, de Tayrac R, Huel C, Bottero J, Gervaise A, Bonnet K, Frydman R, Fernandez H: **Vaginal mesh erosion after transvaginal repair of cystocele using Gynemesh or Gynemesh-Soft in 138 women: a comparison study.** *Int Urogynecol J* 2007, **18:**73–79.
18. Blandon RE, Gebhart JB, Trabuco EC, Klingele CJ: **Complications from vaginally placed mesh in pelvic reconstructive surgery.** *Int Urogynecol J* 2009, **20:**523–531.
19. Yamada BS, Govier FE, Stefanovic KB, Kobashi KC: **Vesicovaginal fistula and mesh erosion after Perigee (transobturator polypropylene mesh anterior repair).** *Urology* 2006, **68:**1121. e5–7.
20. Margullies RU, Lewicky-Gaupp C, Fenner DE, McGuire JE, Clemens Q, DeLancey JOL: **Complications requiring reoperation following vaginal mesh kit procedures for prolapse.** *Am J Obstet and Gynecol* 2008, **199:**678.e1–678.e4.
21. Siegel AL, Kim M, Goldstein M, Levey S, Ilbeigi P: **High incidence of vaginal mesh extrusion using the intravaginalslingplasty sling.** *Urology* 2005, **174:**1308–1311.
22. Kaufman Y, Singh SS, Alturki H, Lam A: **Age and sexual activity are risk factors for mesh exposure following transvaginal mesh repair.** *Int Urogynecol J* 2011, **22:**307–313.

23. Savary DJ: **What about transvaginal mesh repair of pelvic organ prolapse? Review of the literature since the HAS (French Health Authorities) report.** *Gynecol Obstet Biol Reprod* 2009, **38**(1):11–41.

24. US Food and Drug Administration: *FDA public health notification: serious complications associated with transvaginal placement of surgical mesh in repair of pelvic organ prolapse and stress urinary incontinence*; 2011. http://www.fda.gov/MedicalDevices/Safety/Alertsand Notices/ucm262435.htm.

25. Brubaker L, Bump RC, Fynes M: **Surgery for pelvic organ prolapse.** In *3rd International Consultation in Incontinence*. Edited by Abrams P, Cardozo L, Koury S. Paris: Health; 2005:1371–1402.

26. Kapoor DS, Nemcova M, Pantazis K, Brockman P, Bombieri L, Freeman RM: **Reoperation rate for traditional anterior vaginal repair: analysis of 207 cases with a median 4-year follow-up.** *Int Urogynecol J* 2010, **21**:27–31.

27. Young SB, Daman JJ, Bony LG: **Vaginal paravaginal repair: one-year outcomes.** *Am J Obstet Gynecol* 2001, **185**:1360–1366.

28. Corton MM: **Anatomy of pelvic floor dysfunction.** *Obstet Gynecol Clin North Am* 2009, **36**:401–419.

29. Maarten JP, De Ruiter MC, August AB: **Anatomy of the arcus tendineus fasciae pelvis in females.** *Clin Anat* 2003, **16**:131–137.

30. Albright TS, DO, Alan P: **Arcus tendineus fascia pelvis: a further understanding.** *Am J Obstet Gynecol* 2005, **193**:677–681.

31. Koukourou A, Lyon W, Rice J, Wattchow DA: **Prospective randomized trial of polypropylene mesh compared with nylon darn in inguinal hernia repair.** *Br J Surg* 2001, **88**:931–934.

5

Vapoenucleation of the prostate using a high-power thulium laser

Ching-Hsin Chang[1,4,5], Tzu-Ping Lin[1,2,3*], Yen-Hwa Chang[1,2,3], William JS Huang[1,2,3], Alex TL Lin[1,2,3] and Kuang-Kuo Chen[1,2,3]

Abstract

Background: Prostate vaporization and enucleation is a novel treatment option for bladder outlet obstruction caused by benign prostate enlargement. This surgical technique, however, has not yet been standardized. We present our findings of using a high-power thulium laser to accomplish vapoenucleation of the prostate (ThuVEP).

Methods: We prospectively collected and analyzed data from 29 patients who underwent ThuVEP between August 2010 and May 2012. The control group included 30 patients who underwent traditional transurethral resection of the prostate (TURP). Operative variables, patient profiles, preoperative and postoperative urine flow rates, prostate volume (measured using transrectal ultrasonography), and the international prostate symptom score (IPSS) were recorded and analyzed using a two-tailed Student's t-test and analysis of variance.

Results: The ages (mean ± SD) of the patients were 76.1 ± 9.4 and 72.6 ± 7.4 years ($p = 0.28$) in the ThuVEP and TURP groups, respectively. The average urinary flow rates before and 12 months after the operation (volume/maximum flow/average flow) were 243.3/10.5/5.0 and 302.8/17.6/9.4 (in mL, mL/s, mL/s, respectively) in the ThuVEP group and 247.2/10.8/4.6 and 369.9/20.8/12.0, respectively, in the TURP group. Preoperative and postoperative IPSSs were 17.1 ± 5.0 and 6.5 ± 3.8, respectively, in the ThuVEP group and 18.2 ± 4.5 and 6.2 ± 3.3, respectively, in the TURP group. The mean ratio of the estimated postoperative residual prostate volume to the preoperative total volume was 0.47 ($p = 0.449$) in both groups. The overall complication rate was 20.7% in the ThuVEP group and 30.0% in the TURP group.

Conclusions: One year of follow-up showed that ThuVEP and TURP effectively alleviated subjective and objective voiding symptoms with a low rate of complications. Thus, vapoenucleation using a high-power laser is feasible in elderly patients.

Keywords: Benign prostate enlargement, Quanta thulium surgical laser system, Thulium laser, Vapoenucleation

Background

Benign prostate enlargement (BPE) with lower urinary tract symptoms is a commonly observed condition in the daily clinical practice of urologists, especially those treating an aging male population. Surgical intervention is indicated for patients who develop complications associated with bladder outlet obstruction. Acute urinary retention is the most frequently reported complication, occurring in 0.5–6.5% of patients [1]. The likelihood of a male patient requiring transurethral resection of the prostate (TURP) increases by 6, 14, and 18 times with each decade of life after 59 years of age [2].

Surgical interventions and second-line measures are the treatments of choice for high-risk patients [3]. Surgical intervention is believed to have the most significant influence on the natural course of BPE and on preventing complications [4]. Surgical interventions include TURP (monopolar or bipolar) and laser treatment of the prostate,

* Correspondence: tplin63@gmail.com
[1]Department of Urology, Taipei Veterans General Hospital, Taipei, Taiwan
[2]Department of Urology, National Yang-Ming University School of Medicine, Taipei, Taiwan
Full list of author information is available at the end of the article

which includes holmium laser enucleation of the prostate (HoLEP), green light laser, and thulium laser [5].

Several studies have shown that TURP is the most common, widely performed, effective, and cost-efficient treatment to date [5-7]. Although TURP is associated with low morbidity [8], we should explore techniques other than TURP that have even lower morbidity rates.

HoLEP is the most commonly performed surgical intervention in recent decades, and the improvements in urodynamic parameters with this technique are comparable to those obtained with other techniques when performed by experienced surgeons [9]. Krambeck et al. showed a satisfactory outcome and low morbidity with HoLEP [10].

The over-deobstruction achieved by HoLEP, however, might induce postoperative incontinence at an early stage [10]. Because of a steep learning curve, the adoption rate for this technique is low, and only a few studies on large series of patients have been performed in limited centers [11,12]. The learning curve may be prolonged, and 50 cases are required for a surgeon to obtain an outcome that is comparable to that reported in the literature [13].

Thulium laser has several theoretical advantages over the holmium laser (e.g., rapid vaporization and coagulation ability, improved spatial beam quality, precise tissue incision) [14,15]. Bach et al. presented the first study on thulium:yttrium aluminum garnet (Tm:YAG) laser prostatectomy using the vaporesection technique with a 70-W Tm:YAG laser [16]. Shao et al. reported less blood loss in the Tm:YAG group, and the outcome in this group was similar to that observed in the group that underwent enucleation of the prostate using the Ho:YAG laser [17].

Xia et al. reported the first prospective randomized study comparing thulium laser resection with the prostate-tangerine technique (TmLRP-TT) and the standard TURP for symptomatic BPE with a 50-W instrument [18]. Both groups showed significant improvement in subjective symptom scores and urodynamic parameters. TmLRP-TT was significantly superior to TURP in terms of duration of catheterization, duration of hospitalization, and decrease in hemoglobin level [19]. The aforementioned thulium laser series with the Tm:YAG laser (RevoLix®; LISA Laser Products, Katlenburg, Germany) showed promising results. With the advancements in their technology, thulium lasers with higher energy output are now available. An example is the Quanta System Cyber Th:YAG laser. This new generation of Th:YAG lasers offers a maximum energy output of 150 W.

To our knowledge, the present study is the first prospective nonrandomized trial of vapoenucleation using the Cyber Th:YAG laser versus TURP with a 1-year follow-up.

Methods
After receiving approval from the institutional review board of the Taipei Veterans General Hospital (VGHIRB

No. 201007014IC), we recruited patients between August 2010 and May 2012 who had BPE that required surgical intervention. All consents were obtained with the method of written. The study was designed as a prospectively nonblind randomized trial. It included 59 patients. The Th:YAG laser vapoenucleation (ThuVEP) group included 29 patients and the TURP group had 30 patients. Informed consents for participation were obtained from the participants.

The inclusion criteria were an international prostate symptom score (IPSS) >7, maximum urinary flow rate (Qmax) <15 mL/s, and normal level of age-specific prostate-specific antigen (PSA) [20]. Patients with abnormal levels of age-specific PSA or positive findings on digital rectal examination underwent transrectal ultrasonography (TRUS)-guided biopsy to rule out prostate cancer. Ten patients underwent TRUS-guided biopsy before the operation. To ensure intraoperative safety, we asked the patients to discontinue all anticoagulants except low-dose aspirin.

Before the operation, we evaluated the IPSS and quality of life score (QoLs) in each patient. Each was administered the five-item international index of erectile function (IIEF-5) questionnaire. Prostate volume (V1) was measured using TRUS and the prolate ellipsoid volume formula. The postvoid residual (PVR) urine volume was measured using bladder scans and uroflowmetry (UFR).

The patients were placed in the lithotomy position under spinal anesthesia. A single surgeon (T.P.L.) performed all of the ThuVEP procedures. TURP was performed by three surgeons. We used 150-W thulium lasers (Quanta Thulium Surgical Laser System: Cyber TM; Quanta Systems, Solbiate Olona, Italy) coupled with a 26-Fr resectoscope sheath (No. A22040A; Olympus, Tokyo, Japan) for this procedure. Energy was delivered via 550-mm end-firing fibers.

The technique utilized in the ThuVEP group was similar to that used for trilobular HoLEP [21]. Briefly, we initiated the procedure by making two Turner–Warwick-like incisions in the 5 and 7 o'clock direction from the bladder neck to the level of the verumontanum. The incision continued to the surgical capsule. Then, we made a third incision from the bladder neck to the level of the verumontanum (the incision was not too distal) in the 12 o'clock direction. The three lobes were then enucleated starting at the median lobe followed by the right and left lobes. We did not perform a high degree of blunt enucleation by using the beak of the resectoscope. Instead, we used laser energy to incise and connect the incisions performed previously. This procedure was facilitated using a guiding tube (No. A00561A; Olympus) made specifically to elevate the incised prostate from the plane between the adenoma and the surgical capsule of the prostate (Figure 1). After all three lobes were

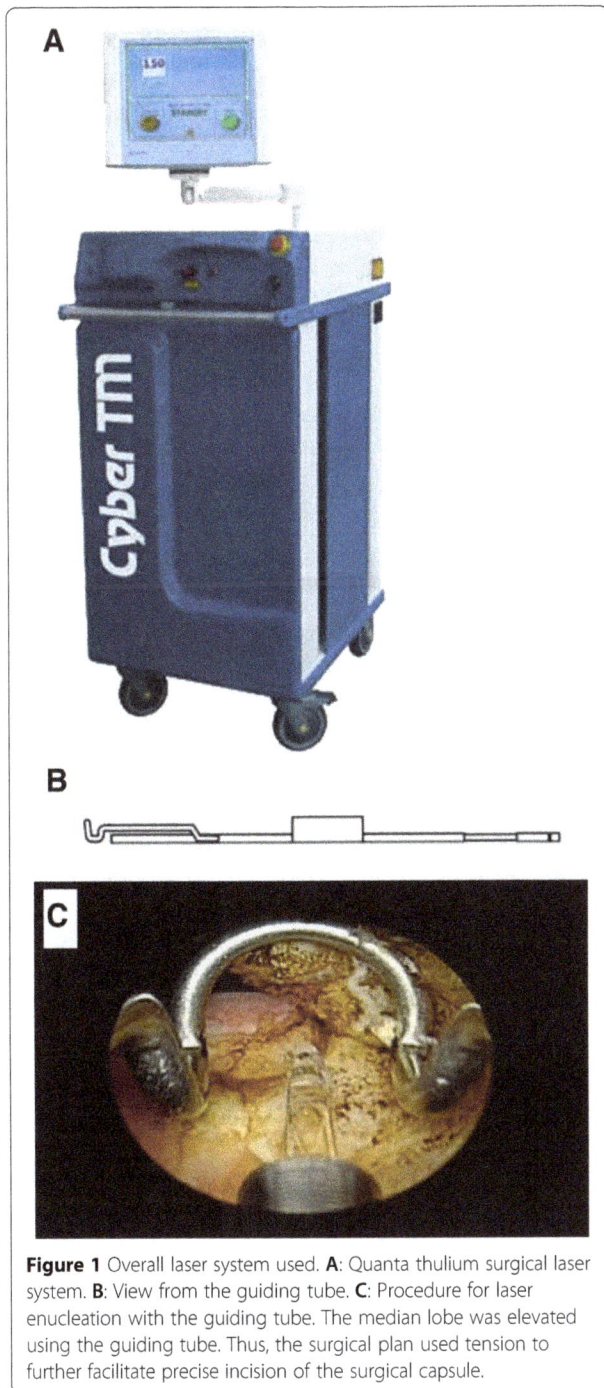

Figure 1 Overall laser system used. **A**: Quanta thulium surgical laser system. **B**: View from the guiding tube. **C**: Procedure for laser enucleation with the guiding tube. The median lobe was elevated using the guiding tube. Thus, the surgical plan used tension to further facilitate precise incision of the surgical capsule.

160 W and a coagulating current of 80 W. All of the prostate chips were removed using a Toomey evacuator.

At the end of both procedures, we inserted a 22-Fr triple-lumen catheter into the bladder and initiated irrigation until hematuria had decreased to a sufficient degree. We performed postoperative histological examination of all the tissues retrieved. Typically, the urethral catheter was removed early on postoperative day 2 or 3 if severe bleeding was not observed in the urine. The voiding pattern was monitored for 1 day, and the patient was discharged home.

The perioperative primary outcomes measured in the two groups included the operative time (interval when the resectoscope sheath was within the urethra), weight of the resected tissue (actual weight of the tissue retrieved), decreased hemoglobin level, decreased serum sodium level, duration of postoperative catheterization, and postoperative hospital stay. We evaluated the IPSS, QoLs, Qmax, and PVR urine in both groups at discharge and at 3, 6, and 12 months after the operation. We recorded all perioperative complications. The IPSS was obtained from the questionnaire and included two subscores: voiding symptoms (incomplete emptying, intermittence, weak stream, straining to void) and storage symptoms (frequency, urgency, nocturia). In addition, preoperative and postoperative sexual function was evaluated from the IIEF-5 [22].

At 6 months after the operation, the prostate volume of each patient was measured using a TRUS procedure using an ultrasonography machine (BK Medical, Herlev, Denmark) with a 7.5-MHz TRUS probe. The estimated residual prostate volume (V2) was calculated as the volume of the entire gland using a prolate elliptical formula (height × width × length × π/6) minus the central defect (also calculated using the prolate elliptical formula). The estimated residual prostate volume ratio was calculated as V2/V1.

All measurement data for the two groups were statistically analyzed using a two-tailed Student's t test. The data are presented as the mean ± standard deviation (SD). The scoring and questionnaire results were analyzed using analysis of variance (ANOVA). Statistical significance was defined as $p < 0.05$.

Results

Baseline characteristics

Most of the baseline characteristics in the two groups showed no differences (Table 1). However, the PVR in the ThuVEP group was higher than that in the TURP group (138.6 ± 127.7 vs. 90.9 ± 66.5, $p = 0.040$). The mean age of the patients in our study was higher than that reported in previous studies [19]. TRUS-guided biopsy was performed in 15.3% of the patients before the procedure because of increased levels of age-specific PSA.

enucleated from the prostate capsule, the three adenomas were pushed into the bladder and morcellated with a mechanical tissue morcellator, then the tissue is evacuated from bladder. At the end of this procedure, the operation site was irrigated with saline in all patients.

In the TURP group, TURP was performed using a standard tungsten wire loop with a cutting current of

Table 1 Baseline characteristics for the groups

Characteristic	ThuVEP	TURP	p
Number	29	30	
Age (years)	76.1 ± 9.4	72.6 ± 7.4	0.280
Anticoagulant*	15(51.7%)	6(20.0%)	0.011
BMI	23.9 ± 2.7	23.7 ± 3.4	0.281
PSA (ng/mL)	5.0 ± 5.4	8.3 ± 7.9	0.076
TRUS estimated weight (g)	57.2 ± 25.1	64.7 ± 32.5	0.758
IPSS	17.1 ± 5.0	17.8 ± 4.3	0.674
Charlson co-morbidity index	1.0 ± 1.0	1.6 ± 2.7	0.639
Qmax (mL/s)	10.5 ± 4.9	10.8 ± 4.7	0.728
PVR vol (mL)*	138.6 ± 127.7	90.9 ± 66.5	0.040

*Statistical difference.

BMI, body mass index; PSA, prostate-specific antigen; TRUS, transrectal ultrasound; IPSS, international prostate symptom score; Qmax, maximum urinary flow rate; PVR, post-void residual volume; ThuVEP, vapoenucleation of the prostate using a high-power thulium laser; TURP, transurethral resection of the prostate.

Perioperative data

The resected tissue was heavier in the TURP group than in the ThuVEP group (37.4 ± 23.0 vs. 21.3 ± 14.3 g, $p = 0.024$), although the estimated residual prostate volume ratio (0.47 ± 0.17 vs. 0.47 ± 0.20, $p = 0.449$) was the same in the two groups. The duration of catheterization (1.8 ± 0.5 vs. 2.3 ± 0.5 days, $p = 0.001$) and postoperative hospital stay (3.0 ± 0.9 vs. 3.4 ± 0.7 days, $p = 0.032$) were shorter for the ThuVEP group than for the TURP group. Other variables, such as total duration of hospitalization, decrease in hemoglobin levels (0.5 ± 1.3 vs. 0.5 ± 1.1, $p = 0.844$), and decrease in serum sodium levels (0.3 ± 2.4 vs. 1.6 ± 2.0, $p = 0.468$) were not statistically different (Table 2). In all, 96.3% patients in the ThuVEP group and 93.3% in the TURP group completed the 1-year follow-up study.

Follow-up of QoLs

The IPSS and QoLs in both groups had decreased significantly postoperatively (Figure 2). The symptoms and QoLs, however, began to improve and continued up to 12 months after the operation. The IPSS, including total scores, subscores of voiding symptoms, and subscores of storage symptoms, all displayed a similar trend of continuing to improve. There were no statistically significant differences in these values between the two groups ($p = 0.551$).

Follow-up of UFR and PVR urine volume

All UFR variables – voided volume, Qmax, mean flow rate – improved significantly in both groups after the operation (not all of the data are shown, Figure 3). The preoperative PVR urine volume was significantly higher in the ThuVEP group. The postoperative PVR urine volume markedly decreased in both groups, with no

Table 2 Perioperative data

Parameter	ThuVEP	TURP	p
Resected weight (g)*	21.3 ± 14.3	37.4 ± 23.0	0.024
Preoperative hemoglobin level (g/dL)	12.9 ± 1.7	13.3 ± 1.6	0.587
Decrease in hemoglobin level (g/dL)	0.5 ± 1.3	0.5 ± 1.1	0.844
Decrease in serum sodium level (mmol/L)	0.3 ± 2.4	1.6 ± 2.0	0.468
Duration of catheterization (day)*	1.8 ± 0.5	2.3 ± 0.5	0.001
Total duration of hospitalization (days)	5.2 ± 1.9	5.2 ± 0.8	0.203
Postoperative duration of hospitalization (days)*	3.0 ± 0.9	3.4 ± 0.7	0.032
Estimated residual prostate volume ratio (V2/V1)	0.47 ± 0.17	0.47 ± 0.20	0.449
PSA ratio (before the operation/12 months after the operation)	2.4 ± 2.9	1.6 ± 1.0	0.180

ThuVEP, vapoenucleation of the prostate using a high-power thulium laser; TURP, transurethral resection of the prostate; PSA, prostate-specific antigen. The duration of catheterization and postoperative hospitalization showed statistical differences. The estimated residual prostate volume (V2) was calculated as the volume of the entire gland using prolate elliptical formula (height × width × length × π/6) minus the central defect (also calculated using the prolate elliptical formula). The estimated residual prostate volume ratio was calculated as V2/V1.
(*Statistical difference).

difference observed in the PVR urine volumes 3 months after the operation in the two groups (68.2 ± 37.5 vs. 69.5 ± 47.9, $p = 0.648$).

Complications

We used the modified Clavien classification system for reporting TURP-related complications in our patients, as proposed by Smith and Patel [23]. Six complications were recorded among the 29 patients in the ThuVEP group: 6.9% patients had grade I complications, and 13.8% had grade II complications. None of the patients exhibited grade III–V complications. Nine complications were recorded in the 30 TURP group patients. Grade I complications were observed in 1.3% of patients and

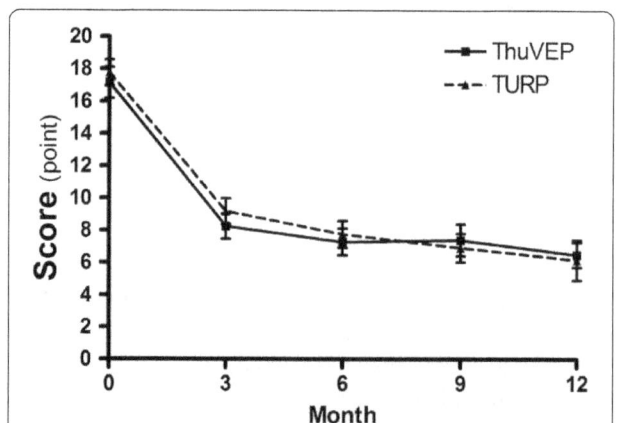

Figure 2 International prostate symptom score (IPSS). No statistical differences were observed between the two groups.

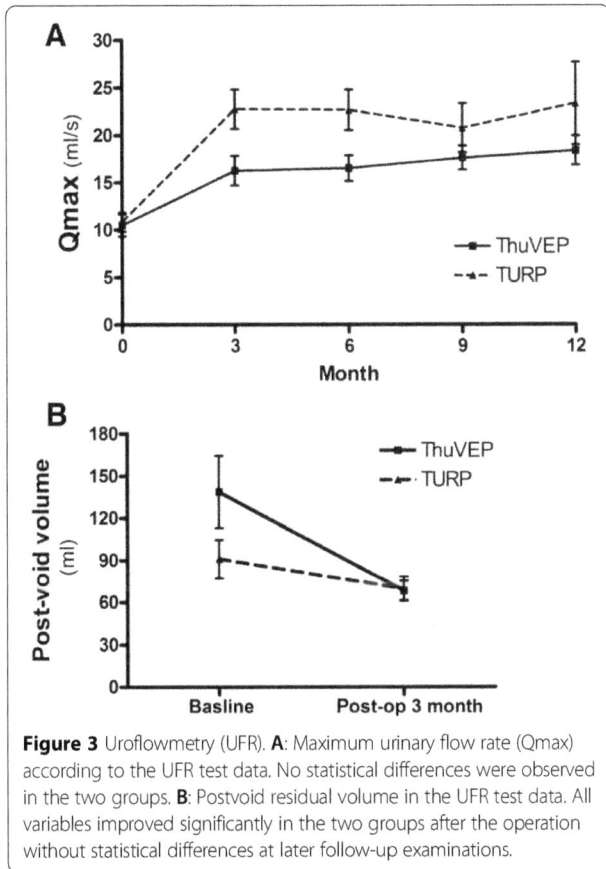

Figure 3 Uroflowmetry (UFR). **A**: Maximum urinary flow rate (Qmax) according to the UFR test data. No statistical differences were observed in the two groups. **B**: Postvoid residual volume in the UFR test data. All variables improved significantly in the two groups after the operation without statistical differences at later follow-up examinations.

Table 3 Modified Clavien classification system for reporting complications of TURP

Criteria	ThuVEP (N = 29)	TURP (N = 30)
Grade 1		
Hematuria clot retention requiring bladder irrigation/clot evacuation/catheter traction	0	1 (3.3%)
Catheter block because of retained TUR chip	0	0
Failed trial without catheter with acute urinary retention requiring bedside recatheterization	2 (6.9%)	0
Transient increase in the serum creatinine level	0	0
Lower urinary tract infection requiring antibiotics	0	0
Grade 2		
Hemorrhage/hematuria requiring transfusion	4 (13.8%)	8 (26.7%)
Urinary tract infection with bacteremia requiring antibiotics	0	0
Supraventricular tachycardia requiring antiarrhythmia drugs	0	0
Pulmonary embolism requiring anticoagulants	0	0
Grade 3		
Extraperitoneal fluid collection caused by subtrigonal catheter requiring endoscopic catheter repositioning and surgical drainage	0	0
Grade 4		
Acute myocardial infarction requiring admission to the ICU	0	0
TUR syndrome requiring admission to the ICU	0	0
Grade 5		
Death	0	0
Total	6	9

ThuVEP, vapoenucleation of the prostate using a high-power thulium laser; TURP, transurethral resection of the prostate.

grade II in 26.7%. No higher-grade complications were observed in this group (Table 3).

Discussion

Surgical techniques used to treat bladder outlet obstruction include Tm:YAG vaporization of the prostate (ThuVAP), Tm:YAG vaporesection of the prostate (ThuVaRP), ThuVEP, and Tm:YAG laser enucleation of the prostate (ThuLEP) [24].

The wavelength of thulium laser matches that of the water absorption peak in tissue at 1.92 mm, which results in sufficient hemostasis, a clear visual field, and rapid incision of the tissues with little thermal damage. Fried et al. reported that continuous-wave 50-W thulium fiber laser vaporized prostate tissue at a rate of 0.45 g/min [8].

Because of the high vaporization inherent in laser–tissue interaction with thulium-YAG laser, the true resected prostate volume was difficult to determine compared to that with other enucleation prostatectomies or TURP. To address this issue, we prospectively measured the prostate volume by TRUS. The estimated residual prostate volume was obtained by subtracting the volume of the entire prostate from that of the central defect, which were calculated using the values of the outer and inner dimensions, respectively. Although the prostate volume differed

significantly after resection, the residual volumes after both approaches (ThuVEP and TURP) were not significantly different. The equal ratio of residual prostate volume was supported by equal symptom improvement and urodynamic improvement. Thus, the ratio of the postoperative prostate volume to the preoperative prostate volume that was estimated from TRUS-guided biopsy samples may better predict symptom alleviation or urodynamic improvement than tissue resected when ThuVEP is utilized.

HoLEP involves a three-lobe technique (median lobe and lateral lobes) for enucleation of the prostate [21]. ThuLEP was introduced by Herrmann et al. [25]. Unlike other techniques that involve determination of the surgical capsule at the apex, this technique involves apical incision of the prostatic tissue down to the surgical capsule. This approach is further facilitated by the superior Th:YAG–tissue interaction and higher vaporizing property. This approach did not compromise the deobstruction as shown by improved urodynamic parameters and alleviated symptoms. Also, this trend toward improvement was still ongoing at the 12-month follow-up.

The perioperative morbidity associated with TURP decreased when the surgical equipment was modified. However, the possibility of TUR syndrome, a common complication, continues to exist. Our study showed that the complication rate, blood transfusion rate, and decrease in the serum sodium and hemoglobin levels were lower with ThuVEP than with other laser instruments or TURP [26].

Laser surgery has been recommended because there is less risk of sexual dysfunction. Xia et al. reported that 3.8% patients in the TmLRP-TT group and 14.6% patients in the TURP group had slightly reduced erectile function at 12 months postoperatively [19]. Preoperatively, about 50% patients who underwent TmLRP-TT and TURP had not had erections sufficient for intercourse [19]. Because of the advanced age of the patients in our study, we did not have a sufficient number of potent patients before the operation in either group to assess this point. Therefore, we were unable to compare the theoretical complications of TUR surgery.

In previous studies, the intraoperative and postoperative complications covered a wide extent of damage and severity: clot retention; significant hematuria that prolongs hospitalization; open cystotomy to remove adenomas; myocardial infarction and atrial fibrillation that require cardioversion; morcellator bladder injury; cerebral vascular accident; sepsis [10]. We used the modified Clavien classification system to report and systematically analyze the complications according to treatment [27]. This method has been adopted in various surgical disciplines as it has improved detection and avoided observation bias. Masumori et al. was the first to use the Clavien classification system to report complications of TURP. The overall perioperative morbidity was 15.8%, including grade I (59.1%) and II (29.5%) complications, those requiring interventions (2.3%, grade III), intensive care unit (ICU) admission (6.8%, grade IV), and one death (0.5%, grade V) [6].

We used the modified Clavien classification system to classify our patients (Table 3). There were no high-grade (grades III–V) complications in either group in our study.

Age and the Charlson co-morbidity index are independent and highly significant ($p < 0.001$) predictors for mortality [7]. Use of oral anticoagulants was regarded as an independent factor for the outcome of TURP as it was associated with significantly longer hospitalization and higher rates of bladder clots, blood transfusions, late hematuria, and thromboembolic events [28].

We prospectively recorded the above factors for our patients (Table 1). A total of 35.6% of the patients in our study took anticoagulants. These patients tended to be

older and had larger prostates with more tissue resected. The blood transfusion rate in this study was higher than that in our previous study, increasing from 2.2% to 4.2% [19,26]. There was a minimal difference, however, in the hemoglobin level before and after the operation (around 0.5 g/dL). These findings indicate that although the thresholds for blood transfusion were low, they would be permissible in these older, fragile patients.

We conducted a nonrandomized controlled study to compare ThuVEP and TURP. We prospectively collected the cohort data and systemically evaluated the Charlson index for co-morbidity and complications reported according to the modified Clavien classification. Our results showed that ThuVEP obtained equal and durable symptomatic and urodynamic improvements at the 12-month follow-up. Preoperative and postoperative TRUS evaluation of prostate size indicated that a uniform amount of tissue was excised. This was especially important in the ThuVEP group because the vaporization rate of the tissue is high using thulium laser. Thus, the tissue resected using ThuVEP cannot represent the exact volume of the resected prostatic tissue.

Our study has several limitations. Most of the procedures were performed by a single surgeon who was responsible for the entire ThuVEP group. Three surgeons were responsible for the TURP group (T.P.L., Y.H.C., W.J.H.). Thus, a comparison of these two groups may be subjected to bias. However, because all participating surgeons had engaged in their clinical practices for more than 10 years, they had accrued surgical experience with 50 patients or more per year. Thus, the operator-related bias was limited. Also, the follow-up duration was not sufficiently long. The outcome of the procedure may differ after a longer follow-up. Finally, our study was not randomized, which lowers the level of evidence-based medicine. Thus, large-scale, prospective, and randomized studies are required to eliminate the possible bias inherent to a nonrandomized study design.

Conclusions

The outcome of high-energy (150 W) ThuVEP in terms of symptom alleviation and improved urodynamic parameters was similar to that obtained using TURP. This laser procedure is well tolerated, and enables efficient excision and rapid organic vaporization. The results indicate the feasibility of high-energy Th:YAG laser vapoenucleation for the treatment of benign prostate hyperplasia.

Abbreviations

ThuVEP: Vapoenucleation of the prostate using high-power thulium laser; TURP: Transurethral resection of the prostate; ANOVA: Analysis of variance; BPE: Benign prostate enlargement; Tm: Thulium; YAG: Yttrium aluminum garnet; PVR: Postvoid residual; UFR: Uroflowmetry.

Competing interests

The authors declare that they have no competing interests.

Authors' contributions

Study conception and design: TPL, ATLL, KKC. Acquisition of data: TPL, YHC, WJSH, ATLL. Analysis and interpretation of data: CHC. Drafting of manuscript: CHC. Critical revision: TPL, ATLL. All authors read and approved the final manuscript.

Acknowledgment

We thank Miss Hui-Chen Lee in the Division of Experimental Surgery for her valuable assistance with the statistical analyses.

Author details

[1]Department of Urology, Taipei Veterans General Hospital, Taipei, Taiwan. [2]Department of Urology, National Yang-Ming University School of Medicine, Taipei, Taiwan. [3]Shu-Tien Urological Science Research Center, Taipei, Taiwan. [4]Department of Urology, Taipei Medical University Hospital, Taipei, Taiwan. [5]Graduate Institute of Medical Sciences, College of Medicine, Taipei Medical University, Taipei, Taiwan.

References

1. Lo KL, Chan MC, Wong A, Hou SM, Ng CF. Long-term outcome of patients with a successful trial without catheter, after treatment with an alpha-adrenergic receptor blocker for acute urinary retention caused by benign prostatic hyperplasia. Int Urol Nephrol. 2010;42:7–12.
2. Merrill RM, Hunter BD. The diminishing role of transurethral resection of the prostate. Ann Surg Oncol. 2010;17:1422–8.
3. Robert G, Descazeaud A, de la Taille A. Lower urinary tract symptoms suggestive of benign prostatic hyperplasia: who are the high-risk patients and what are the best treatment options? Curr Opin Urol. 2011;21:42–8.
4. Flanigan RC, Reda DJ, Wasson JH, Anderson RJ, Abdellatif M, Bruskewitz RC. 5-year outcome of surgical resection and watchful waiting for men with moderately symptomatic benign prostatic hyperplasia: a department of veterans affairs cooperative study. J Urol. 1998;160:12–6. discussion 6–7.
5. Hoekstra RJ, Van Melick HH, Kok ET, Ruud Bosch JL. A 10-year follow-up after transurethral resection of the prostate, contact laser prostatectomy and electrovaporization in men with benign prostatic hyperplasia; long-term results of a randomized controlled trial. BJU Int. 2010;106:822–6.
6. Masumori N, Furuya R, Tanaka Y, Furuya S, Ogura H, Tsukamoto T. The 12-year symptomatic outcome of transurethral resection of the prostate for patients with lower urinary tract symptoms suggestive of benign prostatic obstruction compared to the urodynamic findings before surgery. BJU Int. 2010;105:1429–33.
7. Jeldres C, Isbarn H, Capitanio U, Zini L, Bhojani N, Shariat SF, et al. Development and external validation of a highly accurate nomogram for the prediction of perioperative mortality after transurethral resection of the prostate for benign prostatic hyperplasia. J Urol. 2009;182:626–32.
8. Reich O, Gratzke C, Bachmann A, Seitz M, Schlenker B, Hermanek P, et al. Morbidity, mortality and early outcome of transurethral resection of the prostate: a prospective multicenter evaluation of 10,654 patients. J Urol. 2008;180:246–9.
9. Gilling PJ, Mackey M, Cresswell M, Kennett K, Kabalin JN, Fraundorfer MR. Holmium laser versus transurethral resection of the prostate: a randomized prospective trial with 1-year followup. J Urol. 1999;162:1640–4.
10. Krambeck AE, Handa SE, Lingeman JE. Experience with more than 1,000 holmium laser prostate enucleations for benign prostatic hyperplasia. J Urol. 2010;183:1105–9.
11. Kuntz RM, Lehrich K, Ahyai SA. Holmium laser enucleation of the prostate versus open prostatectomy for prostates greater than 100 grams: 5-year follow-up results of a randomised clinical trial. Eur Urol. 2008;53:160–6.
12. Gnessin E, Mandeville JA, Lingeman JE. An update on holmium laser enucleation of the prostate and why it has stood the test of time. Curr Opin Urol. 2011;21:31–5.
13. Placer J, Gelabert-Mas A, Vallmanya F, Manresa JM, Menéndez V, Cortadellas R, et al. Holmium laser enucleation of prostate: outcome and complications of self-taught learning curve. Urology. 2009;73:1042–8.
14. Fried NM, Murray KE. High-power thulium fiber laser ablation of urinary tissues at 1.94 microm. J Endourol. 2005;19:25–31.
15. Fried NM. High-power laser vaporization of the canine prostate using a 110 w thulium fiber laser at 1.91 microm. Lasers Surg Med. 2005;36:52–6.
16. Bach T, Herrmann TR, Ganzer R, Burchardt M, Gross AJ. RevoLix vaporesection of the prostate: initial results of 54 patients with a 1-year follow-up. World J Urol. 2007;25:257–62.
17. Shao Q, Zhang FB, Shang DH, Tian Y. Comparison of holmium and thulium laser in transurethral enucleation of the prostate]. Zhonghua Nan Ke Xue. 2009;15:346–9.
18. Xia SJ, Zhang YN, Lu J, Sun XW, Zhang J, Zhu YY, et al. Thulium laser resection of prostate-tangerine technique in treatment of benign prostate hyperplasia. Zhonghua Yi Xue Za Zhi. 2005;85:3225–8.
19. Xia SJ, Zhuo J, Sun XW, Han BM, Shao Y, Zhang YN. Thulium laser versus standard transurethral resection of the prostate: a randomized prospective trial. Eur Urol. 2008;53:382–9.
20. Oesterling JE, Kumamoto Y, Tsukamoto T, Girman CJ, Guess HA, Masumori N, et al. Serum prostate-specific antigen in a community-based population of healthy Japanese men: lower values than for similarly aged white men. Br J Urol. 1995;75:347–53.
21. Gilling P. Holmium laser enucleation of the prostate (HoLEP). BJU Int. 2008;101:131–42.
22. Vroege JA. The sexual health inventory for men (IIEF-5). Int J Impot Res. 1999;11:177.
23. Smith RD, Patel A. Transurethral resection of the prostate revisited and updated. Curr Opin Urol. 2011;21:36–41.
24. Bach T, Xia SJ, Yang Y, Mattioli S, Watson GM, Gross AJ, et al. Thulium: YAG 2 mum cw laser prostatectomy: where do we stand? World J Urol. 2010;28:163–8.
25. Herrmann TR, Bach T, Imkamp F, Georgiou A, Burchardt M, Oelke M, et al. Thulium laser enucleation of the prostate (ThuLEP): transurethral anatomical prostatectomy with laser support. Introduction of a novel technique for the treatment of benign prostatic obstruction. World J Urol. 2010;28:45–51.
26. Bach T, Wendt-Nordahl G, Michel MS, Herrmann TR, Gross AJ. Feasibility and efficacy of Thulium:YAG laser enucleation (VapoEnucleation) of the prostate. World J Urol. 2009;27:541–5.
27. Morgan M, Smith N, Thomas K, Murphy DG. Is Clavien the new standard for reporting urological complications? BJU Int. 2009;104:434–6.
28. Descazeaud A, Robert G, Lebdai S, Bougault A, Azzousi AR, Haillot O, et al. Impact of oral anticoagulation on morbidity of transurethral resection of the prostate. World J Urol. 2011;29:211–6.

6

Prediction of open urinary tract in laparoscopic partial nephrectomy by virtual resection plane visualization

Daiki Ueno[1*], Kazuhide Makiyama[1†], Hiroyuki Yamanaka[1†], Takashi Ijiri[2†], Hideo Yokota[2†] and Yoshinobu Kubota[1†]

Abstract

Background: The purpose of this study is presenting a method to predict the presence of an open urinary tract and the position of the opening in laparoscopic partial nephrectomy from three dimensional (3D) computed tomography (CT) images by using novel image segmentation and visualization techniques.

Methods: From CT images of patients who underwent laparoscopic partial nephrectomy, 3D regions of the kidney, urinary tract, and tumor were segmented. For each patient, multiple virtual resection planes of the kidney with different surgical margins (1 mm to 5 mm, every 1 mm) were generated and the presence of an open urinary tract and the position of the opening were predicted from the images.

Results: We compared the predictions with actual operations in 5 cases by using recorded video of the operations and operative notes. In terms of the presence of an open urinary tract, agreement of the predictions and the intraoperative results was obtained in all patients. The expected positions of the openings were close to those in the actual operations.

Conclusions: We have developed a method to virtually visualize the resection plane of laparoscopic partial nephrectomy. Image segmentation methods used in this study were precise and effective. The comparison indicated that our method accurately predicted the presence of an open urinary tract and the position of the opening and provided useful preoperative information.

Keywords: Laparoscopic surgery, Partial nephrectomy, Simulator, Urinary tract opening

Background

Laparoscopic surgery has been preferred by many surgeons and patients because of shorter recovery time and less surgical invasion [1]. A partial nephrectomy shows treatment outcomes equal to those of a radical nephrectomy and preserves postoperative renal function [2-4]. Therefore, laparoscopic partial nephrectomy has become an increasingly common practice for small renal tumors.

To achieve a safe procedure, preoperative information is especially important for laparoscopic surgery. Organs and large vessels around the operated site are difficult to recognize only with the limited two dimensional (2D) view of the laparoscope. It is important to preoperatively understand the anatomical features of the patient.

We developed the three dimensional (3D) image processing software VoTracer to preoperatively obtain significant information from computed tomography (CT) or magnetic resonance imaging (MRI) images. VoTracer supports traditional volume rendering; the user can observe 3D images by modifying local transparency and changing the viewpoint [5]. It also supports various image segmentation methods, such as thresholding [6], region growing [7], graph cut [8,9], and contour-based segmentation [10,11]; the user can quickly segment organ and tumor regions from 3D images with simple interaction.

One of the postoperative complications of partial nephrectomy is urine leakage. If the urinary tract is open during tumor resection, suturing the crack is required

* Correspondence: daikochi810903@yahoo.co.jp
†Equal contributors
[1]Department of Urology, Yokohama City University School of Medicine, 3-9 Fukuura, Kanagawa-ku, Yokohama, Kanagawa 236-0004, Japan
Full list of author information is available at the end of the article

for the prevention of postoperative urine leakage. To formulate an operation strategy, it is useful to predict the margin of the urinary tract opening during the tumor resection.

In this study, we focused on laparoscopic partial nephrectomy and presented a method to predict the presence of an open urinary tract and the position of the opening using VoTracer. We also evaluated our method by comparing our predictions with actual operation results.

Methods

Patients and characteristics

This was a retrospective study including 5 patients who underwent laparoscopic partial nephrectomy at Yokohama City University Hospital by a single surgeon (K.M.) between April 2011 and January 2013. We created virtual resection plane images on another day by accessing medical archives and evaluated it. The study protocol was approved by the Yokohama City University Institutional Review Board. Written informed consent was obtained from all patients. Application of laparoscopic partial nephrectomy was limited to cases where the tumor size was 4 cm or less and the operation could be performed safely. The surgical margin and the angle of cut in were determined by full observation of the tumor by intraoperative ultrasound. Tumor resection was performed by cold cut using scissors with kidney ischemia. Then partial nephrectomy is performed. After the retrograde injection of dilute indigo carmine, the continuous suturing of the opened collecting system

and transected major vessel is performed by 2–0 Vicryl on a SH needle with an intracorporeal knot-tying.

CT image segmentation and virtual-resection-plane

From the delay phase of enhanced CT images of each patient, we segmented three regions: kidney, urinary tract, and tumor. Different segmentation methods were applied for each region. We then generated a virtual resection plane of the kidney by using segmentation. The whole process was performed via VoTracer.

The graph cut image segmentation method [8,9] was applied to segment the kidney region. We roughly specified inside and outside control points on several cross sections of the 3D CT images and the graph cut algorithm segmented the kidney region accurately (Figure 1B). The region growing method [7] was used for the urinary tract. We specified several seeds in the urinary tract region and the method evolves a region from the seeds. We computed the evolution only in voxels of which CT values were larger than r, where $r \in [350, 420]$ was a parameter selected depending on the patient (Figure 1C). The contour-based 3D image segmentation method [11] was employed for segmenting the tumor. We specified several contours on the tumor in the 3D images and the method optimized a segmentation boundary that passed through all contours and had a smooth shape (Figure 1D). This method was useful for regions that did not have obvious high-contrast boundaries.

Given the image segmentation, we generated a virtual resection plane. We first generated polygon surface models of the kidney, urinary tract, and tumor regions

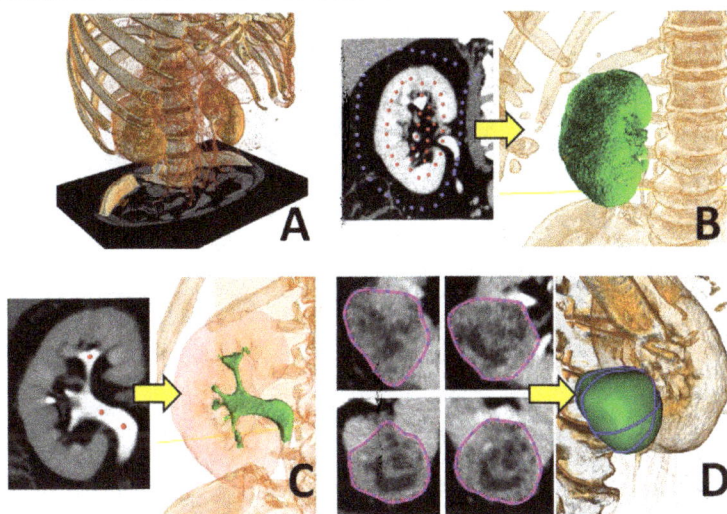

Figure 1 Segmentation of CT image. From an input 3D CT image **(A)**, we segmented the three regions by different methods. **(B)** The kidney region was segmented by the graph cut method [8,9]. We specified several foreground (red) and background (blue) points on a cross section and the method computed the kidney region from the points. **(C)** The urinary tract region was segmented by region growing [7]. The method grew the urinary tract region from several seeds (red points). **(D)** The tumor region was segmented by the contour-based method [11]. The method computed the boundary surface from specified multiple contours.

by Marching cubes algorithm [12] (Figure 2). We then deformed the kidney model so that it had a certain margin from the tumor (Figure 2E-G). We also visualized the CT images on the kidney surface as in Figure 2D. The virtual resection planes visually provided information on the presence of an open urinary tract and the position of the opening in partial nephrectomy.

Prediction and evaluation

A single evaluator (D.U.), who did not know the details of the operation, performed the segmentation of the 3D CT images of the 5 patients using VoTracer. A software developer (T.I.) supported the segmentation process. For each patient, the evaluator created virtual resection planes with 1 mm to 5 mm margins, every 1 mm margin, and predicted whether and where the urinary tract was open during the actual operation (Figure 2).

We compared the predictions and intraoperative results. The presence of an open urinary tract during the actual operation was verified from recorded video of the operation and operative notes. In cases where there was an open urinary tract, the positions of the openings were compared with those in the virtual resection planes.

Results

Table 1 summarizes the backgrounds of the patients, prediction results, and surgical outcomes. Table 1 also shows the minimum margins of the openings the evaluator detected in the virtual resection planes and actual surgical margins measured from the operation samples at the bottom of the tumor.

In terms of presence of an open urinary tract (i.e. minimum opening margin), the predictions and intraoperative results approximately coincided in all patients. However, in patient No. 2, the predicted opening margin was 1 mm greater than the actual margin, and this may be explained by the size of the margin, which was likely to be larger at the site of urinary tract opening than at the bottom. The margin is generally the smallest at the bottom, and becomes larger at the periphery. We think this small difference was not critical for predicting the possible presence of an open urinary tract. The positions of the openings were similar to the predicted positions (Figure 3). In the two cases where the urinary tract was open, the patients were properly treated and no patient had postoperative complications. Surgical pathology reported clear cell renal cell carcinoma with negative margins in all cases.

Discussion

In this study, we focused on open urinary tracts and developed a way to virtually visualize resection planes from CT images. Preoperatively understanding the 3D relationship of organs is particularly important for laparoscopic partial nephrectomy. In the past, surgeons had to infer the relationship of organs from CT slices; they performed 3D shape reconstructions in their heads. This required extensive experience and it was impossible to share ideas with others. In contrast, our method provides visualization that

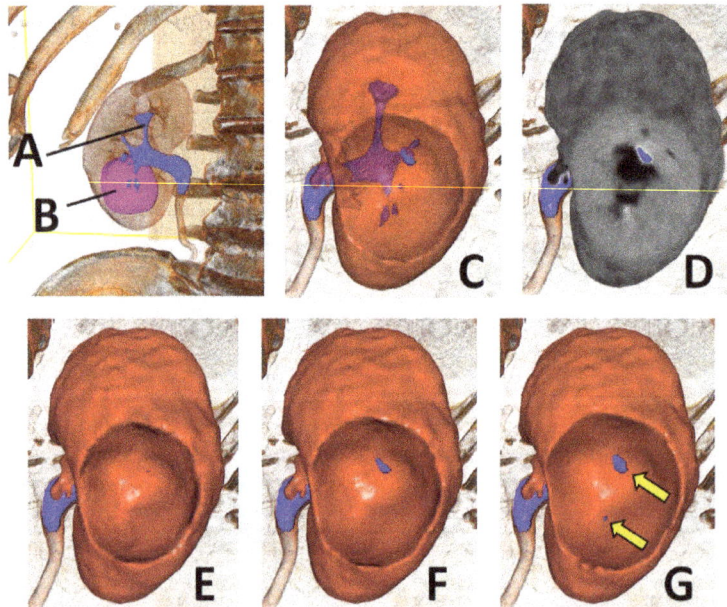

Figure 2 Virtual resection plane. We generated surface models of the urinary tract (**A**) and tumor (**B**) regions. We also generated multiple kidney regions that had 1 mm (**E**), 3 mm (**F**), and 5 mm (**G**) margins from the tumor. We also generated transparent (**C**) and CT-image renderings (**D**) of the kidney model. The CT-image rendering (**D**) allowed observance of the CT value on the resection plane.

Table 1 Patient characteristics and summary of the result

No	Sex	Age	Tumor size (mm)	Tumor location				Prediction of urinary tract status	Intraoperative urinary tract status	Surgical margin (min)	Ischemia time (min)	Operating time (min)
				Right/ Left	Longitudinal location	Arterior/ Posterior	Lateral/ Medial					
1	M	44	19	R	Upper pole	Anterior	Lateral	Not open with 5 mm margin	Not open	3	19	185
2	F	77	26	L	Upper pole	Anterior	Medial	Open with 2 mm margin	Open	1	20	179
3	M	72	35	R	Inferior pole	Posterior	Lateral	Open with 1 mm margin	Open	1	28	206
4	M	65	19	R	Middle pole	Posterior	Medial	Not open with 5 mm margin	Not open	1	13	156
5	M	75	25	R	Middle pole	Posterior	Medial	Open with 4 mm margin	Not open	1	11	158

In the columns, from left to right, we indicate patient information, tumor size, tumor location, prediction of urinary tract status, intraoperative urinary tract status, intraoperative surgical margin, ischemia time, and operating time.

is close to the actual intraoperative view and allows surgeons to easily understand the 3D relationship of important organs. We believe that the preoperative information provided by our visualization method improves the safety of operations.

The major postoperative complications of laparoscopic partial nephrectomy are urine leakage, parenchymal bleeding and acute renal failure. Breda et al. reported that urine leakage of laparoscopic partial nephrectomy occurred in 1.4-2.0% of patients [13]. Thompson et al. reported that ischemia time is the most important factor in predicting renal function preservation [14]. To prevent complications, cracks should be securely sutured and ischemia time should be decreased, which can be accomplished by appropriate preoperative planning. For instance, the approach (trans-abdominal or trans-retroperitoneum), port position, and resection line should be selected depending on the tumor position and surrounding organs. Gill et al. reported on the novel technique of zero ischemia partial nephrectomy with preoperative planning using a visualized 3D view of the renal artery [15]. Our method virtually visualizes the intraoperative view from a different viewpoint. It may allow surgeons to visualize operation procedures in a different preoperative setting and enable them to select a better setting. Nephrometry scoring systems have been developed in an effort to standardize tumor assessment. R.E.N.A.L. Nephrometry Score (NS) has been proposed by Uzzo et al. [16]. Ficarra et al. introduced Preoperative Aspects and Dimensions Used for an Anatomical (PADUA) system. Our visualization technique contributes to more precise scoring of those nephrometry scores [17]. Our study focused on visualization of open urinary tracts, the first such study to have been reported.

Training for laparoscopic surgery is much more difficult than that for open surgery. Since laparoscopic surgery has a steep learning curve, it is important to provide sufficient training. Various laparoscopic surgery training systems have been developed. Some recent systems reproduces the entire procedure of laparoscopic radical nephrectomy [18,19]. However, to the best of our knowledge, no other system provides an actual operative view of the individual patient. In contrast, our method provides visualization similar to the actual laparoscopic operative view using individual patient data.

The image segmentation software VoTracer, which we developed for this study, is useful in creating simulation

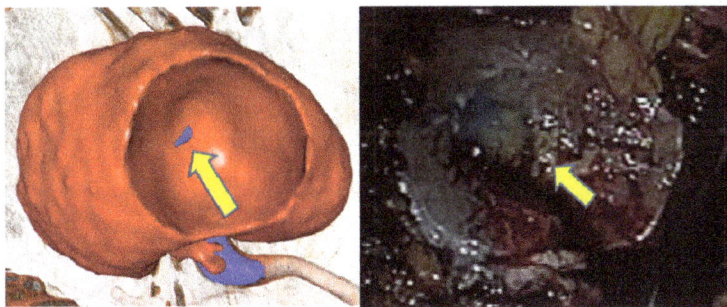

Figure 3 Side-by-side comparison. The right panel is a representative scene from a recorded video of an operation and the left panel shows a virtual resection plane similar to the viewpoint of the actual operation.

models. Our research group has published studies on a mission rehearsal type surgical simulator that uses patient-specific models [20-22]. In these studies, we reported that the patient-specific surgical simulator is useful for less-experienced doctors in practicing standard operations and for experts in developing new surgical procedures. However, one of the biggest obstacles of such a simulator is the process of creating simulation models from 3D images of patients. The image segmentation method presented in this study allowed us to segment each region (kidney, urinary tract, and tumor) in a few minutes. This drastically accelerates the model creation process. Combining the surgical simulator and the image segmentation method is an ongoing project that we hope to realize in the future.

The major limitation of our current method is that the segmentation process requires user operation. The user has to set region growing parameters to correctly segment the urinary tract region. The user also has to specify contours to segment tumor regions based on his or her subjective knowledge (Figure 1D). Thus, segmentation results may vary depending on the user. Notice that this is retrospective study and the number of cases is also restricted. Larger population study is required in order to raise the accuracy of prediction. In the future, we would like to conduct a large-scale study and develop a segmentation method that minimizes user operation as much as possible. In this study, we used the delay phase of contrast enhanced CT in order to precisely segment the urinary tract. Due to CT imaging timing issues, we had several cases in which it was difficult to precisely segment the urinary tract. It is necessary to determine the best timing of CT imaging in order to stably segment urinary tract regions.

Conclusions

In this study, we developed a method to predict the presence of an open urinary tract and the position of the opening in laparoscopic partial nephrectomy from 3D CT images. The results revealed that we could make accurate predictions in 5 cases. This was a retrospective study and the number of cases was small. A larger scale study is required in order to confirm the accuracy of the predictions.

Abbreviations
3D: Three dimensional; 2D: Two dimensional; CT: Computed tomography; MRI: Magnetic resonance imaging; NS: Nephrometry score.

Competing interests
The authors declare that they have no competing interests.

Authors' contributions
DU made conception and desingn and drafted the manuscript. KM participated in the design of the study, and revised the manuscript. HY collected and assemble the data. TI and HY developed the software used in this study. YK conceived of the study, and helped to draft the manuscript. All authors read and approved the final manuscript.

Acknowledgements
This works was supported by Grant-in-Aid for Scientists (No.30550347) from Japan Society for the Promotion of Science. We thank Dr. N Nakaigawa (Yokohama City University) to assist us in the operations.

Author details
[1]Department of Urology, Yokohama City University School of Medicine, 3-9 Fukuura, Kanagawa-ku, Yokohama, Kanagawa 236-0004, Japan. [2]Image Processing Research Tea, RIKEN, Wako, Japan.

References
1. Gaur DD: **Laparoscopic operative retroperitoneoscopy: use of new device.** *J Urol* 1992, **148**:1137–1139.
2. Lee CT, Katz J, Shi W, Thaler HT, Reuter VE, Russo P: **Surgical management of renal tumors 4 cm. or less in a contemporary cohort.** *J Urol* 2000, **163**:730.
3. Lau WK, Blute ML, Weaver AL, Torres VE, Zincke H: **Matched comparison of radical nephrectomy vs nephron- sparing surgery in patients with unilateral renal cell carci- noma and a normal contralateral kidney.** *Mayo Clin Proc* 2000, **75**:1236.
4. McKiernan J, Simmons R, Katz J, Russo P: **Natural history of chronic renal insufficiency after partial and radical nephrectomy.** *Urology* 2002, **59**:816.
5. Kniss J, Kindlmann G, Hansen C: **Multi-dimensional transfer functions for interactive volume rendering.** *IEEE Trans Vis Comput Graph* 2002, **8**(4):270–285.
6. Otsu N: **A threshold selection method from gray-level histograms.** *IEEE Trans Sys Man Cyber* 1979, **9**(1):62–66.
7. Adams R, Bischof L: **Seeded region growing.** *IEEE Trans PAMI* 1994, **16**(6):641–647.
8. Boykov Y, Veksler O, Zabih R: **Fast approximate energy minimization via graph cuts.** *IEEE Trans PAMI* 2001, **23**(11):1222–1239.
9. Li Y, Sun J, Tang CK, Shum HY: **Lazy snapping.** *ACM Trans Graph* 2004, **23**(3):303–308.
10. Ijiri T, Yokota H: **Contour-based interface for refining volume segmentation.** *Comput Graph Forum* 2010, **29**(7):2153–2160.
11. Ijiri T, Yoshizawa S, Sato Y, Ito M, Yokota H: **Bilateral hermite radial basis functions for contour-based volume segmentation.** *Comput Graph Forum* 2013, **32**(2):123–132.
12. Lorensen WE, Cline HE: **A high resolution 3D surface construction algorithm.** *Comput Graph* 1987, **21**(3):163–169.
13. Breda A, Finelli A, Janetschek G: **Complication of laparoscopic surgery for renal masses: prevention, management, and comparison with the open experience.** *Eur Urol* 2009, **55**:836–850.
14. Thompson RH, Lane BR, Lohse CM, Leibovich BC, Fergany A, Frank I, Gill IS, Blute ML, Campbell SC: **Every minute counts when the renal hilum is clamped during partial nephrectomy.** *Eur Urol* 2010, **58**:340–345.
15. Gill IS, Patil MB, Desai MM: **Zero ischemia anatomical partial nephrectomy: a novel approach.** *J Urol* 2012, **187**:807–815.
16. Kutikov A, Uzzo RG: **The R.E.N.A.L. nephrometry score: a comprehensive standardized system for quantitating renal tumor size, location and depth.** *J Urol* 2009, **182**:844–853.
17. Ficarra V, Novara G, Secco S, Macchi V, Porzionato A, De Caro R, Artivani W: **Preoperative aspects and dimensions used for an anatomical (PADUA) classification of renal tumours in patients who are candidates for nephron-sparing surgery.** *Eur Urol* 2009, **56**:786–793.
18. Brewin J, Nedas T, Challacombe B, Elhage O, Keisu J, Dasgupta P: **Face content and construct validation of the first virtual reality laparoscopic nephrectomy simulator.** *BJU Int* 2010, **106**:850–854.
19. Wijn RP, Persoon MC, Schout BM, Martens EJ, Scherpbier AJ, Hendrikx AJ: **Virtual reality laparoscopic nephrectomy simulator is lacking in construct validity.** *J Endourol* 2010, **24**:117–122.

20. Makiyama K, Sakata R, Yamanaka H, Tatenuma T, Sano F, Kubota Y:
Laparoscopic nephroureterectomy in renal pelvic urothelial carcinoma
with situs inversus totalis:preoperative training using a patient-specific
simulator. *Urol* 2012, **80**(6):1375–1378.
21. Yamanaka H, Makiyama K, Tatenuma T, Sakata R, Sano F, Kubota Y:
Preparation for pyeloplasty for ureteropelvic junction obstruction using
a patient-specific laparoscopic simulator:a case report. *J Med Case Reports*
2012, **6**:338.
22. Makiyama K, Nagasaka M, Inuiya T, Takanami K, Ogata M, Kubota Y:
Development of a patient-specific simulator for laparoscopic renal
surgery. *Int J Urol* 2012, **19**:829–835.

Treatment by a nurse practitioner in primary care improves the severity and impact of urinary incontinence in women

Doreth T.A.M Teunissen[*], Marjolein M. Stegeman, Hans H. Bor and Toine A.L.M Lagro-Janssen

Abstract

Background: Urinary Incontinence (UI) is a common problem in women. The management of UI in primary care is time consuming and suboptimal. Shift of incontinence-care from General Practitioners (GP's) to a nurse practitioner maybe improves the quality of care. The purpose of this observational (pre/post) study is to determine the effectiveness of introducing a nurse practitioner in UI care and to explore women's reasons for not completing treatment.

Methods: Sixteen trained nurse practitioners treated female patients with UI. All patients were examined and referred by the GP to the nurse practitioner working in the same practice. At baseline the severity of the UI (Sandvik-score), the impact on the quality of life (IIQ) and the impressed severity (PGIS) was measured and repeated after three months Differences were tested by the paired t and the NcNemar test.
Reasons for not completing treatment were documented by the nurse practitioner and differences between the group that completed treatment and the drop-out group were tested.

Results: We included 103 women, mean age 55 years (SD 12.6). The Sandvik severity categories improved significantly (P < 0.001), as did the impact on daily life (2.54 points, P = 0.012). Among the IIQ score the impact on daily activities increased 0.73 points (P = 0.032), on social functioning 0.60 points (P = 0.030) and on emotional well-being 0.63 points (P = 0.031). The PGIS-score improved in 41.3 % of the patients.
The most important reasons for not completing the treatment were lack of improvement of the UI and difficulties in performing the exercises. Women who withdraw from guidance by the nurse practitioner perceived more impact on daily life (P = 0.036), in particular on the scores for social functioning (P = 0.015) and emotional well-being (P = 0.015).

Conclusion: Treatment by a trained nurse practitioner seems positively affects the severity of the UI and the impact on the quality of life. Women who did not complete treatment suffer from more impact on quality of life, experience not enough improvement and mention difficulties in performing exercises.

Keywords: Urinary Incontinence, Nurse Practitioner, Primary care, Quality of life

Background

Urinary Incontinence (UI) is a common problem in women with a prevalence varying from 25 % to 50 % [1, 2]. The impact of UI on daily life differs amongst patients. The highest impact is found on emotional wellbeing and public activities [3]. In addition, in the Netherlands annually €155 million is spent just on incontinence pads [4].

According to the guideline 'Urinary incontinence' of the The Dutch College of General Practitioners the prevalent treatment for stress- and urge-incontinence is pelvic floor exercises and bladder training respectively [5]. In mixed incontinence the treatment starts with the type of incontinence that is experienced by the patient as most disabling.

Adequate UI management according to the guideline is time-consuming. General practitioners (GP's) may experience a lack of time and knowledge to provide adequate care [6]. Another obstacle is the low motivation of patients to perform the above mentioned interventions [7]. The most important factor for a successful treatment however is

* Correspondence: doreth.teunissen@radboudumc.nl
Department Primary and Community Care, Gender & Women's Health, Radboud University Medical Centre Nijmegen, Internal postal code 118, P.O. Box 9101, 6500 HB Nijmegen, The Netherlands

adherence to these interventions [8, 9]. Known factors for non-adherence to the exercises are difficulties in finding time to exercise and to recall the exercises [10]. An additional impediment is that some authors mention less motivation in the elderly patients to seek help and to accept the care required [7]. Therefore we need more insight into the reasons of patients in not accepting or completing treatment. This offers possibilities to improve the management of UI in primary care.

The last few decades there is a shift going on in care from GP's to nurse practitioners to meet the rising demands for primary care. It appears that the nurse practitioners can produce the same quality of care and achieve comparable health outcomes as GP's [11]. At the same time the care by nurse practitioners is patient-friendly and efficiently organized [12]. It was also shown to be cost-effective in general [13].

In a review about the role of a nurse in the care of patients with incontinence, nine of the twelve included studies reported a significant greater reduction of incontinence episode in the intervention group and patients were very satisfied. The nurses in the studies came from different countries and differed from a nurse with a bachelor of science in nursing degree to a nurse practitioner and the education differed from a full 6 weeks course till a short training by a local physiotherapist or behavioral psychologist [14, 15].

Recently also a Dutch study is conducted with nurse involved in the treatment of patients with UI [16]. Local Nurses working in de community and visiting patients at home, were shortly trained in the care of incontinence. They took tasks from the GP related to diagnostics, intervention and monitoring of patients with UI. The GP kept final responsibility. This study showed that involving a local nurse in UI primary care did reduce severity and impact of UI after three months but this improvement did not stay after twelve months. One of the problems mentioned in this study was the cooperation between the local nurse and GPs [12]. It was difficult to reach GPs to discuss patients and the referral rate from GP to the local nurse was low. Because of this we choose in our study to train nurse practitioners to guide patients with UI. A nurse practitioner is also a nurse but with additional a nurse practitioner diploma (after following a one year during education program focused on chronic care in the general practice). In the Netherlands the nurse practitioner is especially involved in the treatment and guidance of patients with chronic diseases such as Diabetes Mellitus en Chronic Pulmonary Disease with the core businesses to assess risk factors, to give health education and to perform motivational interviewing. A major advantage of the Dutch nurse practitioners is that they are part of the primary care team and they are working in the GP's office. Therefore they are familiar to cooperate with the GP. This facilitates nurse practitioners to consult a GP when necessary, lowers thresholds for patients to seek help and possibly increases patient's motivation. Another advantage of nurse practitioners is that they are involved in the treatment and guidance of patients with chronic diseases such as diabetes mellitus en chronic pulmonary diseases [17]. They can actively ask the patient with diabetes or chronic pulmonary disease about UI. Both morbidities are known with a high prevalence of UI.

Nevertheless the effectiveness of nurse practitioner in primary care trained in UI is not clear. Because of this we firstly set up a training program for nurse practitioners to enable them to take care of patients with UI. Secondly we conducted a clinical observational study to establish the effectiveness of both incontinence severity and quality of life. We also study characteristics and reasons of patients not completing the treatment program. Consequently, we formulated the following research questions:

– does the introduction of a nurse practitioner in the treatment of UI in women in primary care lead to an improvement of the UI severity and the quality of life after three months therapy?
– what are reasons for women not to complete the treatment program given by a trained nurse practitioner and are their differences in patient characteristics between the group that completed treatment and the drop-out group?

Methods
Design
We preformed an observational study.

Setting
In this study a total of 16 nurse practitioners, already working with the GP in GP's offices, in the eastern part of the Netherlands, undertook a training program in which they learned how to manage female patients with UI. The training program included 1.5 days course, several home assignments and refresher courses after three weeks, three and six months. The nurse practitioners were trained in tasks related to diagnostics, intervention and monitoring of incontinence based on the guideline 'urinary incontinence' of the The Dutch College of General Practitioners [5]. All nurse practitioners proved their competence after the course in an assessment. After the 1,5 days course the participants started to guide patients with UI within the beginning feedback from the GP and the members of the trainings board till they have proven their competencies in an individual assessment. At the refresher courses the nurse practitioners could discuss cases with experts and share their experiences. The training protocol is available upon request. The GP's of

the practices the nurse practitioners are working got a 3 h during education course to refresh the guideline and to explain with expertise they could expect from the nurse practitioners after the course.

Participants

Women who asked for help in primary care for symptoms of stress-, urge- or mixed UI were included between June 2009 and December 2010. Patients who underwent an incontinence operation in de past, patients with a pelvic organ prolapse grade IV (Baden Walker), a gynecologic malignancy, a neurological disease or unstable mental disorder were excluded from the study.

Data collection

The GP diagnosed prior to the referral to the nurse practitioner, the type of incontinence and excluded other causes of urinary incontinence like urinary tract infections or malignancies. After explanation about the study and informed consent of the patient to participate in the study the GP gave the patients information about the type of incontinence but did not explain treatment option. Because co-morbidities and use of medication can influence UI we also registered them. We compared these data with the prevalence of the same co-morbidities in a standard primary care population according to the Continuous Morbidity Registration Nijmegen (CMR) to known if our study population is a presentation of a general population. The CMR is a very reliable registration system which determines epidemiological numbers according to the incidence and prevalence of diseases in primary care for scientific research and education [18]. Because the CMR does not register medication for the aim of research we compared the use of diuretics and antidepressants with the corresponding diseases such as hypertension/heart failure and depression as registered in the CMR.

A view days after the consultation with the GP the patients had an appointment with the nurse practitioner. Prior to the first meeting with the nurse practitioner (T0), patients filled out questionnaires to assess the severity of the UI (Sandvik-score and the Patient Global Impression of Severity (PGIS) [19, 20] and its impact on the quality of life (Incontinence Impact Questionnaire) [21]. Patients' variables like age and variables that may impact UI negatively like mobility constraints, micturition habits (taking time, have a good position on the toilet, do not postpone, voiding frequency 5 to 6 times a day), caffeine and alcohol intake were also mapped. Patients received information and advice and started with conservative treatment according to the Dutch guideline 'urinary incontinence' [5]. After six weeks, the patients returned to the nurse practitioner to evaluate the effect until then. The patients were motivated by the nurse to continue practicing and to follow the given advice. After

three months (T1), patients filled out the same questionnaires as they did prior to the first meeting to evaluate the effect of the treatment (Fig. 1). We chose for a follow up of three months because the aim of the study is to study if the intervention seems to be effective and to study the feasibility of the intervention. The dutch guideline 'Urinary incontinence' of the The Dutch College of General Practitioners advise to evaluate the effectiveness of the therapy after three months. If the incontinence isn't improved enough a referral to a physiotherapist of urologist/gynecologist can be considered. If the patient is satisfied with the effectiveness of the therapy it is important to explain that continuing exercises is needed to sustain this effect.

Outcome measures
Primary outcome

The primary outcome measure was the severity of involuntary urine loss. . The severity of involuntary loss of urine was measured by the total Sandvik-score (i.e. quantity of urine loss multiplied by the frequency) [19]. The Sandvik-score of frequency are: never = 0, < 1 time a month = 1, a few times a month = 2, a few times a week = 3 and every day/night = 4. The Sandvik-score of quantity are: none = 0, drops = 1, little amount = 2 and more = 3. The total Sandvik-score can be divided into five categories of severity; none = total Sandvik score 0, mild = total score 1–2, moderate = total score 3–6, severe = total score 8–9 and very severe = total score 12.

Secondary outcome

The secondary outcome measures were the impact of quality of life and patients appraisal of the severity of incontinence.

The impact on the quality of life was measured by the Incontinence Impact Questionnaire (IIQ), a questionnaire highly recommended by the International Consultation on Incontinence (= ICI) and is rated as Grade A [21] The IIQ measures the impact of the UI on daily activities (6 questions), social functioning (10 questions), emotional wellbeing (8 questions) and travelling/mobility (6 questions). For each question the patient can choose between: not at all (0 points), mild (1 point), moderate (2 points) and severe (3 points) [21]. Patients missing 6 or more questions in the IIQ were excluded from further analyses (N = 1).

To evaluate women's overall appraisal of the severity of their UI we asked the patients to rate their experience of the severity of their incontinence problem with the Patient Global Impression of Severity (PGIS) into one of four categories (negligible, mild, moderate, severe) [20].

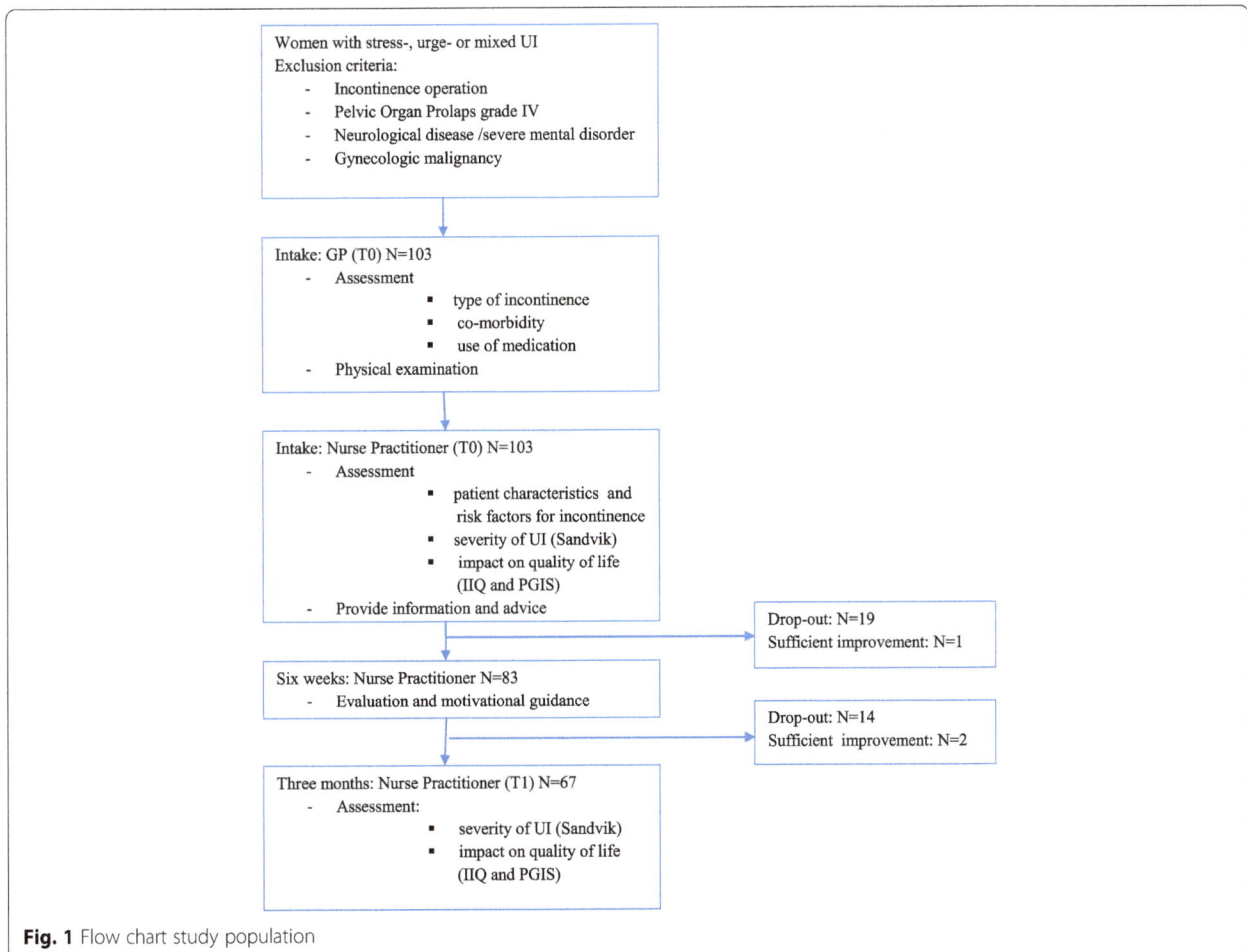

Fig. 1 Flow chart study population

Sample size calculation

Improvement in the severity of the incontinence was estimated to occur in 40 % of those in the treatment group compared to 5 % in the group without intervention. Giving a significance level of 3 % and a power of 80 %, 40 participants were needed. We expected a drop out during the trial of 30 % and therefore we set our target at 60 patients.

Statistical methods

To test for the changes on the total IIQ-scores between T0 and T1 we used paired t-tests. To assess the effect of the treatment on the Sandvik subgroups- and PGIS-scores we used the McNemar test. [22] In order to test for the possible influence of age, the type of incontinence on the effect measures of the treatment we used a General Linear Model (univariate analyse of variance) with the dependent variables age and type of incontinence and the independent variables total Sandvik-. IIQ- and the PGIS-scores.

To investigate differences between the drop-out (patients who started the treatment but dropped out during the follow up of three months) and the group patients

who completed treatment we used a General Linear Model (univariate analyse of variance) with the dependent variables age, the total Sandvik- and IIQ-scores and Chi-square tests for variables type of incontinence, co-morbidity, use of medication and PGIS-scores.

Ethical approval

Upon consultation, the Medical Ethics Committee (CMO region Nijmegen Arnhem) stated that ethical approval was not necessary because of the non-invasive character of the study (CMO-nr 2010/460).

Results

Descriptive data

One hundred and three women entered the treatment program. Thirty-three of them dropped out before the 3 months appointment. Additionally, three patients stopped treatment before the three month appointment because the UI sufficiently improved or they didn't fill out the T1 questionnaires (Fig. 1). The age of the study populations varied between 24–87 years (mean 55.0, SD 12.6). Fifty two (50.2 %) patients were diagnosed with stress-incontinence, 15 (14.7 %) with urge incontinence and 36 (34.8 %) with mixed incontinence (Table 1). Most patients (78 %) suffered from a mild to moderate severity, in 22 % the UI was (very) severe. Thirty five percent of the patients experienced a negligible impact of the UI on daily life, 59 % a mild to moderate impact and two percent a severe impact. Despite the negligible impact of the UI in a part of the women they chose to undergo a treatment because the kind of treatment was not invasive. Table 1 summarizes the co-morbidities and use of medication. For reasons of comparison Table 1 also shows the

Table 1 Patient characteristics N = 103

Characteristic	N (%)	Presented morbidity in women (age 45–65) in standard population (CMR)[a] (%)
Age mean (SD)	55.0 (±14.6)	
Incontinence		
Stress	52 (50.5)	
Urge	15 (14.7)	
Mixed	36 (34.8)	
Severity of UI (Sandvik score)		
Mild	11 (10,7)	
Moderate	69 (67,0)	
Severe	22 (21,4)	
Very severe	1 (0,9)	
Impact on daily life (IIQ)		
Activities	1.61 (SD 2.50)	
Social	1.32 (SD 2.62)	
Emotional	1.37 (SD 2.07)	
Travelling	1.76 (SD 2.54)	
Impression of severity (PGIS)		
Negligible	36 (34,9)	
Mild	40 (39,2)	
Moderate	23 (19,8)	
Severe	4 (2,1)	
Co-morbidity		
Neurologic disease	8 (7.5)	(1.9)[b]
COPD/chronic cough/asthma	10 (9.4)	(6.8)
Diabetes mellitus	8 (7.5)	(4.3)
Heart failure	4 (3.8)	(2,0)
Hypertension	25 (23.6)	(14.5)
Obesity	27 (25.5)	(11.9)
Use of medication		
Diuretics	15 (14.2)	(14.7)[c]
Antidepressants	12 (11.3)	(2.1)[d]
Other	29 (27.4)	–

[a]CMR: Continuous Morbidity Registration Nijmegen
[b]TIA/CVA, Parkinson's disease, epilepsy, [c]Hypertension, heart failure, [d]Depressive disorder

prevalence of co-morbidities and use of medication in a Dutch standard population according to the CMR. Co-morbidities and the use of antidepressants were more prevalent in the study population compared to the standard population.

Sixteen percent of the women declared they were not taking their time for micturition and thirty-seven (34.9 %) patients regularly postponed micturition. In addition, seven (6.8 %) patients had mobility constraints. The average number of caffeine intake was 3.6 cups a day (SD 2.6) and the average number of alcohol intake was 0.8 units a day (SD 1.5), which is quite common in the Netherlands.

Not all patients completed all questionnaires. Fifty-seven (85.1 %) patients completed the Sandvik-score at intake and 3 months. Forty-eight (71.6 %) and 46 (68.7 %) patients completed the IIQ and PGIS at both measurements.

Outcome data

Between baseline and 3 months treatment the Sandvik categories of severity significant improvement *(P = 0.005)*: 23 patients (40.4 %) improved, 3 patients (5.3 %) deteriorated and 31 patients (54.4 %) stayed in the same sub group (Fig. 2). The total IIQ-score improved 2.54 points *(P = 0.012)* (Table 2), whereas the impact on daily activities improved 0.73 points *(P = 0.032)*, on social functioning 0.60 points *(P = 0.030)* and on emotional well-being 0.63 points *(P = 0.031)*. Although the impact on travelling and mobility improved, this difference was not significant *(P = 0.082)*. Also the PGIS-score improved significantly *(P = 0.029)*: there was an improvement for 19 patients (41.3 %), a deteriorated in 4 patients (8.7 %) and in 23 patients (50.0 %) the PGIS did not change (Fig. 3). Age or type of incontinence did not influence the effect of treatment.

We compared the drop-out group with the group that completed treatment to determine whether there were any differences in patient's characteristics, severity of involuntary urine loss and impact of UI on the quality of life. No differences were found between the group that competed treatment and the drop-out group according to age, type of incontinence, co-morbidity, use of medication, Sandvik-scores, IIQ-scores and PGIS-scores. The group that competed treatment contained significantly more patients with hypertension *(P = 0.023)*. The total IIQ-score was significantly higher in the drop-out group *(P = 0.036)* compared to the group that completed treatment. The same applied for the IIQ-scores for social functioning *(P = 0.015)* and emotional well-being *(P = 0.015fig.*

Women mentioned several reasons for not completing treatment (Table 3). Ten patients were not satisfied about the improvement of UI; five of them were referred to a physiotherapist and five to an urologist/gynecologist. Five patients experienced difficulties in performing the

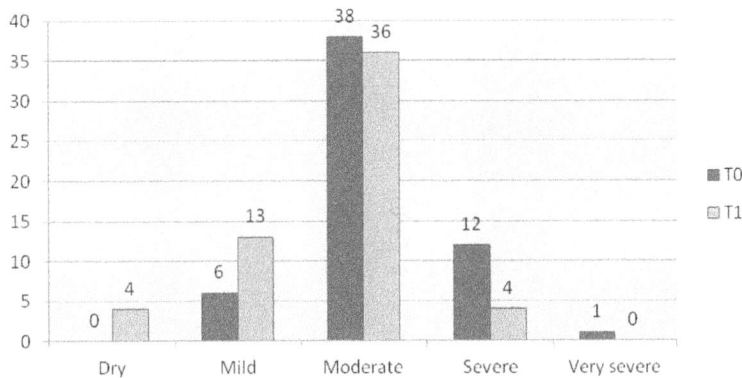

Fig. 2 Number of patients by severity categories (Sandvik) at T0(baseline) and T1(3 months) N=57

exercises or in adherence to the treatment program. Five patients stopped the program because of other health problems or others priorities, like being strongly involved in the care of a sick husband or too busy with the revalidation after a total hip replacement. Lastly, 12 patients did not show up for control without a known reason.

Discussion

Key results
Our first important finding is that treatment by trained nurse practitioners seems to improve the severity of the incontinence and quality of life especially on social functioning and emotional well being after three months of therapy.

Secondary, patients who dropped out from treatment did not differ in age and type of UI compared to the observational group but experience more social and emotional impact of the incontinence. The most important reason for discontinuing treatment is lack of improvement. The in our study group experienced minimal impact of the UI will also be a reason why patients are not always motivated to do exercises for a long time.

Finally, inadequate micturition habits are very common in the observational group Fortunately the nurse practitioner has time to discuss these risk factors and time to give health education and advice specially focused on UI.

Interpretation of the results
The improvement of UI after a nurse practitioner treatment is according to previous studies but the differences

with our study are that these studies are conducted outside primary care practices [14–16, 23, 24]. Our results are also in line with a systematic review stating that nurse practitioners involved in the care of patients in general lead to an improvement of health outcomes and patients satisfaction [24].

Concerning the drop-out one can expect that especially older women or women with more serious incontinence or women who perceive more impact of UI on daily life will not complete treatment. Our study supports this hypothesis only for the impact of UI on quality of life. The total IIQ-score and the IIQ-scores for social functioning and emotional well-being are significantly higher in the drop-out group meaning that they strongly suffer from their incontinence. It takes time to achieve any improvement by treatment and because of the severe impact it may be too difficult or not appropriate to them to wait for improvement.

The lack of improvement as reason for drop-out seems to be quite logical but is scarcely mentioned in the literature [10, 24–28]. Patients also experience difficulties in performing exercises or have to face other health problems. These finding are in line with other studies [10, 25–28].

Concerning the high prevalence of inadequate micturition habits. As already mentioned the nurse practitioner is competent and has the time to discuss these risk factor. Moreover the nurse practitioner is trained to perform motivational interviewing to motivate patients to change life style like micturition habits. The prevalence

Table 2 Impact on quality of life (IIQ-scores) at T0(baseline) and T1(3 months) N = 48

	Intake (T0) (SD)	3 months (T1) (SD)	Change	Paired T-test (p-value)
IIQ total	6.05 (8.41)	3.51 (6.03)	2.54	0.012*
IIQ activities	1.61 (2.50)	0.88 (1.57)	0.73	0.032*
IIQ Social	1.32 (2.62)	0.72 (1.72)	0.60	0.030*
IIQ emotional	1.37 (2.07)	0.74 (1.56)	0.63	0.031*
IIQ travelling	1.76 (2.54)	1.19 (2.00)	0.57	0.082

* P < 0.05

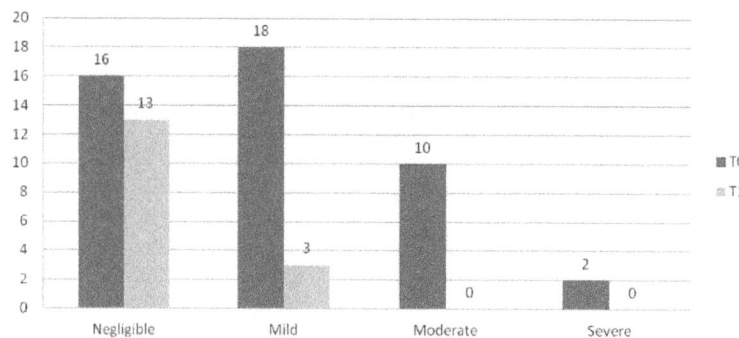

Fig. 3 Number of patients by impressed severity categories (PGIS) at T0 (baseline) and T1 (3 months) N=46

of mobility constraints and the intake of caffeine and alcohol are not extremely high. It's important to take attention to these factors because they negatively affect incontinence.

Limitations

Before drawing any conclusions on the basis of our findings the following needs to be considered.

The dropout rate in this observational study of (32 %) is high but comparable with other studies in which the drop-out rates vary from 11 % to 50 % [14, 15, 23].

A limitation of the current study is that there is no control group involved as in a randomized controlled trial which received usual care from the GP. Several published randomized controlled trial conclude that a control-group without treatment shows no or a slightly improvement of the incontinence [29]. Further research needs to be done to determine whether the nurse practitioner guidance is superior to usual care.

Furthermore as our study focused on the short term effect of the nurse practitioner guidance, more research needs to be done to determine the long term effects.

Generalisability

A trained nurse practitioner involved in the guidance of women with UI seems to have a positive effect on the severity of the UI and the impact of the UI on the quality of life after three months therapy. A major advantage

Table 3 Reasons for non completing treatment N = 33

Reason	N
Lack of improvement, referral to physiotherapist	5
Lack of improvement, referral to urologist/gynaecologist	5
Difficulties performing exercises or adherence to the program	5
Other health problems	4
Other priorities	1
Unrealistic expectations of the program	1
Reasons unknown	12

of the Dutch nurse practitioners is that they are working in the GP's office. Therefore they are familiar to cooperate with the GP. This facilitates nurse practitioners to consult a GP easier when necessary, probably lowers thresholds for patients to seek for help and possibly increases patient's motivation. Former research shows that patient's motivation is one of the most important factors for a successful treatment of UI [9]. Nurse Practitioners can enhance this motivation and thereby increase the effect of treatment. Another advantage of nurse practitioners is that they actively can ask the patient with diabetes or chronic pulmonary disease about UI. Both morbidities are known with a high prevalence of UI and both morbidities are in the Netherlands mostly in care of the nurse practitioner [17].

One of the biggest problems of conservative treatment in case of UI is the high withdrawal of the patients. There are several options to improve the approach of UI by involving a trained nurse practitioner. First of all, exercises should be discussed with patients in a comprehensive way. Nurse practitioners should check several times whether patients still know how to perform the exercises and feel comfortable about it. It is also important that nurse practitioners keep in mind that the training program for patients with UI is time-consuming, not always easy to sustain and difficult to implement in daily life. This applies particularly patients with other health related problems.

Secondly, it is also important to discuss patient's expectations about the aim of the guidance by the nurse practitioner. This provides an opportunity to prevent patients for having unrealistic expectations, thereby avoiding possible disappointments and referrals to specialists before the treatment is finished.

Conclusion

In conclusion a trained nurse practitioner involved in the guidance of women with UI seems to have a small positive effect on the severity of the UI and the impact of the UI on the quality of life after three months of therapy, especially in patients with little complains. Patients who do not complete treatment experience more impact of the UI on social function and emotional well being. We have to keep in mind the high rate of drop-out. Most important reasons for drop out are lake of improvement and difficulties in performing exercises. Also it is not clear if the improvement is due the nurse practitioner or the 'treatment' itself. More research needs to be done in order to determine the long term effects of the nurse practitioner guidance and to determine whether the guidance is superior to a control group with for example usual care.

Abbreviations
GP: General Practitioner; IIQ: Incontinence impact questionnaire; PGIS: Patient global impression of severity; UI: Urinary incontinence; CMR: Continues morbidity registration nijmegen; ICI: International consultation on incontinence.

Competing interests
The authors declare that they have no competing interests.

Authors' contributions
DT concept and design of the study, data collection, data analysis, drafting the article, critical revision and approval of the article; MS data analysis, drafting the article, critical revision and approval of the article; HB data analysis and critical revision and approval of the article; TL concept and design of the study, data analysis, drafting the article, critical revision and approval of the article. All authors read and approved the final manuscript.

Acknowledgements
The development of the training for nurse practitioners was funding by health insurance ENO.

References
1. Melville JL, Katon W, Delaney K, Newton K. Urinary incontinence in US women: a population-based study. Arch Internal Med. 2005;165(5):537–42.
2. Teunissen TA, van den Bosch WJ, van den Hoogen HJ, Lagro-Janssen AL. Prevalence of urinary, fecal and double incontinence in the elderly living at home. Int Urogynecol J Pelvic Floor Dysfunct. 2004;15(1):10–3.
3. Teunissen D, Van Den Bosch W, Van Weel C, Lagro-Janssen T. "It can always happen": the impact of urinary incontinence on elderly men and women. Scand J Prim Health Care. 2006;24(3):166–73.
4. GIP/Health Insurance Board: total cost 2005–2009. 2009. http://www.gipdatabank.nl (the drug information system of national health care institute).
5. Lagro-Janssen ABBH, Van Dongen J, Lemain T, Teunissen D, Van Pinxteren B. Practice guideline 'Urinary incontinence' (first revision) from the Dutch College of General Practitioners. Huisarts Wet. 2006;49(10):10.
6. Albers-Heitner P, Berghmans B, Nieman F, Lagro-Janssen T, Winkens R. Adherence to professional guidelines for patients with urinary incontinence by general practitioners: a cross-sectional study. J Eval Clin Pract. 2008;14(5):807–11.
7. Teunissen D, van den Bosch W, van Weel C, Lagro-Janssen T. Urinary incontinence in the elderly: attitudes and experiences of general practitioners. A focus group study. Scand J Prim Health Care. 2006;24(1):56–61.
8. Alewijnse D, Mesters I, Metsemakers J, Adriaans J, van den Borne B. Predictors of intention to adhere to physiotherapy among women with urinary incontinence. Health Educ Res. 2001;16(2):173–86.
9. Lagro-Janssen AL, Smits AJ, van Weel C. Beneficial effect of exercise therapy in urinary incontinence in family practice depends largely on therapy compliance and motivation. Ned Tijdschr Geneesk. 1994;138(25):1273–6. Gunstig effect van oefentherapie bij urine-incontinentie in de huisartspraktijk vooral afhankelijk van therapietrouw en motivatie.
10. Borello-France D, Burgio KL, Goode PS, Markland AD, Kenton K, Balasubramanyam A, et al. Adherence to behavioral interventions for urge incontinence when combined with drug therapy: adherence rates, barriers, and predictors. Phys Ther. 2010;90(10):1493–505.
11. Laurant M RD, Hermens R, Braspenning J, Grol R, Sibbald B. Substitution of doctors by nurses in primary care. Cochrane database Syst Rev. 2005;2:CD001271.
12. Albers-Heitner PC, Lagro-Janssen TA, Venema PP, Berghmans BL, Winkens RR, de Jonge AA, et al. Experiences and attitudes of nurse specialists in primary care regarding their role in care for patients with urinary incontinence. Scand J Caring Sci. 2010;25(2):303–10.
13. Dierick-van Daele AT, Steuten LM, Metsemakers JF, Derckx EW, Spreeuwenberg C, Vrijhoef HJ. Economic evaluation of nurse practitioners versus GPs in treating common conditions. Br J Gen Pract. 2010;60(570):e28–35.
14. De Moulin M, Hamers J, Paulus A, Berendsen C, Halfens R. The tole of the nurse in community continence care: a systematic review. Int J Nurs Studies. 2005;42(4):479–92.
15. Williams KS, Assassa RP, Cooper NJ, Turner DA, Shaw C, Abrams KR, et al. Clinical and cost-effectiveness of a new nurse-led continence service: a randomised controlled trial. Br J Gen Pract. 2005;55(518):696–703.
16. Albers-Heitner PC, Lagro-Janssen TA, Joore MM, Berghmans BL, Nieman FF, Venema PP, et al. Effectiveness of involving a nurse specialist for patients with urinary incontinence in primary care: results of a pragmatic multicentre randomised controlled trial. Int J Clin Pract. 2011;65(6):705–12.
17. van Gerwen M, Schellevis F, Lagro-Janssen T. Comorbidities associated with urinary incontinence: a case–control study from the Second Dutch National Survey of General Practice. J Am Board Fam Med. 2007;20(6):608–10.
18. van Weel C. The Continuous Morbidity Registration Nijmegen: Background and history of a Dutch general practice database. Eur J Gen Pract. 2008;14 Suppl 1:5–12.
19. Sandvik H, Seim A, Vanvik A, Hunskaar S. A severity index for epidemiological surveys of female urinary incontinence: comparison with 48-h pad-weighing tests. Neurourol Urodyn. 2000;19(2):137–45.
20. Yalcin I, Bump RC. Validation of two global impression questionnaires for incontinence. Am J Obstet Gynecol. 2003;189(1):98–101.
21. Abrams P, Cardozo L, Koury S, Wein A. Incontinnence. http://www.ics.org/Publications/ICI_4/book.pdf.
22. Feuer EJ, Kessler LG. Test statistic and sample size for a two-sample McNemar test. Biometrics. 1989;45(2):629–36.
23. Du Moulin MF, Hamers JP, Paulus A, Berendsen CL, Halfens R. Effects of introducing a specialized nurse in the care of community-dwelling women suffering from urinary incontinence: a randomized controlled trial. J Wound Ostomy Continence Nurs. 2007;34(6):631–40.
24. Du Moulin MF, Hamers JP, Paulus A, Berendsen C, Halfens R. The role of the nurse in community continence care: a systematic review. In J Nurs Stud. 2005;42(4):479–92.
25. Alewijnse D, Mesters I, Metsemakers J, van den Borne B. Predictors of long-term adherence to pelvic floor muscle exercise therapy among women with urinary incontinence. Health Educ Res. 2003;18(5):511–24.
26. Alewijnse D, Mesters IE, Metsemakers JF, van den Borne BH. Program development for promoting adherence during and after exercise therapy for urinary incontinence. Patient Educ Couns. 2002;48(2):147–60.
27. Holley RL, Varner RE, Kerns DJ, Mestecky PJ. Long-term failure of pelvic floor musculature exercises in treatment of genuine stress incontinence. South Med J. 1995;88(5):547–9.
28. Sarma S, Hawthorne G, Thakkar K, Hayes W, Moore KH. The development of an Incontinence Treatment Motivation Questionnaire for patients undergoing pelvic floor physiotherapy in the treatment of stress incontinence. Int Urogynecol J Pelvic Floor Dysfunct. 2009;20(9):1085–93.
29. Hay-Smith CDJ. Pelvic floor muscle training versus no treatment, or inactive control treatments, for urinary incontinence in women. Cochrane Database Syst Rev. 2010;20(1):CD005654.

Simultaneous retrograde intrarenal surgery for ipsilateral asymptomatic renal stones in patients with ureteroscopic symptomatic ureteral stone removal

Dehui Lai[1,2*], Meiling Chen[1], Yongzhong He[1] and Xun Li[1,2]

Abstract

Background: Ipsilateral asymptomatic renal stone associated with symptomatic ureteral stone is not a rare event, and the recommended treatment policy was not declared clearly. This study was conducted to compare the outcomes of simultaneous retrograde intrarenal surgery (RIRS) and ureteroscopy to ureteroscopy alone for this clinical event.

Methods: 415 patients with symptomatic ureteral stone and ipsilateral asymptomatic renal stones were reviewed to obtain two match groups, who were treating with simultaneous modality (group A, N = 72), or ureteroscopy alone (group B, N = 72). Matching criteria were ureteral and renal stone side, duration and location, the presence of pre-stented. Perioperative and postoperative characteristics were compared between the two groups.

Results: Mean stone burdens were similar between group A and B. Mean operative duration for group A and B were 72.4 ± 21.3 and 36.4 ± 10.2 min, respectively ($P < 0.001$). Mean hospital duration was 6.4 ± 2.9 and 5.3 ± 2.1 days in group A and B, respectively ($P = 0.521$). Ureteral SFR was 100% in each group. Renal SFR for RIRS was 86.1%. Complication rates in group A were higher (22.2% vs 13.9%), but the differences were not statistically significant ($P = 0.358$). In group A, complications were significantly less in pre-stented patients (3/25 vs 5/11, $P = 0.04$). Auxiliary treatment rate was significant higher in group B (69.4% vs 5.6%, $P < 0.001$) during follow-up (mean >18 months).

Conclusions: Simultaneous RIRS for ipsilateral asymptomatic renal stones in patients with ureteroscopic symptomatic ureteral stone removal can be performed safely and effectively. It promises a high SFR with lower auxiliary treatment rate, and does not lengthen hospital duration and increase complications.

Keywords: Retrograde intrarenal surgery, Asymptomatic renal stone, Simultaneous treatment

Background

Asymptomatic renal stones are common in urological patients. They would be symptomatic without a complete retrieval at a certain time and required surgical treatment [1]. Although the current recommended method is active surveillance with an option for 2–3 years in EUA guidelines, it will be associated with a higher risk of surgical intervention [2,3]. Ipsilateral asymptomatic renal stone associated with symptomatic ureteral stone is not a rare event, and the recommended treatment policy was not declared clearly in any guidelines, especially in patients who had already removed symptomatic ureteral stone by ureteroscopy.

Retrograde intrarenal surgery (RIRS) is rapidly popular, benefited from the advance in flexible ureteroscopic instrumentation and holmium laser lithotripsy. It had been reported as an effective and definitive therapeutic option for patients with small to mid-size renal stones [4-6]. It is also recommended in some endourological centers for its high stone free rate (SFR) and low complications, when comparing with shock wave lithotripsy (SWL) and

* Correspondence: dehuilai@hotmail.com
[1]Urology Department, Fifth Affiliated Hospital, Guangzhou Medical University, 621 Gangwan Road, Huangpu District, Guangzhou, Guangdong 510700, China
[2]Translational Medical Center, Minimally Invasive Technology and Product, Guangzhou Medical University, Guangzhou, Guangdong, China

percutaneous nephrolithotomy (PCNL) in treating renal stones in size of <2 cm [4,7-9]. Although a high success rate has been showed independently for endoscopic treatment of ureteral and renal stones, there are few reports in the literature on simultaneous RIRS for asymptomatic renal stones in patients with ipsilateral ureteroscopic symptomatic ureteral stone removal.

The aim of this study was to evaluate the effectiveness and associated complications of this policy.

Methods

We obtained approval for this study from the ethics committee of the fifth affiliated hospital of Guangzhou Medical University. Written informed consent was obtained from all the participants. This study was designed as a retrospective controlled study, approved by our hospital review board. The computerized files of 415 patients with ipsilateral symptomatic ureteral stone and asymptomatic renal stones between March 2009 and July 2013 were reviewed and a database was constructed. 72 patients who underwent simultaneous RIRS for ipsilateral asymptomatic renal stones after ureteroscopic symptomatic ureteral stone removalwas defined as group A. The matched group was 72 patients, who underwent ureteroscopic laser lithotripsy (URL) for the symptomatic ureteral stone alone (group B). Matching criteria were stone side, burden and location, as well as the presence of a pre-placed D-J stent.

Patients with congenital renal anomalies, pelvi-ureteral junction obstruction, ureteral strictures, previous SWL treatment, and urinary tract infection were excluded. Ureteral and renal stone side and location were assessed preoperatively by noncontrast spiral CT scanning. Stone burden was defined as the surface area and calculated according to the European Association of Urology guidelines. Preoperative laboratory tests included blood and urinary routine test, serum creatinine estimation, and prothrombin concentration.

Surgical procedure

Prophlactic parenteral antibiotics were administrated in all patients. Patients were placed in the lithotomy position under continual epidural anesthesia. After retrograde pyelography, a 0.035 inch guidewire was placed in the upper tract. Ureter stones were treated using 8.0/9.8 French ureteroscope (Richard Wolf). Large stones were fragmented with holmium laser and the fragments were removed with the stone basket or grasping devices. After the ureteral stone was completely removed, a 12/14 F ureteral access sheath (UAS) (COOK) was placed with appropriate length in the patients who will undergo RIRS. The flexible ureteroscope (7.5Fr Karl Storz Flex-X, or 6/9.9Fr Richard Wolf Cobra) was inserted through the guidewire to the renal pelvis. Complete inspection of the entire collecting system was performed and small stones were removed by nitinol basket. Large stones were fragmented with holmium laser. Adequate stone fragmention was considered when fragments could remove by the stone basket or smaller than 2 mm in diameter. At the end of the procedure, the entire collecting system was inspected for the residual stones under the fluoroscopic guidance and a D-J stent was left for 4 weeks.

One month after procedure, all patients were assessed by noncontrast spiral CT to confirm the SFR. Complete stone-free was defined as the absence of any fragments. A visual analogue pain scale (VAS) was used to quantify the degree of pain. Preoperative and postoperative characteristics, complication rate, hemoglobin drop, hospital duration, SFR, auxiliary treatment rate (ATR), medical cost were compared between two groups. Auxiliary treatments were defined as the treatment for managing the residual renal stone or sever complication. Auxiliary procedure was defined as using surgical methods in the treatment during follow-up.

After the first follow-up evaluation, patients returned for an assessment with urinalysis, KUB or urinary ultrasound every 3 months during the first year and every 6 months thereafter.

Statistical analysis was done using SPSS 17.0® for Windows®. Continuous variables were compared with student t test and Wilcoxon test, and Univariable analysis was conducted using the Pearsonχ^2 statistic or Fisher's exact test for categorical data. Differences resulting in $p < 0.05$ were considered significant.

Results

Patients' demographic and preoperative characteristics were summarized in Table 1. There were no significant differences between two modalities. Perioperative and Postoperative characteristics were compared in Table 2. Mean operative duration for group A and B were 72.4 ± 21.3 (range 42.5–100) and 36.4 ± 10.2 (range 24–50) min, respectively (P < 0.001). Mean fluoroscopy time was significantly longer in group A (P < 0.001). Mean drop in the postoperative hemoglobin level was 0.5 ± 0.21 (range 0.1–0.7) g/dL in group A, which was found to be statistically significant (P < 0.001) compared with the corresponding decrease (0.2 ± 0.11, range 0.1–0.4 g/dL) in group B. However, no blood transfusion was required in both groups. VAS was higher in group A at postoperative 6 h, 12 h and 24 h, but the difference was not statistically significant at postoperative 24 h (P = 0.477). Mean hospital duration was 6.4 ± 2.9 days (range 3–12) in group A, and 5.3 ± 2.1 days (range 2–12) in group B (P = 0.521).

Complication rates in group A were higher (22.2% vs 13.9%), but the differences were not statistically significant (P = 0.358). Four patients in each group were administrated by oral analgesics for post-operative pain

Table 1 Demographic data of patient

Variable	Group A (URL + RIRS)	Group B (URL alone) (URL alone)	P
	72 patients	72 patients	
Age, year, mean (SD), range	48.2 (11.4),19–65	50.4 (13.2),22–71	0.296
Gender, no. (%)			0.468
Males	42 (58.3)	48 (66.7)	
Females	30 (41.7)	24 (33.3)	
BMI, kg/m2, mean (SD), range	22.98 (3.51),19–32	25.32 (5.12),20–31	0.084
Stone side, no. (%)			0.481
Left	30 (41.7)	36 (50)	
Right	42 (58.3)	36 (50)	
Grade of hydronephrosis, no. (%)			0.659
None	8 (11.1)	10 (13.9)	
Mild	46 (63.9)	38 (52.8)	
Moderate	18 (25)	24 (33.3)	
Ureteral stone location, no. (%)			0.405
proximal	20 (27.8)	24 (33.3)	
middle	8 (11.1)	12 (16.7)	
distal	44 (61.1)	36 (50)	
Ureteral stone burden, mm^2, mean (SD), range	67.4 (27.2),40.2–110.3	71.3 (31),39.2–102.3	0.884
Renal stone location			0.981
Upper pole	22 (30.6)	20 (27.8)	
Middle pole	20 (27.8)	24 (33.3)	
Lower pole	30 (41.6)	28 (38.9)	
Renal stone burden, mm^2, mean (SD), range	110.1 (42.2),68.3–170.1	124.5 (36.7),75.2–174.3	0.589
Pre-procedural placement of D-J stent, no. (%)	50 (69.5)	52 (72.2)	0.802

(Clavien). Four patients had post-operative vomit (Clavien) in group A was treated by oral antiemetic. Transient post-operative fever was developed in four patients in each group and could be successfully treated with antibiotics and antipyretics (Clavien). Of group A and B, four and two, respectively, had minor ureteral perforations (Clavien a). They were successfully treated by D-J stent for 8 weeks and did not have any subsequent sequelae at follow-up. In group A, complications were significantly less in patients with pre-procedural D-J stent placement (3/25 vs 5/11, P = 0.04). Also, ureteral perforation was only encountered in patients without pre-procedural D-J placement.

One-month ureteral SFR was 100% in each group. In group A, one-month renal SFR was 86.1%. Eight failures of RIRS were due to impossible to reach the calyx containing stone. Residual fragments were seen in two patients, which were passed spontaneously during follow-up. Statistically significant was not found in stone composition between group A and B.

Follow-up data was recorded in all patients (Table 3). Mean follow-up time for all patients was 18.6 ± 9.6 months (range 12–36). The ATR was significant higher in group B

(69.4% vs 5.6%, p < 0.001). In group A, two patients underwent PCNL for renal stone, while 62 auxiliary procedures were performed in 46 patients in group B, including URL (n = 10), RIRS (n = 22), ESWL (n = 26), PCNL (n = 4). Of 46 patients, Four had obstructing steinstrasse after ESWL were treated by URL, ten underwent RIRS because of significant residual stone after ESWL and two underwent PCNL for the renal stone due to failure in RIRS. Therefore, mean number of procedures per patient was significantly higher in group B (1.86 vs 1.03, p < 0.001). But mean medical cost per patient was still higher in group A (16431.2 ± 3425.3 vs 13125.1 ± 2165.4 RMB, P < 0.001).

Discussion

Asymptomatic renal stone associated with ipsilateral symptomatic ureteral stone is not a rare event [10,11]. URL has equivalent or superior results comparing with ESWL in treating symptomatic ureteral stone. [12] When encountering a coexisted ipsilateral asymptomatic renal stone, no established guidelines are available. Active observation, ESWL, PCNL as well as RIRS should be discussed. Previous research had showed that active observation will be associated with a higher risk of

Table 2 Perioperative and postoperative characteristics of patients

Variable	Group A (URL + RIRS) 72 patients	Group B (URL alone) 72 patients	P
Operative duration, mean (SD), range (min)	72.4 (21.3),42.5–100	36.4 (10.2),24–50	<0.001
Haemoglobin drop (g/dL), mean (SD)	0.5 (0.21),0.1–0.7	0.2 (0.11),0.1–0.4	<0.001
Hospital duration, mean, (SD), range (days)	6.4 (2.9),3–12	5.3 (2.1),2–12	0.521
Complication rate, no. (%)	8 (22.2)	5 (13.9)	0.358
Modified Clavien classification			
GradeI	8 (11.1)	4 (5.6)	
Grade II	4 (5.6)	4 (5.6)	
Grade IIIa	4 (5.6)	2 (2.8)	
Pain visual analogue score (1 – 10), mean, (SD), range			
At 6 h	4.3 (1.3),4–7	3.1 (1.1),2–6	<0.001
At 12 h	2.8 (0.9),2–5	2.1 (0.7),1–4	<0.001
At 24 h	2.0 (0.3),1–4	1.8 (0.1),1–3	0.477
Ureteral stone free rate (U-SFR), no. (%)	72 (100)	72 (100)	-
Renal stone free rate (R-SFR), no. (%)	62 (86.1)	0 (0)	<0.001
Stone composition, no. (%)			0.872
Calcium oxalate	34 (47.2)	30 (41.7)	
Calcium oxalate and phosphate	20 (27.8)	24 (33.3)	
Uric acid	16 (22.2)	14 (19.4)	
Struvite	2 (2.8)	4 (5.6)	

Table 3 Follow-up data of patients

Variable	Group A (URL + RIRS) 72 patients	Group B (URL alone) 72 patients	P
Follow-up, mean, (SD), range (months)	18.9 (10.2),14–32	18.5 (9.4),12–34	0.675
Auxiliary treatment rate, no. (%)	4 (5.6)	50 (69.4)	<0.001
Cause of auxiliary treatment in follow-up, no. (%)			
Renal colic	2 (2.8)	10 (13.9)	
Repetatus urinary tract infection	0	6 (8.3)	
Stone induced hematuria	2 (2.8)	10 (13.9)	
Increase in creatinine levels	0	4 (5.6)	
Patient's desire (increased stone duration)	0	20 (27.8)	
Medical expulsive treatment, no. (%)	2 (2.8)	4 (5.6)	<0.001
Patients required auxiliary procedures, no (%).	2 (2.8)	46 (63.9)	<0.001
Auxiliary procedures, no	2	62	-
URL	0	10	
FURL	0	12	
ESWL	0	26	
PCNL	2	4	
Procedure per patient, mean, (SD), range	1.03 (0.17),1–2	1.86 (0.76),1–3	<0.001
Medical cost per patient, mean, (SD), range (RMB)	16431.2 (3425.3) 14985.3–21325.4	13125.1 (2165.4) 9105.1–15143.2	<0.001

surgical intervention [2,3]. Patients choosing ESWL often needed multiple sessions to achieve higher SFR [13]. PCNL, a favoured treatment for stone >2 cm, is associated with higher potential risks, such as bleeding, urosepsis, and urine leakage [2]. Recently, simultaneously RIRS becomes feasible in treating ipsilateral renal stone and seems to be an attractive option. We compare the outcomes of this simultaneous modality to URL alone in this study.

Ureteral stone was completely removed in each group. In simultaneous RIRS group, the overall renal SFR after 1 month was 86.1%, which was similar to that of previous reports. Goldberg H et al. showed that patients with pre-procedural D-J stent can achieve a higher renal SFR (93.3% VS 71%) [14]. However, the difference was not found in this study. Inability to reach the lower pole calyx may be the main reason of RIRS failure [15,16]. We observed that eight cases were due to this. Also, the other predictive factor of renal SFR was stone size. Grasso and Ficazzola reported that RIRS can achieved an SFR of 82%, 71% and 65% with stone size of <1 cm, 1–2 cm and >2 cm, respectively [15]. RIRS may be required to clear a large stone by multiple procedures [17]. In our center, it is often performed for renal stone in size of <2 cm, which can achieved a higher SFR in one session. In this study, the simultaneous RIRS achieved 86.1% renal SFR for treating this size stone.

The other important results were lower ATR, while complications were not significantly increased. The causes of the higher ATR in URL alone group were often stone induced (Table 3). In Streem's and Glowacki's study, respectively, Patients with active observation, more than 70% and 48.5% required treatment due to increased stone duration or clinical symptomatic episode in next 5 years [18,19]. Although our mean follow-up period were >18 months, the ATR was 69.4% in URL alone group comparing to only 5.6% in simultaneous RIRS group. Few patients with residual stone may be one of the reasons. And the other reason was that causes of auxiliary treatment after RIRS were unexpected incidents such as complications or flexible ureteroscope damage, which is low in current reports Therefore, it is important to emphasize the possibility of auxiliary treatment in patients with URL alone is up to 70%, and with simultaneous RIRS is only required in unpredictable situation during preoperative conversation.

UAS is becoming increasingly popular worldwide because of facilitating the access, decreasing intrarenal pressure and protecting the scope [20]. However, several studies had shown that the over distention created by UAS may induce ureteral ischemia and wall injuries [21]. In this study, we found that ureteral perforations were developed in two patients in simultaneous RIRS group, who were not pre-stented. Traxer O and Thomas A reported that D-J

prestenting significantly decreases the incidence of severe access sheath related injuries [22]. Moreover, overall complications were significantly less in patients with pre-procedural D-J stent (6/50 vs 10/22, P = 0.04). Thereby, it is wisdom to place DJ stent pre-procedurally in patients who were planned to undergo simultaneous RIRS.

Although RIRS had minimal invasive nature, the low morbidity was probably due to greater expertise in high-volume RIRS center. When a surgeon is still in his learning curve of RIRS, more attention should be paid in performing simultaneous modality.

Beside the invasive nature of RIRS, another disadvantage included the consumption of expensive instruments such as fragile flexible ureteroscope, nitinol basket and UAS. Large studies showed the need for repair flexible ureteroscope after an average of 18 cases [23]. Obviously, the costs for RIRS are higher than URL. In our study, although mean procedure per patient was significantly more in URL alone group, the mean medical cost per patient was still higher in simultaneous RIRS group during follow-up (mean >18 months). Simultaneous modality does not appear to be cost effective. However, SH Lee et al. reported that patients benefited from cost-effectiveness when choosing RIRS simultaneously, with respect to their health insurance system [24]. Rencently, repair for a new generation flexible ureteroscopes was needed after 20–22 procedures [25,26]. Moreover, flexible ureteroscopes can have a significantly longer lifespan (10.6 vs 21.6 uses before damage), by following guidelines and with training. [27]. Thus, we believed that the results may be changed with the developments of instruments, techniques and national health insurance system.

An interesting observation from study was that 47.8% patients in URL alone group underwent ESWL. Despite higher retreatment rates, it remains a preferred option because of non-invasive nature and high level of acceptance by patients and doctors. Although Keeley FX et al. demonstrated that ESWL for small asymptomatic renal stones does not offer any advantage to patients in terms of SFR comparing to observation (28% vs 17%, P = 0.06) [1], we found it can partly eliminate apprehensiveness of patients, and can achieve a higher SFR in upper pole renal stone. However, A policy of treating asymptomatic renal stones with ESWL may be still associated with a high risk of requiring invasive procedures > 50% patients were required additional URL, RIRS or even PCNL for obstructing steinstrasse and residual stone.

The main limitation of this study is its retrospective design. Allocation to a treatment modality depended on the surgeon's preference. We tried to overcome this possible selection bias by comparing match groups of patients and stones. Another limitation was the small number of patients and a single center study. Therefore, a prospective randomized controlled study with a larger sample of multiple centers with a long time follow-up is needed.

Conclusions

Simultaneous RIRS for ipsilateral asymptomatic renal stones in patients with ureteroscopic symptomatic ureteral stone removal can be performed safely and effectively.

It promises a high SFR with lower auxiliary treatment rate, and dose not lengthen hospital duration and increase complications.

Pre-procedurally Placing DJ stent in patients planned to undergo RIRS simultaneously may reduce the complication rate.

Abbreviations

RIRS: Retrograde intrarenal surgery; URL: Ureteroscopic laser lithotripsy; ESWL: Extracorporeal shock wave lithotripsy; PCNL: Percutaneous nephrolithotomy; SFR: Stone free rate; ATR: Auxiliary treatment rate; UAS: Ureteral access sheath; VAS: Visual analogue pain scale; CT: Computed tomography.

Competing interests

The authors declare that they have no competing interests.

Authors' contributions

Conceived and designed the experiments: DHL. Performed the experiments: DHL, XL, YZH. Analyzed the data: DHL, MLC. Contributed reagents/materials/analysis tools: DHL, MLC. Wrote the paper: DHL, MLC. All authors read and approved the final manuscript.

References

1. Keeley Jr FX, Tilling K, Elves A, Menezes P, Wills M, Rao N, et al. Preliminary results of a randomized controlled trial of prophylactic shock wave lithotripsy for small asymptomatic renal calyceal stones. BJU Int. 2001;87(1):1–8.
2. Turk C, Knoll T, Petrik A, Sarica K, Straub M, Seitz C. Guidelines on urolithiasis. 2012. p. 1–102. Available at: http://www.uroweb.org/gls/pdf/20_Urolithiasis.pdf.
3. Koh LT, Ng FC, Ng KK. Outcomes of long-term follow-up of patients with conservative management of asymptomatic renal calculi. BJU Int. 2012;109(4):622–5.
4. Sabnis RB, Jagtap J, Mishra S, Desai M. Treating renal calculi 1-2 cm in diameter with minipercutaneous or retrograde intrarenal surgery: a prospective comparative study. BJU Int. 2012;110(8 Pt B):E346–9.
5. Sabnis RB, Ganesamoni R, Doshi A, Ganpule AP, Jagtap J, Desai MR. Micropercutaneous nephrolithotomy (microperc) vs retrograde intrarenal surgery for the management of small renal calculi: a randomized controlled trial. BJU Int. 2013;112(3):355–61.
6. Resorlu B, Unsal A, Ziypak T, Diri A, Atis G, Guven S, et al. Comparison of retrograde intrarenal surgery, shockwave lithotripsy, and percutaneous nephrolithotomy for treatment of medium-sized radiolucent renal stones. World J Urol. 2013;31(6):1581–6.
7. Ozturk U, Sener NC, Goktug HN, Nalbant I, Gucuk A, Imamoglu MA. Comparison of percutaneous nephrolithotomy, shock wave lithotripsy, and retrograde intrarenal surgery for lower pole renal calculi 10-20 mm. Urol Int. 2013;91(3):345–9.
8. Ho CC, Hafidzul J, Praveen S, Goh EH, Bong JJ, Lee BC, et al. Retrograde intrarenal surgery for renal stones smaller than 2 cm. Singapore Med J. 2010;51(6):512–5.
9. Srisubat A, Potisat S, Lojanapiwat B, Setthawong V, Laopaiboon M. Extracorporeal shock wave lithotripsy (ESWL) versus percutaneous nephrolithotomy (PCNL) or retrograde intrarenal surgery (RIRS) for kidney stones. Cochrane Database Syst Rev. 2009;7(4):CD007044.
10. Kanao K, Nakashima J, Nakagawa K, Asakura H, Miyajima A, Oya M, et al. Preoperative nomograms for predicting stone-free rate after extracorporeal shock wave lithotripsy. J Urol. 2006;176(4 Pt 1):1453–6.
11. Abdel-Khalek M, Sheir KZ, Mokhtar AA, Eraky I, Kenawy M, Bazeed M. Prediction of success rate after extracorporeal shock-wave lithotripsy of renal stones–amultivariate analysis model. Scand J Urol Nephrol. 2004;38(2):161–7.
12. Galvin DJ, Pearle MS. The contemporary management of renal and ureteric calculi. BJU Int. 2006;98(6):1283–8.
13. Sarkissian C, Noble M, Li J, Monga M. Patient decision making for asymptomatic renal calculi: balancing benefit and risk. Urology. 2013;81(2):236–40.
14. Goldberg H, Holland R, Tal R, Lask DM, Livne PM, Lifshitz DA. The impact ofretrograde intrarenal surgery for asymptomatic renal stones in patients undergoing ureteroscopy for a symptomatic ureteral stone. J Endourol. 2013;27(8):970–3.
15. Grasso M, Ficazzola M. Retrograde ureteropyeloscopy for lower pole caliceal calculi. J Urol. 1999;162(6):1904–8.
16. Resorlu B, Oguz U, Resorlu EB, Oztuna D, Unsal A. The impact of pelvicaliceal anatomy on the success of retrograde intrarenal surgery in patients with lower pole renal stones. Urology. 2012;79(1):61–6.
17. Riley JM, Stearman L, Troxel S. Retrograde ureteroscopy for renal stones larger than 2.5 cm. J Endourol. 2009;23(9):1395–8.
18. Streem SB, Yost A, Mascha E. Clinical implications of clinically insignificant store fragments after extracorporeal shock wave lithotripsy. J Urol. 1996;155:1186.
19. Glowacki LS, Beecroft ML, Cook RJ, Pahl D, Churchill DN. The natural history of asymptomatic urolithiasis. J Urol. 1992;147(2):319–21.
20. Stern JM, Yiee J, Park S. Safety and efficacy of ureteral access sheaths. J Endourol. 2007;21(2):119–23.
21. Lallas CD, Auge BK, Raj GV, Santa-Cruz R, Madden JF, Preminger GM. Laser Doppler flowmetric determination of ureteral blood flow after ureteral access sheath placement. J Endourol. 2002;16(8):583–90.
22. Traxer O, Thomas A. Prospective evaluation and classification of ureteral wall injuries resulting from insertion of a ureteral access sheath during retrograde intrarenal surgery. J Urol. 2013;189(2):580–4.
23. Monga M, Best S, Venkatesh R, Ames C, Lee C, Kuskowski M, et al. Durability of flexible ureteroscopes: a randomized, prospective study. J Urol. 2006;176(1):137–41.
24. Lee SH, Kim TH, Myung SC, Moon YT, Kim KD, Kim JH, et al. Effectiveness of flexible ureteroscopic stone removal for treating ureteral and ipsilateral renal stones: a single-center experience. Korean J Urol. 2013;54(6):377–82.
25. Binbay M, Yuruk E, Akman T, Ozgor F, Seyrek M, Ozkuvanci U, et al. Is there a difference in outcomes between digital and fiberoptic flexible ureterorenoscopy procedures? J Endourol. 2010;24(12):1929–34.
26. Multescu R, Geavlete B, Georgescu D, Geavlete P. Conventional fiberoptic flexible ureteroscope versus fourth generation digital flexible ureteroscope: a critical comparison. J Endourol. 2010;24(1):17–21.
27. Karaolides T, Bach C, Kachrilas S, Goyal A, Masood J, Buchholz N. Improving the durability of digital flexible ureteroscopes. Urology. 2013;81(4):717–22.

9

Does visualisation during urethrocystoscopy provide pain relief?

J. Koenig[†], S. Sevinc, C. Frohme, H. Heers, R. Hofmann and A. Hegele[*†]

Abstract

Background: To measure the effects of real-time visualisation during urethrocystoscopy on pain in patients who underwent ambulatory urethrocystoscopy.

Methods: An observational study was designed. From June 2012 to June 2013 patients who had ambulatory urethrocystoscopy participated in the study. In order to measure pain perception we used a numeric rating scale (NRS) 0 to 10. Additional data was collected including gender, reason for intervention, use of a rigid or a flexible instrument and whether the patient had had urethrocystoscopy before.

Results: 185 patients were evaluated. 125 patients preferred to watch their urethrocystoscopy on a real-time video screen, 60 patients did not. There was no statistically relevant difference in pain perception between those patients who watched their urethrocystoscopy on a real-time video screen and those who did not ($p = 0.063$). However, men who were allowed to watch their flexible urethrocystoscopy experienced significantly less pain, than those who did not ($p = 0.007$). No such effects could be measured for rigid urethrocystoscopy ($p = 0.317$). Furthermore, women experienced significantly higher levels of pain during the urethrocystoscopy than men ($p = 0.032$).

Conclusions: Visualisation during urethrocystoscopy procedures in general does not significantly decrease pain in patients. Nevertheless, men who undergo flexible urethrocystoscopy should be offered to watch their procedure in real-time on a video screen. To make urethrocystoscopy less painful for both genders, especially for women, should be subject to further research.

Keywords: Cystoscopy, Pain, Bladder, Real-time visualisation

Background

Pain relief is one of the most important tasks of every doctor. It is one of the most common reasons for consultation and a basic skill of the medical profession. Therefore, pain relief is something patients expect from their doctors. Unfortunately, it is also one of the most complicated tasks and often the best medical practice requires procedures that are not only uncomfortable, but inflict pain.

One such a procedure is the urethrocystoscopy. It is not invasive enough to justify the risk of complete anaesthesia but also too uncomfortable to be not taken seriously. As a frequently used tool in diagnosis and a treatment of various urological conditions such as bladder carcinoma, tumour infiltration and haematuria, the significance of urethrocystoscopies in everyday urological practice has increased [1].

Various attempts have been made in the past to make urethrocystoscopy less painful. The biggest achievement in patient comfort probably presents the invention of the flexible urethrocystoscope. Before, men and women alike were examined with a rigid instrument. Due to gender related anatomical differences rigid urethrocystoscopy on men was quite painful [2]. This changed with the invention of the flexible instrument. Since then repeated effort was made to further improve patients comfort. The application of lidocaine gel was introduced.

---

* Correspondence: hegele@med.uni-marburg.de
[†]Equal contributors
Department of Urology and Pediatric Urology, University hospital Marburg, Philipps University, Marburg, Germany

Unfortunately, its benefit remains uncertain [3]. Several other attempts to reduce pain during uerthrocystoscopy have been made, as a technique called a bag squeeze [4], the inhalation of nitrous oxide gas during the procedure [5], application of Midazolam [6] or transcutaneous electrical nerve stimulation [7].

Over the past few years evidence occurred that patients might benefit from watching their urethrocystoscopy real-time on a video screen [8–11].

Up to now only specific parts of the patient population were investigated. Men who were to undergo flexible urethrocystoscopy and women who had rigid urethrocystoscopy. Results of previous studies show [8–11], that visualisation during urethrocystoscopy decreases pain in certain patient populations in randomised controlled trails. As pain is a composite of an entire experience influenced by many different factors, we wanted to test the outcomes in every day clinical practice.

We generated a prospective observational study in everyday clinical practice to measure the pain patients experienced during urethrocystoscopy while visualising the procedure on a real-time video screen compared with the pain patients who did not visualise their procedure experienced. The aim was to test whether visualisation aided in increasing patient comfort during urethrocystoscopy.

We expected that distraction would decrease the level of pain patients experienced during the procedure [12].

Methods
Observational study design
To access the differences in pain perception between patients who were able to watch their urethrocystoscopy real-time on a video screen and patients who were not, we conducted a prospective observational study. Our aim was to stay as close as possible to everyday clinical practice to provide a clear image of patients' pain perception in an everyday clinical setting. Everyday clinical practice is influenced by many different factors which have to be eliminated in a randomised controlled trial. Therefore what has been evaluated in a randomised controlled study cannot necessarily be applied to everyday clinical practice. Hence, we decided not to randomise our study. As the study was done to investigate clinical data of patients treated solely at our institution, and data obtained was anonymized concurrently, approval of the local ethics committee (Ethics Committee, Faculty of Medicine Marburg) was therefore not required according to the German Ethics Committees regulations.

Patients
The patient population consisted of all patients who underwent an ambulatory urethrocystoscopy from June 2012 to June 2013 in the urological outpatient clinic of the Department of Urology and Paediatric Urology at the university hospital of Marburg. Exclusion criteria were the necessity of systemic or local anaesthesia and the use of sedatives or analgesics other than Instillagel®. In total 185 patients were included.

Urethrocystoscopy
The procedure patients received was not randomized. They could choose whether they wanted to visualise the procedure on a real-time video monitor along with the urologist or whether they preferred not to.

Pain perception and pain control depend on various factors and differ greatly between individuals [12]. To take individual differences in account we decided to let the patient choose which option he or she felt more comfortable with. The monitor was then positioned according to patient's wishes.

The urethrocystoscopy was performed according to the standardised scope technique of the Department of Urology and Paediatric Urology of the University hospital, Marburg. The procedure was performed in lithothomy position. Pelvis and legs were covered and anus and genitals were disinfected. For rigid urethrocystoscopy Storz, Wolf or Olympus 70/120° instruments were used and the flexible urethrocystoscopy was also performed with Storz, Wolf and Olympus instruments.

Instillagel® was applied 10 min before the procedure as recommended in recent studies [3]. In male patients a penile clamp was used to ensure proper instillation.

In order to avoid limitations in our results based on the skill of a single urologist, the urethrocystoscopy was performed by different urologists. Therefore interindividual differences in technique and skill were taken into account, as they are a part of everyday clinical practice.

Data
After the procedure patients were asked by the attending nurse to quantify their pain on a numeric rating scale (NRS) from 0 to 10. 0 was defined as no pain, 1–4 mild pain, 5–7 moderate pain and 8–10 as severe pain [13].

Additional data was collected including the patients gender, reasons for intervention, the use of a rigid or flexible instrument, whether the patient had had urethrocystoscopies before and what kind of instrument was used. Furthermore we assessed whether patients thought themselves to be sensitive to pain or no. All data was computerised on Microsoft Excel® 2013 (Microsoft, USA) and analysed with IBM SPSS® Statistics for Windows Version 22 (Ehningen, Germany) using the Mann – Whitney – U – test. A p value of < 0.05 was considered statistically significant.

Results

General Data

185 patients were evaluated (age 17 to 91 years). The mean age of the 44 female patients was 59 years (17 – 91 years). The mean age of the 141 male patients was 65 years (26 – 89 years). 125 patients (66 %) wanted to follow their urethrocystoscopy in real – time on video with the urologist, 60 (34 %) patients preferred not to. 131 had flexible urethrocystoscopies. 91 (69,5 %) of these patients watched their procedure real-time and 40 (30,5 %) did not. Of the 54 patients who underwent rigid urethrocystoscopy 34 (63 %) wanted to watch the procedure on the video screen and 20 (37 %) did not. 105 (55 %) patients had undergone an urethrocystoscopy before and for 80 (45 %) patients it was the first time they had had the procedure. Patient data is summarised in Table 1.

Pain

The median value on the numeric rating scale was 2 ($\pm$2.2, range 0–9) for patients who watched their procedure in real-time on a video screen and 3 ($\pm$2.1, range 0–9) for those who did not without statistical difference (p = 0.063, see Table 2).

When analysed separately patients who had flexible urethrocystoscopies, had significantly less pain when they were allowed to watch the procedure (2 ($\pm$2.0, range 0–8) vs 3.5 ($\pm$2.1, range 0–8), p = 0.007; see Fig. 1).

When using the rigid urethrocystoscope no significant differences could be shown.

Experience with the procedure proved to be significant in pain perception. Patients who had had the procedure before had significantly less pain (p < 0.005). Women who had had experience with urethrocystoscopy still had significantly more pain than their male counterparts (p = 0.031). Pain perception was not significantly lower in patients with experience who watched the procedure than in those who did not (p = 0.165).

Gender differences

Of the 127 patient who had flexible urethrocystoscopies only 2 (1.6 %) were women. Therefore, no valid results could be obtained about the benefit of real-time visualisation in women who had flexible urethrocystoscopies. In contrast, 41 patients who had rigid urethrocystoscopies were women (74,5 %) and 14 were men.

Analysed separately women who could watch their rigid urethrocystoscopy on a real-time video screen did not feel significantly less pain than women who did not (3 vs 2, p = 0.290). No valid results could be obtained regarding men who had rigid urethrocystoscopies, as only two men decided not to watch their urethrocystoscopy.

Female patients (3.5, $\pm$ 2.4, range 0–9) had significantly more pain than male patients (2.7, $\pm$ 2.2, range 0–9) during urethrocystoscopies (p = 0.032, see Fig. 2), although there was no significant difference in the self – assessment of pain between both genders (p = 0.092).

Discussion

In our observational study we investigated the differences in pain during urethrocystoscopy between patients who could watch their procedure on a real-time video screen and patients who could not in an everyday clinical setting. We found that only men who underwent flexible urethrocystoscopy and wanted to watch their procedure on a real-time video screen perceived their urethrocystoscopy as significantly less painful. For other patients this effect was not observed. Furthermore, women who underwent urethrocystoscopy have significantly more pain than men.

To our knowledge only a few studies so far have examined the impact of real – time visualisation on pain perception during urethrocystoscopy. Clement et al. [8] conducted a prospective randomized study in 2004 with patients who had flexible urethrocystoscopy. Four further randomised studies on male patients who underwent flexible urethrocystoscopy were conducted by Patel [9] in 2006, Cornel [14] in 2007, Soomro [10] in 2010 and Zhang [11] in 2011. Patel also analysed the impact of real – time visualisation on pain in women who underwent rigid urethrocystoscopies in another randomised study in 2008 [15].

So far only Clements et al. [8] showed the impact of real – time visualisation on urethrocystoscopy on patients of both genders.

A number of differences between the randomised controlled studies and this observational study make direct comparison difficult.

First, in our study we used a numeric rating scale 0 to 10 to measure perceived pain. Patel et al. used a 100 mm visual analogue scale in both of his studies [9, 15]. Clements et al., Cornel et al., Soomro et al. and Zhang et al. used a

Table 1 Summarized patient data

	Number	Average age(range)	Flexible/rigid	Video yes/no	Experience yes/no	Tumor/follow up	Prone to feel pain yes/no
Total	185	64(17–91)	127/54	125/60	103/82	97/88	43/142
Men	141	69 (26–89)	125/14	100/42	85/56	82/59	29/112
Women	44	64 (17–91)	2/41	25/17	18/26	15/29	14/30

Table 2 Influence of visualisation/no visualisation on individual pain scores separated by kind of urethrocystoscopy

	Visualisation (n)	No visualisation (n)	p value
Urethrocystoscopy in general	125	60	0.063
	NRS = 2	NRS = 3	
Flexible urethrocystoscopy	91	40	0.007
	NRS = 2	NRS = 3.5	
Rigid urethrocystoscopy	34	20	0.317
	NRS = 3	NRS = 3	

visual analogue scale 0 to 10 [8, 10, 11, 14]. According to Williamson et al.'s review on pain scales both scales provide the same information but cannot be converted into one another [16]. Given that the different scales transfer the same information the results of the different studies can be compared.

Second, inclusion and exclusion criteria were different in the studies mentioned. In order to best approximate everyday clinical practice our exclusion criteria were broadly defined as the use of general or local anaesthesia and analgesics. In the other studies exclusion criteria were more narrowly defined [8–11, 14, 15].

Third, different numbers of urologists performed urethrocystoscopies on the included patients. In Soomro study and our study more than one urologist performed the urethrocystoscopy, so that the results would not be limited to the skill of one person [10]. In Clements et al., Patel et al. and Zhang et al. studies only one urologist performed the procedure [8, 9, 11]. We think both

approaches could include possible bias. Assessing the results of more than one urologist mixes different skills and difference in performance which might influence pain. Limiting the results to the performance of one urologist means that the pain score can only be related to this one urologist's performance. We decided to have more than one urologist perform urethrocystoscopy as it is closer to everyday clinical practise, even though we are aware that this approach might include possible bias. As this study was done in an outpatient clinic to assess pain during urethrocystoscopy in everyday clinical practise, we believed the results could be better related to everyday clinical practise if more than one urologist performed the procedure.

The greatest limitation of our study is that it was not randomised. Patients could choose whether they wanted to observe their own urethrocsytoscopy or not. Pain is a very subjective parameter. Therefore, it is difficult to assess and to generalise [17]. We tried to create the most

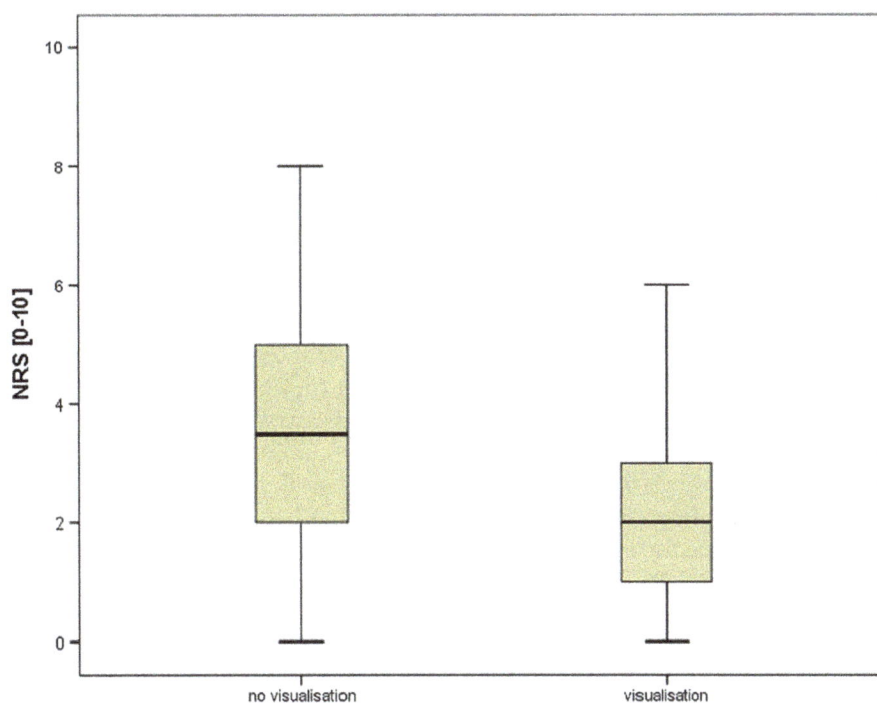

Fig. 1 Significant different pain scores in patients undergoing flexible urethrocystoscopy with or without visualisation (p=0.007)

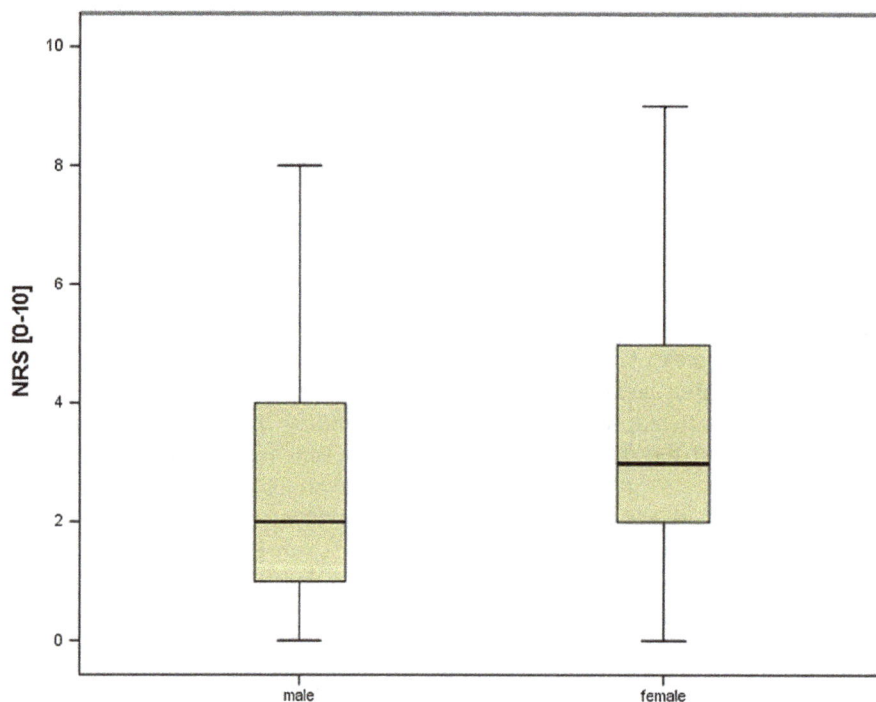

Fig. 2 Female patients had signficant more pain during urethrocystoscopy than male patients (p=0.032)

comfortable setting for our patients, which included letting them choose what they felt most at ease with. In letting the patient choose whether they wanted to watch the procedure on a real-time screen, we were closer to everyday clinical practice, where no patient who does not want to watch his or her own procedure on real time video is forced to do so.

Our data showed that visualisation on a real-time screen does not make urethrocsytoscopy less painful for patients in general. Kesari et al. investigated the role of visualisation on a real-time video screen with thorough explanation during the procedure [18]. In this small cohort (n = 51) patients who watched their procedure real time on a video screen did not benefit regarding their anxiety or their pain. In this study visualisation was examined as an addition to explanation and not as a measure to decrease pain on its own [18].

Focusing on flexible urethrocystoscopies our results confirm the results found by Clements et al., Patel et al., Soomro et al. and Zhang et al. [8–11]. Men who are able to watch their urethrocystoscopy in real-time on a video screen find it significantly less painful. Cornel et al.'s results oppose these findings [14]. Soomro et al. suggested that this might be due to the fact that the lithotomy position is less comfortable than the supine position [10] In Zhang et al.'s study and in our observational study all patients were examined in the lithotomy position, nevertheless our results showed that the procedure was significantly less painful for those who could watch it on a

real – time video screen. Cultural differences between European and American men are offered as a possible explanation [11]

In our patient cohort only 2 women had flexible urethrocystoscopy. Therefore based on this data no assumptions can be made about the effect real time visualisation has on pain during flexible urethrocystoscopy on women. This might be due to the recommendations regarding flexible urethrocystoscopy on women based on the recent findings of Gee et al. and Quiroz et al. [19, 20]. They state that there is no difference in comfort for women regardless of whether or not a rigid or a flexible instrument is used. For rigid urethrocystoscopies our results concerning women were similar to those of Patel et al. regarding the use of real-time visualisation in women who had rigid urethrocystoscopies. It has to be pointed out, that our observational study also included men who had rigid urethrocystoscopies. But as only two men did not watch their rigid urethrocystoscopy on a real-time video screen, no valid statistical analysis could be performed.

Cornel et al. found that patients who had experience with urethrocystoscopy did not find it more comfortable than those who had not [14]. We found that patients who had had urethrocystoscopy before had significantly less pain than those who did not. These finding are in line with recently published data in over 1300 consecutive procedures showing that pain levels during first cystoscopy is higher than for repeated cystoscopies [21]. Again, this might be due to cultural differences but it could also be due to the smaller number of patients Cornel et al. included in their study. Anatomy suggests that urethrocystoscopy should be more painful for men than for women given the difference in length of the urethra. In our observational study this was not the case. Women experienced significantly more pain than men. This suggests that the invention of flexible urethrocystoscopy made the procedure more comfortable for men. No such benefit occurred in women. Patel et al. presume that this is the case because women are not able to visualise the most painful part of urethrocystoscopy: the passage of the urethra as it is performed blindly in women [15]. It is however not clear what the most painful part in urethrocystoscopy on women is, because the study generated by Taghizadeh et al. included only men [22]. To our knowledge, no such study about the most painful part in urethrocystoscopy in women exists. As Patel et al. points out, there is probably more than one factor that makes urethrocystoscopy more painful for women [15]. The results of a recent study suggest that by using flexible instruments it is possible to reduce pain in women during flexible urethrocystoscopy [21]. Therefore the use of a flexible instrument on women should be encouraged.

Conclusions

In regard to pain prevention in urethrocystoscopy three valuable conclusions can be drawn from this study. First, men who undergo flexible urethrocystoscopies should be offered to watch their procedure in real – time on video along with the urologist. If they agree to watch they will benefit from their decision. Second, more effort should be put into making urethrocystoscopy more comfortable for women, especially because female patient's pain threshold might be lower than the pain threshold of male patients [17]. It is therefore important that sufficient pain control is administered on both genders. Third, real-time visualisation alone does not make the urethrocystoscopy less painful. On its own it is not sufficient enough.

New efforts should be made to improve patients' comfort level during urethrocystoscopy procedure. An example of such efforts can be found in the new observations made by Yeo et al. and Zhang et al. who found that using music to help patients relax during urethrocystoscopy may lead to benefical results [23, 24].

Competing interests
The authors declare that they have no competing interests.

Authors' contributions
JK Data collection, data analysis, manuscript writing, SS Data collection, manuscript editing, CF data collection, manuscript editing, HH Data collection, manuscript editing, RH Data collection, Manuscript editing, AH Project development, data collection, data analysis, manuscript writing

References

1. Hofmann R. Endoskopische Urologie, Atlas und Lehrbuch. 2. Aufl. Heidelberg: Springer; 2009. p. p. 29.
2. Flannigan GM, Gelister JS, Noble JG, et al. Rigid versus flexible cystoscopy. A controlled trial of patient tolerance. Br J Urol. 1988;62(6):537–40.
3. Patel AR, Jones JS, Babineau D. Lidocaine 2 % gel versus plain lubricating gel for pain reduction during flexible cystoscopy: a meta-analysis of prospective, randomized, controlled trials. J Urol. 2008;179(3):986–90.
4. Gunendran T, Briggs RH, Wemyss-Holden GD, et al. Does increasing hydrostatic pressure ("bag squeeze") during flexible cystoscopy improve patient comfort: a randomized, controlled study. Urology. 2008;72(2):255–8. discussion 258–9.
5. Calleary JG, Masood J, Van-Mallaerts R, et al. Nitrous oxide inhalation to improve patient acceptance and reduce procedure related pain of flexible cystoscopy for men younger than 55 years. J Urol. 2007;178(1):184–8. discussion 188.
6. Song YS, Song ES, Kim KJ, et al. Midazolam anesthesia during rigid and flexible cystoscopy. Urol Res. 2007;35(3):139–42.
7. Hruby G, Ames C, Chen C, et al. Assessment of efficacy of transcutaneous electrical nerve stimulation for pain management during office-based flexible cystoscopy. Urology. 2006;67(5):914–7.
8. Clements S, Sells H, Wright M. Use of video in flexible cystoscopy: a prospective randomised study of effect on patient experience. Ambul Surg. 2004;11(1–2):45–6.
9. Patel AR, Jones JS, Angie S, et al. Office based flexible cystoscopy may be less painful for men allowed to view the procedure. J Urol. 2007;177(5):1843–5.
10. Soomro KQ, Nasir AR, Ather MH. Impact of patient's self-viewing of flexible cystoscopy on pain using a visual analog scale in a randomized controlled trial. Urology. 2011;77(1):21–3.
11. Zhang Z, Tang L, Wang X, et al. Seeing is believing: a randomized controlled study from China of real-time visualization of flexible cystoscopy to improve male patient comfort. J Endourol. 2011;25(8):1343–6.
12. Malloy KM, Milling LS. The effectiveness of virtual reality distraction for pain reduction: a systematic review. Clin Psychol Rev. 2010;30(8):1011–8.
13. Serlin RC, Mendoza TR, Nakamura Y, et al. When is cancer pain mild, moderate or severe? Grading pain severity by its interference with function. Pain. 1995;61(2):277–84.
14. Cornel EB, Oosterwijk E, Kiemeney LA. The effect on pain experienced by male patients of watching their office-based flexible cystoscopy. BJU Int. 2008;102(10):1445–6.
15. Patel AR, Jones JS, Babineau D. Impact of real-time visualization of cystoscopy findings on procedural pain in female patients. J Endourol. 2008;22(12):2695–8.
16. Williamson A, Hoggart B. Pain: a review of three commonly used pain rating scales. J Clin Nurs. 2005;14(7):798–804.
17. Miller C, Newton SE. Pain perception and expression: the influence of gender, personal self-efficacy, and lifespan socialization. Pain Manag Nurs. 2006;7(4):148–52.
18. Kesari D, Kovisman V, Cytron S, et al. Effects on pain and anxiety of patients viewing their cystoscopy in addition to a detailed explanation: a controlled study. BJU Int. 2003;92(7):751–2.
19. Quiroz LH, Shobeiri SA, Nihira MA, et al. Randomized trial comparing office flexible to rigid cystoscopy in women. Int Urogynecol J. 2012;23(11):1625–30.
20. Gee JR, Waterman BJ, Jarrard DF, et al. Flexible and rigid cystoscopy in women. JSLS. 2009;13(2):135–8.
21. Greenstein A, Greenstein I, Senderovich S, Mabjeesh NJ. Is diagnostic cystoscopy painful ? Analysis of 1,320 consecutive procedures. Int Braz J Urol. 2014;40(4):S.533–8.
22. Taghizadeh AK, El Madani A, Gard PR, et al. When does it hurt? Pain during flexible cystoscopy in men. Urol Int. 2006;76(4):301–3.
23. Yeo JK, Cho DY, Oh MM, et al. Listening to music during cystoscopy decreases anxiety, pain, and dissatisfaction in patients: a pilot randomized controlled trial. J Endourol. 2013;27(4):459–62.
24. Zhang Z, Wang X, Xu C et al.: Music Reduces Panic: An Initial Study of Listening to Preferred Music Improves Male Patient Discomfort and Anxiety During Flexible Cystoscopy. J. Endourol. 2014; ahead of print

10

Protocol for a randomized, placebo-controlled, double-blind clinical trial investigating sacral neuromodulation for neurogenic lower urinary tract dysfunction

Stephanie C Knüpfer[1], Martina D Liechti[1], Livio Mordasini[2], Dominik Abt[2], Daniel S Engeler[2], Jens Wöllner[3], Jürgen Pannek[3], Bernhard Kiss[4], Fiona C Burkhard[4], Marc P Schneider[1], Elena Miramontes[1], Alfons G Kessels[5], Lucas M Bachmann[6] and Thomas M Kessler[1]*

Abstract

Background: Sacral neuromodulation has become a well-established and widely accepted treatment for refractory non-neurogenic lower urinary tract dysfunction, but its value in patients with a neurological cause is unclear. Although there is evidence indicating that sacral neuromodulation may be effective and safe for treating neurogenic lower urinary tract dysfunction, the number of investigated patients is low and there is a lack of randomized controlled trials.

Methods and design: This study is a prospective, randomized, placebo-controlled, double-blind multicenter trial including 4 sacral neuromodulation referral centers in Switzerland. Patients with refractory neurogenic lower urinary tract dysfunction are enrolled. After minimally invasive bilateral tined lead placement into the sacral foramina S3 and/or S4, patients undergo prolonged sacral neuromodulation testing for 3–6 weeks. In case of successful (defined as improvement of at least 50% in key bladder diary variables (i.e. number of voids and/or number of leakages, post void residual) compared to baseline values) prolonged sacral neuromodulation testing, the neuromodulator is implanted in the upper buttock. After a 2 months post-implantation phase when the neuromodulator is turned ON to optimize the effectiveness of neuromodulation using sub-sensory threshold stimulation, the patients are randomized in a 1:1 allocation in sacral neuromodulation ON or OFF. At the end of the 2 months double-blind sacral neuromodulation phase, the patients have a neuro-urological re-evaluation, unblinding takes place, and the neuromodulator is turned ON in all patients. The primary outcome measure is success of sacral neuromodulation, secondary outcome measures are adverse events, urodynamic parameters, questionnaires, and costs of sacral neuromodulation.

Discussion: It is of utmost importance to know whether the minimally invasive and completely reversible sacral neuromodulation would be a valuable treatment option for patients with refractory neurogenic lower urinary tract dysfunction. If this type of treatment is effective in the neurological population, it would revolutionize the management of neurogenic lower urinary tract dysfunction.

Keywords: Urinary bladder, Neurogenic lower urinary tract dysfunction, Sacral neuromodulation, Randomized, Placebo-controlled, Double-blind trial

* Correspondence: tkessler@gmx.ch
[1]Neuro-Urology, Spinal Cord Injury Center & Research, University of Zürich, Balgrist University Hospital, Forchstrasse 340, 8008 Zürich, Switzerland
Full list of author information is available at the end of the article

Background

Neurogenic lower urinary tract dysfunction (LUTD) is highly prevalent and affects the lives of millions of people worldwide. It has a major impact on quality of life and, besides the debilitating manifestations for patients, it also imposes a substantial economic burden for every healthcare system. Neurogenic LUTD is a challenge because all available treatment modalities (i.e. conservative, minimally invasive and surgical therapies) may either fail or be invasive causing considerable complications and/or side effects.

Sacral neuromodulation (SNM) [1] has become a well-established and widely accepted treatment for patients with refractory LUTD such as non-obstructive chronic urinary retention, urgency frequency syndrome, and urgency incontinence [2-6] and it has been incorporated into the guidelines of the European Association of Urology (EAU) (www.uroweb.org), the International Consultation on Incontinence (ICI) [7], and the National Institute for Health and Clinical Excellence (NICE) (www.nice.org.uk). Originally, SNM was not considered an option for neurogenic LUTD but some studies suggested that it is also effective in neurological patients [3,8]. Considering that SNM is minimally invasive and completely reversible, it is of great interest whether this is a valuable treatment option for patients with neurogenic LUTD. In a recent systematic review and meta-analysis [9], we found that there is evidence indicating that SNM may be effective and safe for the treatment of this group of patients. However, the number of investigated patients is low with high between-study heterogeneity and there is a lack of randomized controlled trials [9].

We therefore designed a prospective, randomized, placebo-controlled, double-blind multicenter clinical trial to assess the efficacy and safety of SNM for treating patients with neurogenic LUTD. The study hypothesis is that in patients with refractory neurogenic LUTD, SNM leads to an at least 35% increase in success rate as compared to placebo (i.e. sham) stimulation within 2 months, i.e. SNM is considerably more effective than placebo (i.e. sham) stimulation.

Methods and design

Study design

This study is a prospective, randomized, placebo-controlled, double-blind multicenter trial including 4 SNM referral centers in Switzerland: Neuro-Urology, Spinal Cord Injury Center & Research, University of Zürich, Balgrist University Hospital, Zürich; Department of Urology, Cantonal Hospital St. Gallen, St. Gallen; Neuro-Urology, Swiss Paraplegic Center Nottwil, Nottwil; Department of Urology, University of Bern, Bern.

In case of successful prolonged SNM, the neuromodulator is implanted and patients are randomized using a computer program considering 3 strata according to the neuro-urological diagnosis, i.e. a) urgency frequency syndrome and/or urgency incontinence, b) chronic urinary retention, and c) combination of urgency frequency syndrome and/or urgency incontinence and chronic urinary retention. After a 2 months SNM optimization phase following neuromodulator implantation, the neuromodulator is turned ON or OFF in a 1:1 allocation by an investigator not involved in the assessment of the clinical outcome.

The Figure 1 gives an overview of the procedures that the patients will undergo during the course of the study.

Study population and recruitment

According to the inclusion and exclusion criteria (Table 1), we will investigate patients with refractory neurogenic LUTD. The following variables will be considered: gender, age, neurological disease, duration of neurological disease, previous treatment, bladder diary variables, urinalysis, urethro-cystoscopy, bladder washing cytology, urodynamic investigations, and questionnaires, i.e. Female Sexual Function Index (FSFI) [10]/International Index of Erectile Function (IIEF) [11] and Qualiveen [12].

Determination of sample size

We are planning a study of independent cases and controls with 1 control per case. Prior data indicate that the (spontaneous) success rate among controls is 0.15. If the true success rate for experimental subjects (SNM ON) is at least 0.5, we will need to study 27 experimental subjects (SNM ON) and 27 control subjects (SNM OFF) to be able to reject the null hypothesis that the failure rates for experimental (SNM ON) and control subjects (SNM OFF) are equal with probability (power) 0.8. The type I error probability associated with this test of this null hypothesis is 0.05. Taking into account potential dropouts, we will include 30 patients per group.

Study location and partners

- Neuro-Urology, Spinal Cord Injury Center & Research, University of Zürich, Balgrist University Hospital, Zürich, Switzerland
- Department of Urology, Cantonal Hospital St. Gallen, St. Gallen, Switzerland
- Neuro-Urology, Swiss Paraplegic Center, Nottwil, Switzerland
- Department of Urology, University of Bern, Switzerland
- Department of Clinical Epidemiology and Medical Technology Assessment, Maastricht University Medical Center, Maastricht, The Netherlands
- Medignition Inc., Research Consultants, Zug, Switzerland

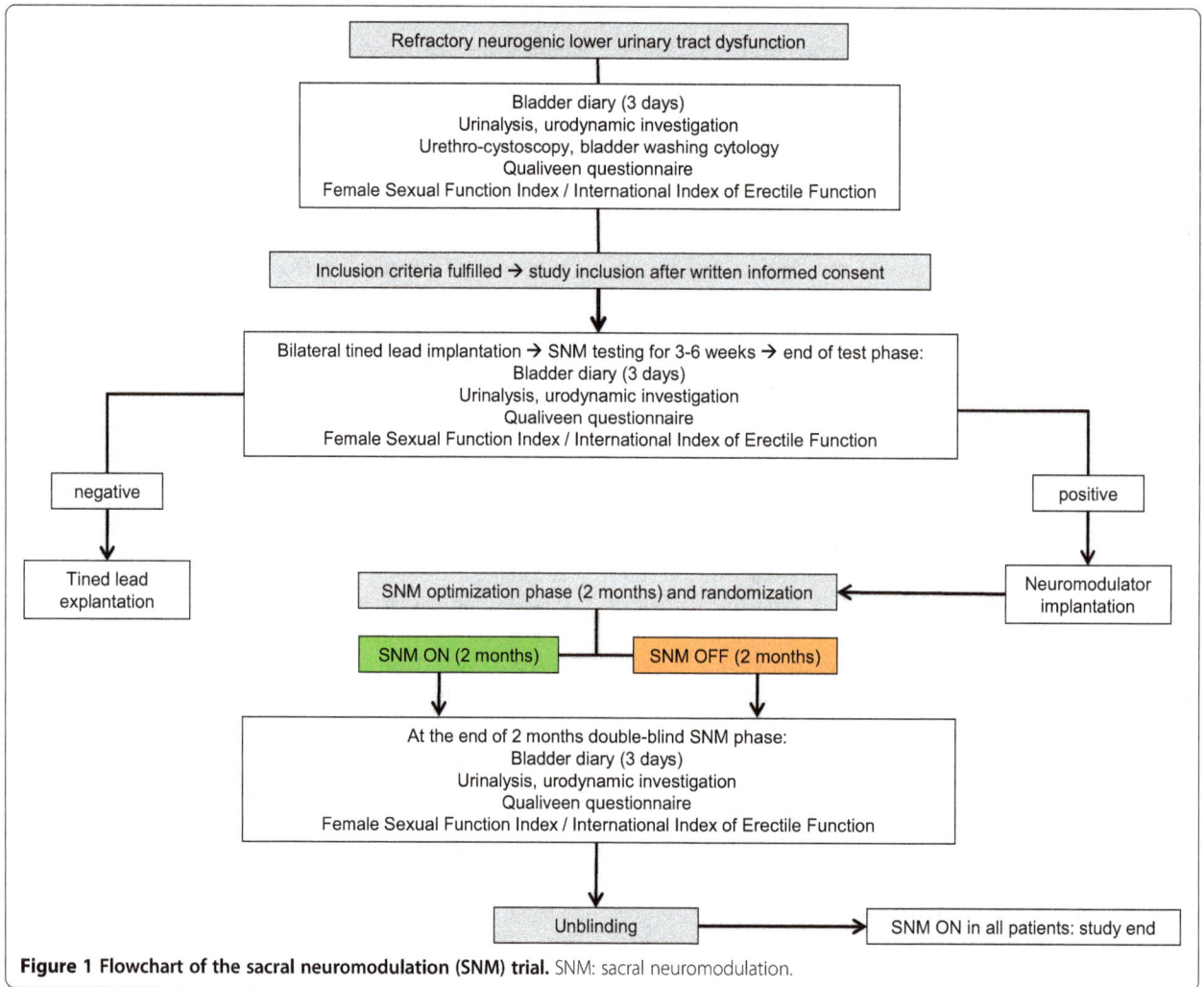

Figure 1 Flowchart of the sacral neuromodulation (SNM) trial. SNM: sacral neuromodulation.

Investigations

In case the patients with refractory neurogenic LUTD fulfill the study inclusion criteria following neuro-urological evaluation (bladder diary for at least 3 days, urinalysis, urodynamic investigation, urethro-cystoscopy and bladder washing cytology, Qualiveen questionnaire [12], FSFI [10]/IIEF [11], they are included after providing written informed consent. The Figure 1 gives an overview of the procedures that the patients will undergo during the course of the study. After minimally invasive bilateral

Table 1 Inclusion and exclusion criteria for patients with refractory neurogenic lower urinary tract dysfunction (LUTD)

Inclusion criteria	Exclusion criteria
• Age >18 years	• Age <18 years
• Refractory neurogenic LUTD	• Non-neurogenic LUTD
• Urgency frequency syndrome and/or urgency incontinence refractory to antimuscarinics (pharmacotherapy for at least 4 weeks with at least 2 antimuscarinics)	• Botulinum toxin injections into the detrusor and/or urethral sphincter in the last 6 months
• Chronic urinary retention refractory to alpha-blocker (pharmacotherapy with an alpha-blocker for at least 4 weeks)	• Pregnancy or breast feeding
• Combination of urgency frequency syndrome and/or urgency incontinence refractory to antimuscarinics (pharmacotherapy for at least 4 weeks with at least 2 antimuscarinics) and chronic urinary retention refractory to alpha-blocker (pharmacotherapy with an alpha-blocker for at least 4 weeks)	• Individuals especially in need of protection (according to Research with Human Subjects published by the Swiss Academy of Medical Sciences (www.samw.ch/en/News/News.html))
• Written informed consent	• No written informed consent

tined lead placement into the sacral foramina S3 and/or S4 (stage one), patients undergo prolonged SNM testing for 3–6 weeks completing a bladder diary to assess the response to treatment. In accordance with the literature [5,6], an improvement of at least 50% in the key bladder diary variables (i.e. number of voids and/or number of leakages, post void residual) compared to the baseline values is considered a positive test and an indication for neuromodulator implantation. At the end of the test phase, the patients have a neuro-urological re-evaluation (bladder diary for at least 3 days, urinalysis, urodynamic investigation, Qualiveen questionnaire [12], FSFI [10]/IIEF [11]). In case of negative prolonged SNM testing, the tined leads are explanted. In case of successful prolonged SNM testing, the neuromodulator is generally implanted in the upper buttock (rarely in the anterior abdominal wall) (stage two). After neuromodulator implantation, each patient has a 2 months phase when the neuromodulator is turned ON using sub-sensory threshold stimulation (SNM optimization phase) to optimize the effectiveness of neuromodulation by determining the most effective stimulation parameters (choice of stimulation electrodes, intensity of stimulation) for each patient. At the end of the SNM optimization phase, patients are randomized in a double-blind parallel design to SNM ON or OFF. During an outpatient visit, neuromodulation parameters and bladder diary parameters are checked and the neuromodulator is turned ON or OFF by an investigator not involved in assessment of the clinical outcome. Considering that sub-sensory stimulation is used for SNM, the patients do not feel if the stimulation is ON or OFF. At the end of the 2 months double-blind SNM phase, the patients have a neuro-urological re-evaluation (bladder diary for at least 3 days, urinalysis, urodynamic investigation, Qualiveen questionnaire [12], FSFI [10]/IIEF [11]). During this visit, unblinding takes place and the neuromodulator is turned ON in all patients.

Safety

The investigators will inform the patients, the study monitoring board, and the ethics committee if it becomes evident that the disadvantages of participation may be significantly greater than was foreseen in the research proposal. The study will be suspended pending further review by the study monitoring board, except insofar as suspension would jeopardize the patients' health. The investigators will take care that all patients are kept informed.

Adverse events will be assessed and categorized according to the National Cancer Institute Common Terminology Criteria for Adverse Events (CTCAE) version 4 in grade 1 to 5 (http://ctep.cancer.gov/protocolDevelopment/electronic_applications/ctc.htm). All adverse events will be

followed until they have abated, or until a stable situation has been reached. Depending on the event, follow-up may require additional tests or medical procedures as indicated, and/or referral to the general physician or a medical specialist.

In the case of withdrawal of consent to participate in the study, all possible efforts will be made to convince the patient to continue to have safety follow-up evaluations.

In the event one of the following situations arises among treated patients during the conduct of the study, the study will be temporarily suspended and a comprehensive safety review conducted evaluating if the study has to be terminated prematurely:

- Any death secondary to rapid unexpected progression of an underlying medical condition.
- Severe clinical or neurological deterioration in more than one subject.
- Any other serious adverse event determined by the study monitoring board to be a reason to suspend the study.

Study outcome measures

Primary: Success of SNM: Defined in accordance with the literature [5,6] as improvement of at least 50% in the key bladder diary variables (i.e. number of voids and/or number of leakages, post void residual) compared to the baseline values (i.e. patients with urgency frequency syndrome and/or urgency incontinence: at least 50% decrease in number of voids and/or number of leakages; patients with chronic urinary retention: at least 50% decrease in post void residual; patients with a combination of urgency frequency syndrome and/or urgency incontinence and chronic urinary retention: at least 50% decrease in number of voids and/or number of leakages, and/or at least 50% decrease in post void residual).

Secondary: A) Adverse events: Categorization according to the National Cancer Institute Common Terminology Criteria for Adverse Events (CTCAE) version 4 in grade 1 to 5 (http://ctep.cancer.gov/protocolDevelopment/electronic_applications/ctc.htm).

B) Urodynamic parameters: cystometric capacity (mL), compliance (mL/cmH$_2$O), detrusor overactivity (if yes: bladder volume (mL) at detrusor overactivity, maximum detrusor pressure amplitude (cmH$_2$O), detrusor leak point pressure (cmH$_2$O)), maximum detrusor pressure (cmH$_2$O), detrusor pressure at maximum flow rate (cmH$_2$O), maximum flow rate (mL/s), voided volume (mL), post void residual (mL), pelvic floor electromyographic activity (normal/detrusor sphincter dyssynergia).

C) Questionnaires, i.e. Qualiveen and FSFI/IIEF.

D) Costs of SNM.

Data analysis

Statistics

Interval scaled variates will be summarized with means and standard deviations (SD) or medians and interquartile ranges where appropriate. Dichotomous variates will be described as ratios and percentages.

Univariate analysis

T-tests will be used to compare means between groups and chi-squared tests to compare dichotomous variables.

Multivariate analysis

To adjust for unequal distribution of parameters at baseline, multivariate regression models, linear models in case of an interval scaled outcome and logistic regression in case of a dichotomous outcome will be performed.

Ethics and dissemination

This trial will be performed in accordance with the World Medical Association Declaration of Helsinki [13], the guidelines for Good Clinical Practice [14] and the guidelines of the Swiss Academy of Medical Sciences [15]. Handling of all personal data will strictly comply with the federal law of data protection in Switzerland [16]. The trial has been registred at clinicaltrials.gov (www.clinicaltrials.gov/ct2/show/NCT02165774).

Discussion

First-line treatment for neurogenic LUTD includes antimuscarinics and some form of catheterization if necessary, preferably intermittent self-catheterization [17]. However, the treatment effect is often unsatisfactory, so that other options have to be considered, including onabotulinumtoxinA injections into the detrusor [18] or more invasive procedures such as bladder augmentation or urinary diversions. Thus, it is of utmost importance to know whether the minimally invasive and completely reversible SNM, a well established and widely accepted therapy for refractory non-neurogenic LUTD, would be a valuable treatment option for patients with refractory neurogenic LUTD. In addition, SNM may enable voiding without intermittent catheterization, the standard technique for chronic neurogenic urinary retention today. As a significant number of patients cannot perform this technique due to the underlying neurological disorder, SNM may not only prevent major surgery but also life-long treatment with indwelling catheters, which are related to significant long-term complications.

Assessing efficacy and safety of SNM for neurogenic LUTD, it is essential to be aware of the fact that these patients usually have undergone multiple failed previous treatments. In the case that SNM is also effective in the neurological population, this would have major implications for daily practice and would completely revolutionize the management of neurogenic LUTD.

This trial is multidisciplinary and will significantly influence all involved disciplines, i.e. neuro-urology, urology, and neurology. Especially in neurology, this project will increase the awareness of LUTD in neurological disorders and the related effective treatment options including SNM.

Ethics approval

This study has been approved by the local ethics committees (Kantonale Ethikkommission Zürich KEK-ZH-Nr. 2011–0048, St. Gallen KEK-SG-Nr. 12/069, Luzern KEK-LU-Nr. 12047, Bern KEK-BE-Nr. 094/12).

Abbreviations

CTCAE: Common Terminology Criteria for Adverse Events; EAU: European Association of Urology; FSFI: Female Sexual Function Index; ICI: International Consultation on Incontinence; IIEF: International Index of Erectile Function; LUTD: Lower urinary tract dysfunction; NICE: National Institute for Health and Clinical Excellence; SNM: Sacral neuromodulation.

Competing interests

The authors declare that they have no competing interests.

Authors' contributors

TMK, DSE, AGK, and LMB created the study design. SCK and TMK drafted the manuscript. MDL, LM, DA, DSE, JW, JP, BK, FCB, MPS, EM, AGK, and LMB critically reviewed the manuscript. TMK obtained the funding of this study. All the authors read and approved the final manuscript.

Acknowledgements

The authors would like to acknowledge the Swiss National Science Foundation, Vontobel-Stiftung, Gottfried und Julia Bangerter-Rhyner-Stiftung, Dr. Urs Mühlebach, and Swiss Continence Foundation for financial support.

Funding

Swiss National Science Foundation, Vontobel-Stiftung, Gottfried und Julia Bangerter-Rhyner-Stiftung, Dr. Urs Mühlebach, and Swiss Continence Foundation.

Author details

[1]Neuro-Urology, Spinal Cord Injury Center & Research, University of Zürich, Balgrist University Hospital, Forchstrasse 340, 8008 Zürich, Switzerland. [2]Department of Urology, Cantonal Hospital St. Gallen, St. Gallen, Switzerland. [3]Neuro-Urology, Swiss Paraplegic Center, Nottwil, Switzerland. [4]Department of Urology, University of Bern, Bern, Switzerland. [5]Department of Clinical Epidemiology and Medical Technology Assessment, Maastricht University Medical Center, Maastricht, The Netherlands. [6]Medignition Inc., Research Consultants, Zug, Switzerland.

References

1. Wöllner J, Hampel C, Kessler TM: **Surgery illustrated - surgical atlas sacral neuromodulation.** *BJU Int* 2012, 110(1):146–159.
2. Brazzelli M, Murray A, Fraser C: **Efficacy and safety of sacral nerve stimulation for urinary urge incontinence: a systematic review.** *J Urol* 2006, 175(3 Pt 1):835–841.
3. Chartier-Kastler EJ, Ruud Bosch JL, Perrigot M, Chancellor MB, Richard F, Denys P: **Long-term results of sacral nerve stimulation (S3) for the treatment of neurogenic refractory urge incontinence related to detrusor hyperreflexia.** *J Urol* 2000, 164(5):1476–1480.
4. Herbison GP, Arnold EP: **Sacral neuromodulation with implanted devices for urinary storage and voiding dysfunction in adults.** *Cochrane Database Syst Rev* 2009, 2:CD004202.

Protocol for a randomized, placebo-controlled, double-blind clinical trial investigating sacral neuromodulation...

69

5. Kessler TM, Buchser E, Meyer S, Engeler DS, Al-Khodairy AW, Bersch U, Iselin CE, Roche B, Schmid DM, Schurch B, Zrehen S, Burkhard FC: **Sacral neuromodulation for refractory lower urinary tract dysfunction: results of a nationwide registry in Switzerland.** *Eur Urol* 2007, **51**(5):1357–1363.

6. van Kerrebroeck PE, van Voskuilen AC, Heesakkers JP, Lycklama a Nijholt AA, Siegel S, Jonas U, Fowler CJ, Fall M, Gajewski JB, Hassouna MM, Cappellano F, Elhilali MM, Milam DF, Das AK, Dijkema HE, van den Hombergh U: **Results of sacral neuromodulation therapy for urinary voiding dysfunction: outcomes of a prospective, worldwide clinical study.** *J Urol* 2007, **178**(5):2029–2034.

7. Abrams P, Andersson KE, Birder L, Brubaker L, Cardozo L, Chapple C, Cottenden A, Davila W, de Ridder D, Dmochowski R, Drake M, Dubeau C, Fry C, Hanno P, Smith JH, Herschorn S, Hosker G, Kelleher C, Koelbl H, Khoury S, Madoff R, Milsom I, Moore K, Newman D, Nitti V, Norton C, Nygaard I, Payne C, Smith A, Staskin D, *et al*: **Fourth International Consultation on Incontinence Recommendations of the International Scientific Committee: evaluation and treatment of urinary incontinence, pelvic organ prolapse, and fecal incontinence.** *Neurourol Urodyn* 2010, **29**(1):213–240.

8. Wallace PA, Lane FL, Noblett KL: **Sacral nerve neuromodulation in patients with underlying neurologic disease.** *Am J Obstet Gynecol* 2007, **197**(1):96. e91-95.

9. Kessler TM, La Framboise D, Trelle S, Fowler CJ, Kiss G, Pannek J, Schurch B, Sievert KD, Engeler DS: **Sacral neuromodulation for neurogenic lower urinary tract dysfunction: systematic review and meta-analysis.** *Eur Urol* 2010, **58**(6):865–874.

10. Kriston L, Gunzler C, Rohde A, Berner MM: **Is one question enough to detect female sexual dysfunctions? A diagnostic accuracy study in 6,194 women.** *J Sex Med* 2010, **7**(5):1831–1841.

11. Kriston L, Gunzler C, Harms A, Berner M: **Confirmatory factor analysis of the German version of the international index of erectile function (IIEF): a comparison of four models.** *J Sex Med* 2008, **5**(1):92–99.

12. Costa P, Perrouin-Verbe B, Colvez A, Didier J, Marquis P, Marrel A, Amarenco G, Espirac B, Leriche A: **Quality of life in spinal cord injury patients with urinary difficulties. Development and validation of qualiveen.** *Eur Urol* 2001, **39**(1):107–113.

13. Association WM: **World Medical Association Declaration of Helsinki: ethical principles for medical research involving human subjects.** *JAMA* 2013, **310**(20):2191–2194.

14. International conference on harmonisation: *Good clinical practice guideline*; 1996 [http://www.ich.org/products/guidelines/efficacy/article/efficacy-guidelines.html]

15. Swiss Academy of Medical Sciences: *Guideline - Concerning scientific research involving human beings*; 2009 [www.samw.ch/dms/de/Publikationen/Leitfaden/d_Forschung-mit-Menschen.pdf]

16. The Federal Authorities of the Swiss Confederation: *Bundesgesetz über den Datenschutz (DSG) vom 19. Juni 1992*; 1992 [http://www.admin.ch/ch/d/sr/2/235.1.de.pdf]

17. Pannek J, Blok B, Castro-Diaz D, Del Popolo G, Groen J, Karsenty G, Kessler TM, Kramer G, Stöhrer M: *EAU guidelines on neuro-urology*; 2014 [http://www.uroweb.org/gls/pdf/21%20Neuro-Urology_LR.pdf]

18. Wöllner J, Kessler TM: **Botulinum toxin injections into the detrusor.** *BJU Int* 2011, **108**(9):1528–1537.

Wide-neck renal artery aneurysm: parenchymal sparing endovascular treatment with a new device

Michele Rossi[1], Gianluca Maria Varano[1*], Gianluigi Orgera[1], Alberto Rebonato[2], Florindo Laurino[1] and Cosimo De Nunzio[3]

Abstract

Background: Renal artery aneurysm is a rare disorder with a high mortality rate in the event of rupture, the most frequent complication, which can also occur in lesions smaller than those indicated for treatment by current criteria. Surgery is still the first-line treatment, although a growing trend toward endovascular management of visceral artery aneurysms has emerged because of the high efficacy and low invasiveness that has been demonstrated by several authors. Treatment of wide-necked aneurysms and, depending on location, those at renal artery bifurcations or distal branches is more complex and may require invasive surgical techniques, such as bench surgery.

Case presentation: We describe the successful use of a new neurointerventional coil to treat an enlarging wide-necked segmental-branch renal aneurysm in an elderly woman who was not a candidate for surgery because of several comorbidities.

Conclusions: The technique described allowed safe, successful treatment of a wide-necked aneurysm in an unfavorable vascular territory, reducing the risk of downstream artery embolization and consequent parenchymal damage and decreased renal function. In similar cases, other endovascular devices have often proven to be ineffective at nephron sparing. To validate the safety and efficacy of this system, more cases treated in this manner should be studied.

Keywords: Renal artery aneurysm, Visceral artery aneurysm, Wide-neck aneurysm, Embolization, Penumbra, Microcoil embolization

Background

Renal artery aneurysm (RAA) is a rare disorder, occurring in 0.01%–1.3% of the general population. It represents 1% of all aneurysms but is the second most common visceral artery aneurysm, accounting for approximately 25% [1,2].

RAAs are classified into four categories: saccular (70%); fusiform (22.5%); dissecting (7.5%); and mixed, including microaneurysms [3]. Saccular aneurysms, the most common, typically occur at the primary or secondary bifurcations of renal arteries [4]; more rarely they are located intraparenchymally in a segmental artery or more distal branches. Etiologies for saccular aneurysms include atherosclerosis, fibromuscular dys-

plasia, and neurofibromatosis. RAAs are often noted incidentally but can also be accompanied by hypertension, hematuria, or pain. Hypertension related to RAA remains a controversial topic; however, most case series on RAA treatment report improvement or resolution of hypertension after treatment [2].

The indication for treatment is currently based on a size threshold that continues to be debated, although most authors believe that aneurysms 2 cm or less in diameter do not require treatment. However, the decision to treat an aneurysm should be made not only on the basis of size, but also after considering other issues, such as the presence of clinical symptoms (hematuria, hypertension, back pain, and renal infarction), anatomical and morphological characteristics (location, wall calcification, enlarging lesion), and general clinical features (life expectancy, comorbidities, planned pregnancy). Finally, it should be considered that the mortality rate for spontaneous rupture is about 80% [5]. This outcome has also been described for aneurysms smaller than 1 cm [6,7].

* Correspondence: gianluca.varano@gmail.com
[1]Department of Radiology Interventional Radiology Unit, Ospedale Sant'Andrea, University "La Sapienza", Via di Grottarossa 1035/1039 00189, Rome, Italy
Full list of author information is available at the end of the article

Many treatment options are currently available. Surgical management still represents the standard of care, particularly for aneurysms located at the renal artery bifurcation as well as those involving distal branches [8]. Surgical repair may involve in situ or extracorporeal bench surgery [6], and may require a long operation time and have substantial perioperative complications such as unplanned nephrectomy, with a failure rate of 6.6%. After successful early surgical repair, there is a reintervention rate of 5.8% resulting from such complications as anastomotic stenosis or graft thrombosis [9].

Despite the relative success of surgical repair of symptomatic aneurysms, there is a growing trend toward endovascular alternatives over open procedures because of their low invasiveness and reduced morbidity. A recent review of endovascular treatment reported good clinical and angiographic success rates without major complications, loss of kidney function, or nephrectomy [10]. However, no large case series or case reports with long-term follow-up are currently available.

Several endovascular embolization techniques have recently been developed to manage aneurysms with heterogeneous anatomical features. Indeed, while narrow-necked saccular aneurysms can be successfully treated with transcatheter coil embolization regardless of type [3], endovascular treatment of wide-necked aneurysms is not yet well established and may require the use of more sophisticated techniques. These techniques, originally conceived in neurointerventional practice, are based on balloon- or stent-assisted embolization. During these procedures, a suitable device is released within the feeding vessel across the neck of the aneurysm to prevent coil prolapse during deployment and facilitate denser packing of the aneurysm, with the aim of reducing the likelihood of parent-vessel embolization. Stents employed are either self-expandable (bifurcation and segmental artery) or balloon-expandable (main stem) depending on the reference vessels and operator preference [7,11].

Complications associated with these techniques include artery dissection, thrombosis, and rupture; microthrombi embolization; and renal infarction [8,11]. Endovascular techniques are not often used in distal aneurysms, since the smaller the reference vessel, the harder it is to release a stent or use a balloon without damaging the vessel wall or inducing thrombosis.

The use of stent graft has also been reported for treatment of aneurysms beyond the first renal artery division but has a low success rate in terms of sparing the segmental artery and parenchyma [10,12,13].

Case presentation

A 74-year-old woman presented to our hospital emergency room with sharp left flank pain radiating posteriorly. She had experienced three similar episodes over the last 9 months. During one of the episodes, the patient had undergone clinical examination and abdominal ultrasound, which showed a renal intraparenchymal aneurysm about 10 mm in diameter.

Her medical history was remarkable for severe chronic obstructive pulmonary disease, diabetes, and hypertension, all treated medically. After the patient was admitted, a color Doppler ultrasound (CDUS) and a multidetector computed tomography (MDCT) scan confirmed an 18-mm saccular aneurysm of the left renal anterior segmental artery. The aneurysm was characterized by a wide (12-mm) neck and the absence of intraluminal thrombus or parietal calcification (Figure 1).

A multidisciplinary consultation that included general and vascular surgeons, urologists, and interventional radiologists was held, in which aneurysm morphology, the absence of calcifications, and the propensity of the aneurysm to enlarge were considered. In light of the patient's performance status and comorbidities, the decision was made to treat the aneurysm with endovascular exclusion. After the patient provided informed consent, the embolization was performed under local anesthesia via transaxillary access. After selective catheterization of the left renal artery, digital subtraction angiography (DSA) was performed using a 5-Fr Cobra 1 angiographic catheter (TEMPO®AQUA®, Cordis Corp., Bridgewater, NJ, USA) coaxially introduced into a 6-Fr flexible, long-sheath introducer (Flexor® Check-Flo® Introducer; Cook Medical, Bloomington, IN, USA) to assess the relationship between the aneurysm and the left renal vasculature on multiple projections (Figure 2). After

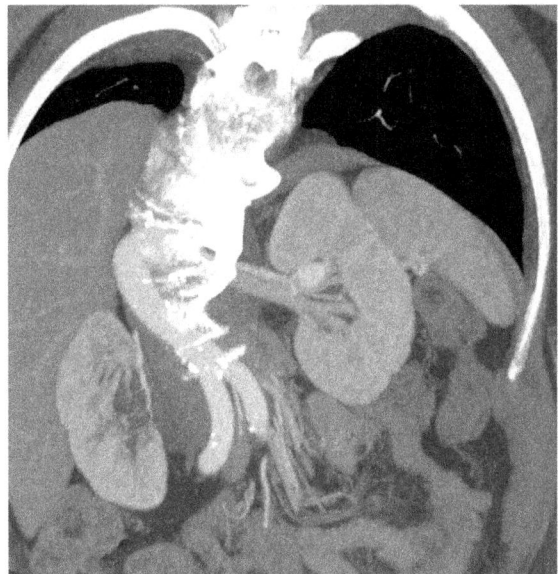

Figure 1 Contrast-enhanced abdominal computed tomography. Oblique coronal multiplanar reconstruction shows the aneurysm in the upper portion of the left kidney, originating from the anterior segmental artery.

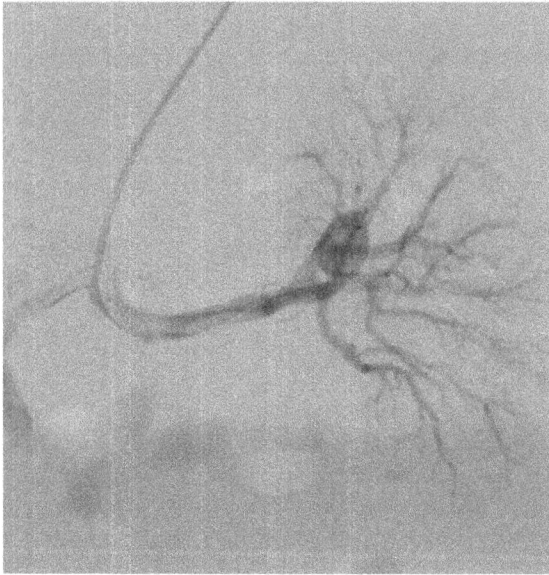

Figure 2 Digital subtraction angiography. Selective left renal injection through a transbrachial multipurpose 5-Fr catheter, with rapid injection of a wide-necked aneurysm originating from an upper-pole anterior segmental artery.

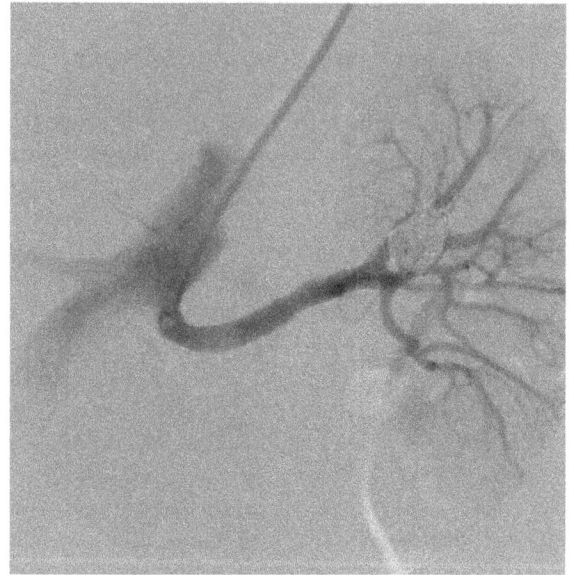

Figure 4 Selective left renal artery angiography after coil deployment and detachment. There is a compact appearance of the coils and complete filling of the aneurysm with downstream vascular-tree preservation.

introducing a coaxial neurointerventional microcatheter (Penumbra PX400™ Delivery Microcatheter; Penumbra Inc., Alameda, CA, USA) into the aneurysmal sac, superselective DSA was performed to confirm the absence of branches originating from within the sac, and a slow, swirling flow inside the sac was observed (Figure 3).

To protect the renal vasculature, three complex-shaped bare nitinol microcoils (Penumbra Coil 400™ 18 mm × 57-cm and 15 mm × 57 cm Complex Standard and 13 mm × 48-cm Complex Soft; Penumbra, Inc.) were then sequentially deployed in the aneurysm until it was densely packed

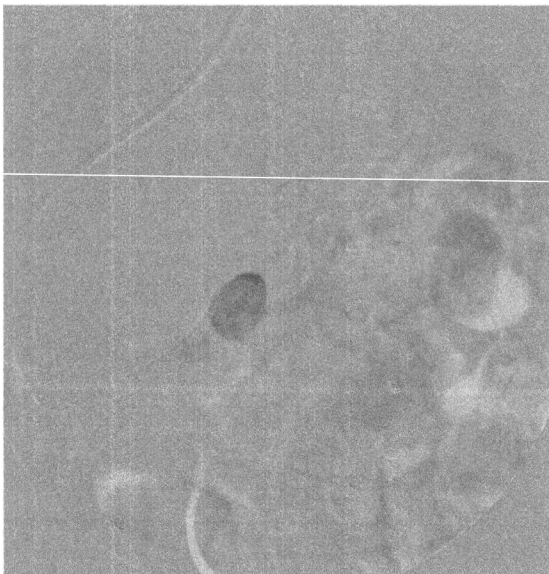

Figure 3 Superselective contrast injection into the aneurysm through a dedicated microcatheter coaxially advanced inside the larger 5-Fr angiographic mother catheter, immediately before the coil deployment.

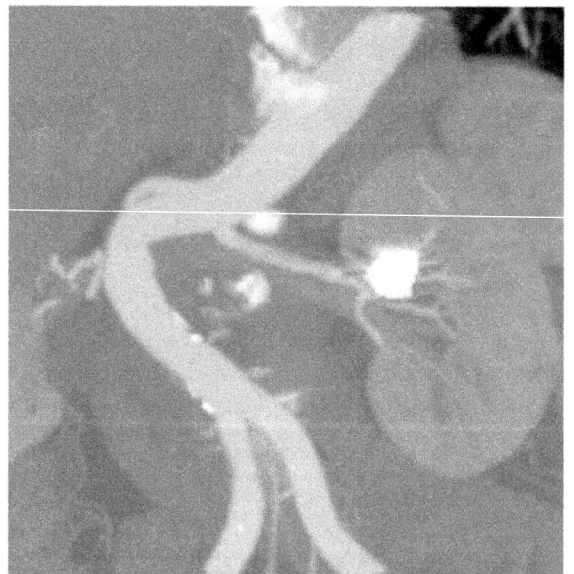

Figure 5 Abdominal contrast-enhanced computed tomography 1 month after the procedure. Oblique coronal multiplanar reconstruction clearly shows the aneurysm exclusion from complete coil filling and normal parenchymal contrast enhancement without evidence of segmental ischemic damage.

to 10.5% of the aneurysm volume. Each coil was detached only when angiography clearly showed complete and exclusive coiling inside the sac. The first coil, which was used to prevent coil migration through the neck into the parent artery, was the stiffest available and was sized slightly larger than the aneurysmal dome, thus creating a cage through which the other, more flexible coils could be safely deployed.

The final DSA demonstrated complete embolization and regular renal parenchymal opacification without parent-vessel embolization or thrombosis (Figure 4). The patient was asymptomatic at the time of discharge, 48 h after the procedure. Renal function, as evaluated by estimated glomerular filtration rate, was similar before (89 mL/min/1.73 m^2) and after the intervention (92 mL/min/1.73 m^2). The patient was followed up monthly with clinical examinations and laboratory tests. Her blood pressure remained unchanged, and her previous therapies were maintained. CDUS performed at 3 months and MDCT performed 1 and 3 years after the intervention confirmed preservation of the superior segmental artery and normal parenchymal perfusion (Figure 5).

Conclusions

In the present case, considering the patient's comorbidities and location of the aneurysm, surgical repair would have been very invasive and would likely have required bench surgery, so endovascular exclusion was preferable. The anatomical features and location of the aneurysm, and the need for accurate coil deployment before release, justified the use of this new type of neurointerventional detachable coil, which has not previously been reported to treat RAA. A high packing density, with fewer coils and shorter procedure time than are required for other procedures using different materials, was also obtained.

To our knowledge, this is the first case of a visceral aneurysm treated with the Penumbra Coil 400™ Embolization System (Penumbra Inc.) that includes 3 years of follow-up. These 0.020-inch coils are larger in diameter than other neurointerventional coils and are inherently softer because of their diameter (softness increases by the third power of the diameter) and because of the different thickness of the nitinol stretch-resistant wire. The coil-within-a-coil design increases the ability of the device to occupy the aneurysmal sac with less risk of misplacement [14].

As previously reported, in the treatment of complex renal aneurysms in difficult locations, a neurointerventional coil system may facilitate complete sac embolization with lower morbidity and less risk of decreased renal function than can be achieved with surgery or other endovascular techniques. The Penumbra system in particular, because of its conformability and greater length-volume ratio, allows rapid and complete embolization with less risk of parent-vessel damage.

More cases should be treated in this manner to validate the safety and efficacy of this system.

Consent

Written informed consent was obtained from the patient for publication of this Case report and any accompanying images. A copy of the written consent is available for review by the Editor of this journal.

Abbreviations
RAA: Renal artery aneurysm; MDCT: Multidetector computed tomography.

Competing interest
The authors declare that they have no competing interests.

Authors' contributions
GMV and MR drafted the report, contributed to concept, and cared for the patient. GO and CDN drafted the report, and approved the final version of the manuscript. AR and FL contributed to concept and design and made relevant corrections. All authors read and approved the final manuscript.

Author details
[1]Department of Radiology Interventional Radiology Unit, Ospedale Sant'Andrea, University "La Sapienza", Via di Grottarossa 1035/1039 00189, Rome, Italy. [2]Department of Surgery, Radiology, and Odontostomatology Sciences, Santa Maria della Misericordia University Hospital, University of Perugia, Sant'Andrea delle Fratte, 06129 Perugia, Italy. [3]Division of Urology, Ospedale Sant'Andrea, University "La Sapienza", Roma Via di, Grottarossa 1035/1039 00189, Rome, Italy.

References
1. Tham G, Ekelund L, Herrlin K, Lindstedt EL, Olin T, Bergentz SE: **Renal artery aneurysms. Natural history and prognosis.** *Ann Surg* 1983, **197**(3):348–352.
2. Henke PK, Stanley JC: **Renal artery aneurysms: diagnosis, management and outcomes.** *Minerva Chir* 2003, **58**:305–311.
3. Poutasse EF: **Renal artery aneurysms.** *J Urol* 1975, **113**:443–449.
4. Hageman JH, Smith RF, Szilagyi S, Elliott JP: **Aneurysms o f the renal artery: problems of prognosis and surgical management.** *Surgery* 1978, **84**:563–572.
5. Rebonato A, Rossi M, Rebonato S, Cagini L, Scialpi M: **Giant hepatic artery aneurysm: a fatal evolution.** *J Emerg Med* 2013, **45**(6):e217–e219.
6. Lupattelli T, Abubacker Z, Morgan R, Belli AM: **Embolization of a renal artery aneurysm using ethylene vinyl alcohol copolymer (Onyx).** *J Endovasc Ther* 2003, **10**:366–370.
7. Clark WIC, Sankin A, Becske T, Nelson PK, Fox M: **Stent-assisted gugliemi detachable coil repair of wide-necked renal artery aneurysm using 3-D angiography.** *Vasc Endovascular Surg* 2008, **41**:528.
8. Somarouthu B, Rabinov J, Wong W, Kalva SP: **Stent-assisted coil embolization of an intraparenchymal renal artery aneurysm in a patient with neurofibromatosis.** *Vasc Endovasc Surg* 2011, **45**(4):368–371.
9. Henke PK, Cardneau JD, Welling TH, Upchurch GR Jr, Wakefield TW, Jacobs LA, Proctor SB, Greenfield LJ, Stanley JC: **Renal artery aneurysms: a 35-year clinical experience with 252 aneurysms in 168 patients.** *Ann Surg* 2001, **234**:454–463.
10. Garg N, Pipinos II, Longo GM, Thorell WE, Lynch TG, Johanning JM: **Detachable coils for repair of extraparenchymal renal artery aneurysms: an alternative to surgical therapy.** *Ann Vasc Surg* 2007, **21**(1):97–110.

11. Xiong J, Guo W, Liu X, Yin T, Jia X, Zhang M: **Renal artery aneurysm treatment with stent plus coil embolization.** *Ann Vasc Surg* 2010, **24**:695. e1–695.e3.

12. Tan WA, Chough S, Saito J, Wholey MH, Eles G: **Covered stent for renal artery aneurysm.** *Catheter Cardiovasc Interv* 2001, **52**:106–109.

13. Rossi M, Rebonato A, Citone M, La Torre M, David V: **Common hepatic artery aneurysm successfully treated with a celiac axis stent graft. Two years of follow up.** *Eur J Rad Extra* 2010, **75**(3):e125–e128.

14. Milburn J, Pansara AL, Vidal G, Martinez RC: **Initial experience using the Penumbra coil 400: comparison of aneurysm packing, cost effectiveness, and coil efficiency.** *J Neurointerv Surg* 2013, in press.

Extravascular stent management for migration of left renal vein endovascular stent in nutcracker syndrome

Lu Tian[1], Shanwen Chen[2*], Gaoyue Zhang[3], Hongkun Zhang[1], Wei Jin[1] and Ming Li[1]

Abstract

Background: Nutcracker syndrome is an entity resulting from left renal vein compression by the aorta and the superior mesenteric artery, which leads to symptoms of hematuria or left flank pain. The alternative option of endovascular or extravascular stenting is very appealing because of the minimal invasive procedures. Stents in the renal vein can cause fibromuscular hyperplasia, proximal migration or embolization.

Case presentation: A 30-year-old female was diagnosed with nutcracker syndrome for severe left flank pain. After failed conservative approach, she underwent endovascular stenting and subsequently developed recurrent symptom for stent migration one month postoperatively. She underwent successful extravascular stenting with complete symptom resolution.

Conclusion: The extravascular stenting is an alternative option after migration of left renal vein endovascular stenting. The computed tomographic imaging was closely correlated to therapeutic interventions and stent migration.

Keywords: Nutcracker syndrome, Stent migration, Management

Background

Left renal vein (LRV) compression by the aorta and the superior mesenteric artery (SMA) leading to symptoms of hematuria or left flank pain has been classically described as nutcracker syndrome (NCS) [1, 2]. Minimal invasive management includes both endovascular stenting and extravascular stenting [1, 2]. We reported a teaching case with NCS who underwent endovascular stenting and subsequently developed recurrent symptom for stent migration one month postoperatively. She underwent successful extravascular stenting with complete symptom resolution.

Case presentation

A 30-year-old female was presented with severe left flank pain for one year. Laboratory data was within normal limits. Her physical examination was unremarkable, with a body mass index of 19 Kg/m^2.

On April 8th, 2011, the computed tomographic angiography (CTA) and magnetic resonance angiography showed narrowing of the LRV in the aortomesenteric portion. On May 25th, 2011, a duplex ultrasound demonstrated the compressed LRV between the aorta and the SMA, varices of left gonadal vein arising from the LRV, and a peak velocity (PV) of 17 cm/s in the renal hilum and 106 cm/s in the aortomesenteric portion of the LRV (the PV ratio of 6.2) (Fig. 1a, b). On June 2th, 2011, left renal venography revealed obstruction of LRV outflow, perihilar varices, and an 8 mm Hg pressure gradient across the suspected narrowing in the LRV (Fig. 1c).

After failed conservative approach, the left renal venography was performed under local anesthesia to confirm and manage the narrowing of the LRV. A 10 mm × 40 mm SmartControl stent (Cordis, Johnson & Johnson, USA http://www.jnj.com) was deployed. The left renal venography showed unobstructed blood outflow, and full stent expansion without obvious protrusion of the stent in the inferior vena cava (Fig. 1d). The patient had nearly immediate resolution of her symptom and was discharged on postoperative day 5.

* Correspondence: chensw123@126.com
[2]Department of Urology, the First Affiliated Hospital of Medical College, Zhejiang University, No. 79 Qing Chun Road, HangZhou 310003, China
Full list of author information is available at the end of the article

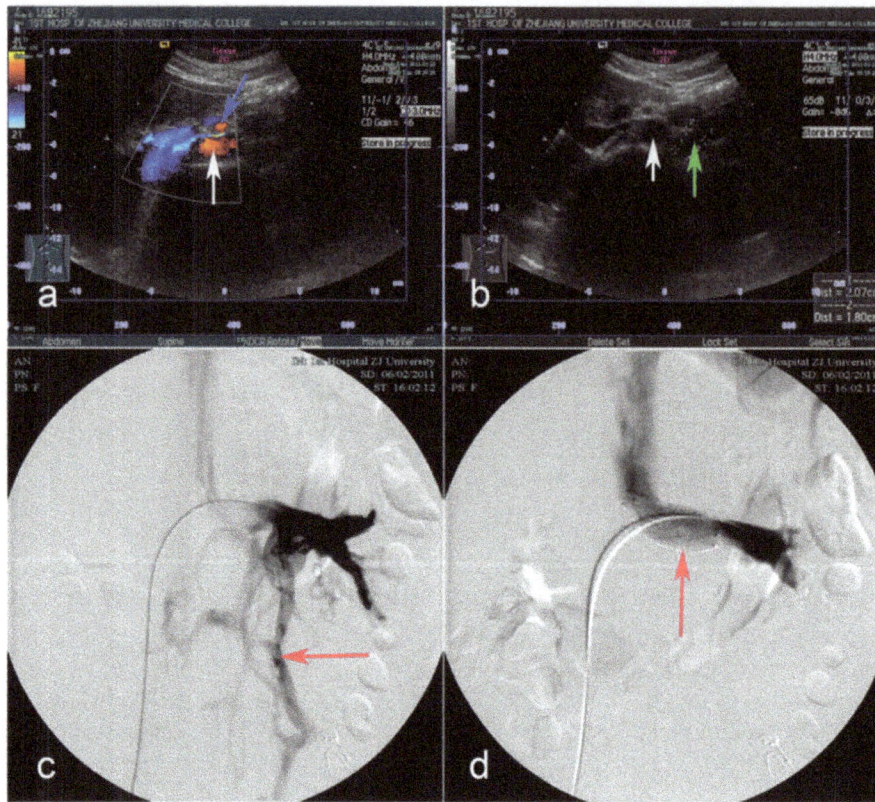

Fig. 1 The images of the duplex ultrasound and the left renal venography. **a**, Right transverse image: Duplex ultrasound demonstrated the compressed left renal vein between the aorta (white arrow) and the superior mesenteric artery (blue arrow), and the left renal vein was pressed like a beak. **b**, Left transverse image: Duplex ultrasound demonstrated a narrowing of the left renal vein at the aortomesenteric portion and varices of left gonadal vein (green arrow) arising from the left renal vein on the left of aorta (white arrow). **c**, Before extravascular stenting, left renal venography demonstrated there was obstruction of left renal venous outflow and perihilar varices (red arrow). **d**, After endovascular stenting (red arrow), left renal venography showed unobstructed blood outflow and full stent expansion without obvious protrusion of the stent in the inferior vena cava

After one month of endovascular stenting, the patient began to experience recurrent left flank pain. On July 5th, 2011, the second CTA demonstrated an endovascular stent migration on the left of SMA (Fig. 2). On July 15th, 2011, the third CTA demonstrated further migration of the endovascular stent on the left of SMA (Fig. 2). Since there was a continuing migration of the stent on computed tomographic imaging within 10 days, the extravascular stent was proposed on July 26th, 2011. The endovascular stent was found migrated to the left of SMA and adhered to the vessel wall tightly, and the stent could not be moved. The varicose gonadal

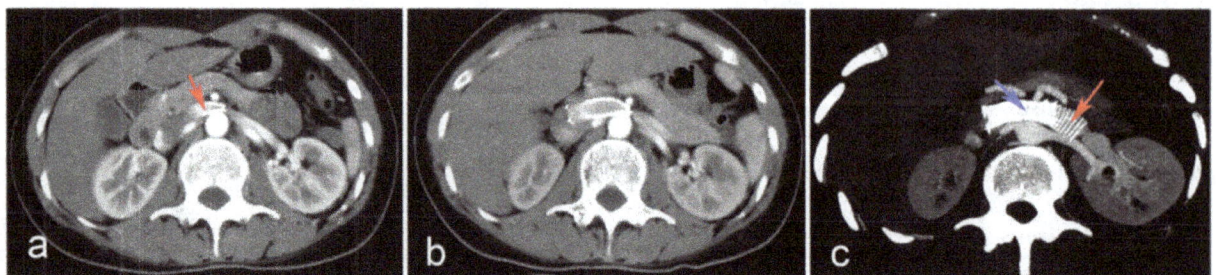

Fig. 2 The images of the computed tomographic angiography (CTA). **a**, The second CTA evaluation was suggestive of an endovascular stent migration (red arrow) on the left of the superior mesenteric artery. **b**, The third CTA demonstrated further migration of the endovascular stent on the left of SMA. **c**, The follow-up CTA demonstrated the extravascular stent (red arrow) was patent and well positioned, and the endovascular stent (blue arrow) remained on the left of the superior mesenteric artery

vein was seen arising from the LRV. Excessive fibrous tissue was found at the origin of the SMA, and excised for adequate decompression of the LRV (Fig. 3a). We estimated and cut the graft to an appropriate length to fit between the inferior vena cava and the gonadal vein or longer. After the left gonadal vein and adrenal central vein were ligated and transected (Fig. 3a), an externally reinforced polytetrafluoroethylene graft (REF F4008, Bard Peripheral Vascular, Inc. http://www.bardpv.com/) of 8 mm diameter was selected to form an extravascular stent around the LRV (Fig. 3b). The graft was wrapped around the LRV and fixed together at each ring (Fig. 3c). The graft was sewn to the adventitia of the abdominal aorta and the endovascular stent was sewn to the wall of the LRV to prevent from the further migration. The patient had nearly immediate resolution of her symptom and was discharged on postoperative day 7.

At 36 months' follow-up, the patient was asymptomatic. The fourth, fifth and sixth CTA demonstrated the extravascular stent was patent and well positioned, and the endovascular stent remained to be on the left of the superior mesenteric artery at the first week, third month, and ninth month after extravascular stent placement respectively (Fig. 2).

Discussion

Endovascular stenting has been used for seventeen years for the treatment of NCS due to its minimally invasive nature. A survey of the published English literature revealed 124 cases treated in this manner including our largest stenting experiences to date [2–9]. Although, the current literature suggests that stenting is a safe and effective procedure, stent migration notes in 7.3 % of all cases [2–5]. The reason of endovascular stent migration may be the effect of cardiac motion, early activity, mismatch between renal vein diameter or stent diameter, or inaccurate positioning of the stent within the lesion.

The clinical implications of migration are significant and can lead to thrombosis, vessel trauma, embolization, and its most disastrous consequence (rupture). It requires prompt and effective diagnosis and management to prevent potentially implications.

Sequence of image for diagnosis or follow-up has more or less been rationalized to duplex ultrasound, computerized tomography or magnetic resonance angiography, and finally left renal venography [2]. Duplex ultrasound is the easiest and the least expensive method. Zhelan Zheng et al. [10] pointed out standards for ultrasonic diagnosis of the disease as follows: (1)the low velocity of stenosis of the LRV at supine position accelerates remarkably, and the acceleration is more obvious after standing for 15 min,which is more than 100 cm/s; (2) the inner diameter ratio between renal hilum and stenosis of the LRV at supine position is more than 3, while it is more than 5 after standing for 15 min. When two index are coincident with the standards, NCS may be primary diagnosed. The CTA (including non-invasive 3-D) may be a useful tool in the diagnosis of the NCS and follow-up testing. CTA provided fine outlines that gave a precise depiction of both endovascular stent migration on the left of the SMA and a compression of the LRV between the aorta and the SMA. Furthermore, the stent migrating distance can be measured, and many distorting collateral veins were seen arising from the LRV in the CTA. The CTA imaging was closely correlated to therapeutic interventions and stent migration.

The typical treatment is percutaneous removal of the migrated stent. However, under certain circumstances, such as stent migration to the heart, special stent, or endothelialization of stent, percutaneous removal may be difficult or even impossible, thus surgery may be required. Hartung et al. described a LRV stent that migrated into the retro hepatic inferior vena cava; an attempt to retrieve it with a Goose Neck failed when the

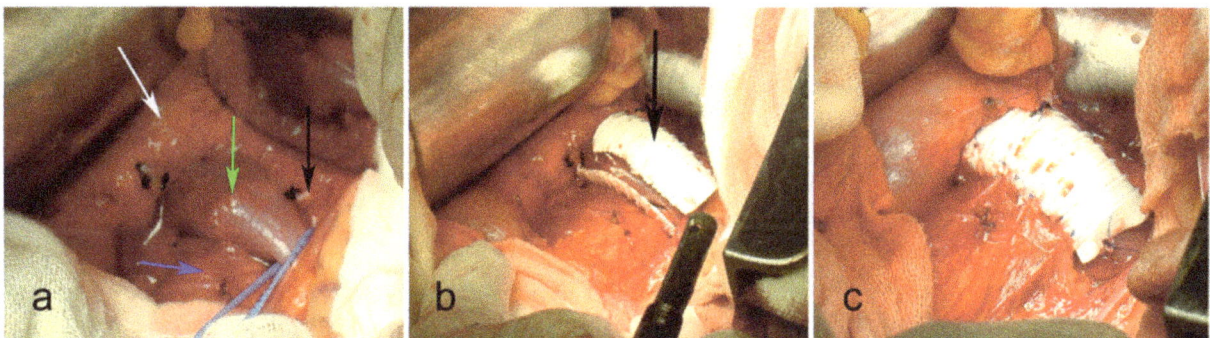

Fig. 3 The images of the extravascular stent placement. **a**, The migrated endovascular stent was inside the left renal vein (green arrow), and the left adrenal central vein (black arrow) was ligated and transected. The aorta (blue arrow); the inferior vena cava (white arrow). **b**, Intraoperative photograph demonstrated the graft (black arrow) was wrapped around the renal vein. **c**, The graft was fixed together at each ring and sewn to the adventitia of the abdominal aorta

stent took a transversal orientation after 5 cm, and further attempts also failed [4]. A patient with a nitinol stent is difficult to manage percutaneously because of its inherent characteristics and probable endothelialization of the stent in 1 year, which makes the procedure more challenging [11]. In our previous case, one stent migrated into the right atrium and the patient required surgery after unsuccessful percutaneous removal [3]. In such cases, surgical removal is a safer and more feasible option. However, surgical removal is associated with high morbidity: Long period of renal congestion and additional anastomoses. Compared with surgical removal, extravascular stenting is a minimally invasive treatment modality.

Compared with vascular displacement, extravascular stenting for NCS is a minimally invasive treatment modality. Especially for children and adolescents, intravascular stenting should be cautiously recommended because the lumen of the LRV may become wider and the stents cannot match any longer during physical development. One may postulate that externally suturing stent could be a way to keep it in place; therefore, Barnes firstly reported extravascular stenting and externally suturing the stent performed by open surgery in 1988 [12]. Currently, sporadic cases of extravascular stenting for the NCS have been reported with excellent outcome at short-term follow up [13–17]. The stent has good conformability to adapt to the vessel wall and adhere to the vessel wall tightly [6]. In our opinion, the extravascular approach to treat endovascular stent migration is favored to avoid the potential complications.

Consideration must also be given to the original stent placement. If removal is not possible or failed, the original stent should be fixed to prevent repeated movements of the stent. Both the new and old stents should be sewn to the vessel wall to ensure that the extravascular and endovascular stents did not migrate, as shown in our case.

Conclusions
The extravascular stenting is an alternative option after migration of left renal Vein endovascular stenting. The computed tomographic imaging was closely correlated to therapeutic interventions and stent migration.

Consent
Written informed consent was obtained from the patient for publication of this manuscript and accompanying images. A copy of the written consent is available for review by the Editor-in-Chief of this journal.

Abbreviations
LRV: Left renal vein; SMA: Superior mesenteric artery; NCS: Nutcracker syndrome; CTA: Computed tomographic angiography; PV: Peak velocity.

Competing interests
The authors declare that they have no competing interests.

Authors' contributions
LT cared for the patients and drafted the report. GZ, HZ,WJand ML cared for the patient. SC revised and approved the final version of the manuscript. All authors reviewed the report and approved the final version of the manuscript.

Acknowledgements
Language editor Keer Chen edited our manuscript.

Author details
[1]Department of Vascular Surgery, the First Affiliated Hospital of Medical College, Zhejiang University, Hangzhou 310003, China. [2]Department of Urology, the First Affiliated Hospital of Medical College, Zhejiang University, No. 79 Qing Chun Road, HangZhou 310003, China. [3]Department of Urology, the Second Affiliated Hospital of Zhejiang Chinese Medical University, Hangzhou 310005, China.

References
1. Ahmed K, Sampath R, Khan MS. Current trends in the diagnosis and management of renal nutcracker syndrome: a review. Eur J Vasc Endovasc Surg. 2006;31(4):410–6.
2. Chen S, Zhang H, Shi H, Tian L, Jin W, Li M. Endovascular stenting for treatment of Nutcracker syndrome: report of 61 cases with long-term followup. J Urol. 2011;186(2):570–5.
3. Chen S, Zhang H, Tian L, Li M, Zhou M, Wang Z. A stranger in the heart: LRV stent migration. Int Urol Nephrol. 2009;41(2):427–30.
4. Hartung O, Grisoli D, Boufi M, Marani I, Hakam Z, Barthelemy P, et al. Endovascular stenting in the treatment of pelvic vein congestion caused by nutcracker syndrome: lessons learned from the first five cases. J Vasc Surg. 2005;42(2):275–80.
5. Wang X, Zhang Y, Li C, Zhang H. Results of endovascular treatment for patients with nutcracker syndrome. J Vasc Surg. 2012;56(1):142–8.
6. Chen S, Zhang H, Tian L, Li M. Endovascular management of nutcracker syndrome after migration of a laparoscopically placed extravascular stent. Am J Kidney Dis. 2012;60(2):322–6.
7. Li H, Sun X, Liu G, Zhang Y, Chu J, Deng C, et al. Endovascular stent placement for nutcracker phenomenon. J Xray Sci Technol. 2013;21(1):95–102.
8. Liu Y, Sun Y, Wu XJ, Jiang Y, Jin X. Endovascular stent placement for the treatment of nutcracker syndrome. Int Urol Nephrol. 2012;44(4):1097–100.
9. Baldi S, Rabellino M, Zander T, Gonzalez G, Maynar M. Endovascular treatment of the nutcracker syndrome: report of two cases. Minim Invasive Ther Allied Technol. 2011;20(6):356–9.
10. Zhelan Zheng ZT, Mou Y, Wang J, Xu Q. Investigations on diagnostic standards of nutcracker syndrome with ultrasonic examination. Chin J Ultrasonography. 2004;13(5):363–5.
11. Gabelmann A, Kramer SC, Tomczak R, Gorich J. Percutaneous techniques for managing maldeployed or migrated stents. J Endovasc Ther. 2001;8(3):291–302.
12. Barnes RW, Fleisher 3rd HL, Redman JF, Smith JW, Harshfield DL, Ferris EJ. Mesoaortic compression of the left renal vein (the so-called nutcracker syndrome): repair by a new stenting procedure. J Vasc Surg. 1988;8(4):415–21.
13. Zhang Q, Zhang Y, Lou S, Liu F, Ye Z, Zhang D. Laparoscopic extravascular renal vein stent placement for nutcracker syndrome. J Endourol Endod Soc. 2010;24(10):1631–5.
14. Scultetus AH, Villavicencio JL, Gillespie DL. The nutcracker syndrome: its role in the pelvic venous disorders. J Vasc Surg. 2001;34(5):812–9.
15. Hartung O, Barthelemy P, Berdah SV, Alimi YS. Laparoscopy-assisted left ovarian vein transposition to treat one case of posterior nutcracker syndrome. Ann Vasc Surg. 2009;23(3):413. e413-416.
16. Chung BI, Gill IS. Laparoscopic splenorenal venous bypass for nutcracker syndrome. J Vasc Surg. 2009;49(5):1319–23.
17. Li P, Shao P, Qin C, Ju X, Meng X, Li J, et al. Retroperitoneal laparoscopic extravascular stent placement for renal nutcracker syndrome: initial experience. Urol Int. 2014;92(4):396–9.

Pain and satisfaction during rigid cystoscopic ureteral stent removal

Jae Heon Kim[1], Sun Young Park[2], Mun Gyu Kim[2], Hoon Choi[3], Dan Song[4], Sung Woo Cho[4] and Yun Seob Song[1*]

Abstract

Background: Cystoscopy evokes discomfort and pain, especially in males. The cystoscopic retrograde approach is standard in the removal of ureteral stents. However the satisfaction and degree of pain during the procedure according to the use of several pain controlling methods are unclear.

Methods: This is a cross-sectional survey of 60 patients who underwent cystoscopic ureteral stent removal under intravenous analgesics (group 1, n = 20), midazolam induction (group 2, n = 20), and propofol (group 3, n = 20). Procedural pain and post-procedure satisfaction were determined, and cost differences between the approaches were clarified.

Results: Group 2 and 3 showed significantly less pain than group 1 (P < 0.001) and significantly higher satisfaction rate than group 1 (P < 0.001). Comparison of groups 2 and 3 revealed showed significantly less pain and higher satisfaction rate in group 3 (P < 0.001 for both). In Group 1, 17 (85.0%) patients wanted other treatment modalities, compared to eight group 2 patients (40.0%) and no group 3 patients.

Conclusions: Considering the potential pain and dissatisfaction of rigid cystoscopic ureteral stent removal, procedures utilizing moderate sedation with midazolam or general anesthesia using propofol without muscle relaxation should be considered.

Keywords: Stent, Stent exchange, Stent removal, Cystscopy, Urolithiasis, Pain

Background

Although the real benefit of ureteral stenting after ureteroscopic removal of stone (URS) is contentious, the chance with ureteral stenting following ureteroscopic removal of stone is frequent [1]. After URS, ureteral stents are removed at post-operative 1 or 2 weeks, typically by cystoscopic retrograde removal [2,3]. However, because of the rigidity and larger diameter of cystoscopes, most patients need analgesia and some patients need deep sedation during the procedure [2,3]. In real practice, those stents are removed mostly in the outpatient setting using urethral lubrication jelly with or without narcotic intramuscular premedication [4-6].

Recently, lubrication jelly and lidocaine injection were reported to be no more effective for pain control during cystoscopy [7-11]. A flexible cystoscopy is a good alternative to rigid cystoscopy to reduce pain during procedure, but flexible cystoscopy is less available in korea and moreover there have been little reports about ureteral stent removal with flexible cystoscopy.

There have been many studies about pain during rigid or flexible cystoscopy, but there have been few studies about pain during cystoscopic stent removal. Although shorter in duration than cystoscopy, cystoscopic stent removal yields a similar pain to cystoscopy, and moreover larger diameter of rigid cystoscopy is needed for use of foreign body forceps. In our previous pilot study, cystoscopy using midazolam produced marginally greater satisfaction among men [6]. This is the main reason why we adapted diverse pain controlling method including propofol. The aim of this prospective, randomized, pilot study was to compare the satisfaction about cystoscopic stent removal according to different pain relief methods and to compare the costs.

* Correspondence: yssong@schmc.ac.kr
[1]Department of Urology, Soonchunhyang University Hospital, 657 Hannam-Dong, Yongsan-Gu, Seoul 140-743, Korea
Full list of author information is available at the end of the article

Methods

Study sample

From September 2012 to March 2013, 60 male patients with a history of prior URS and ureteral stenting due to ureteral stone were enrolled. Informed consent was obtained from all patients. The mean age of patients was 47.45 years. Subjects with severe cardiovascular disease, pulmonary disease, liver disease, and drug abuse history were excluded as were patients with a prior cystoscopy procedure were excluded. The 60 patients were subclassified randomly according to several pain controlling methods: cystoscopy + intravenous (IV) analgesics (group 1, n = 20); cystoscopy + midazolam (group 2, n = 20); and cystoscopy + propofol (group 3, n = 20). This study was approved by Institutional review board of Soonchunhyang University Hospital. *Trial registration* KCT0001260.

Procedures

All patients were placed in the dorsolithotomy position in the operation room. The same two urological surgeons (Jae Heon Kim and Yun Seob Song) performed all cystoscopic ureteral stent removals using a 17.5 Fr rigid cystoscope. Prior to the procedure, the urethra was instilled with 2% lidocaine topical jelly. After 5–10 min, the cystoscope was introduced to the urethra and bladder, and the ureteral stent was removed using foreign body forceps. In the operating room, electrocaridography, noninvasive blood pressure monitoring, and pulse oximetry monitoring were done. Vital signs were checked during the procedure and after the procedure in the day care unit. The presence of complications including oxygen desaturation, autonomic movement, arrythmia, injection pain, and phlebitis were also examined. Before discharge, the patients were asked to rate their comfort level using a visual analog scale (VAS) and satisfaction scale, detailed in the Additional file 1. Recovery from sedation was assessed by the mini-mental state examination (MMSE).

IV administration of ketorolac

Intravenous analgesic administration was performed after lidocaine jelly instillation into the urethra. Intravenous administration of ketorolac 30 mg was used for pain control. Before discharge, the patients were asked to rate their comfort level as described above.

Moderate sedation with midazolam

Midazolam with doses of 3-5 mg (no more than 0.03 mg/kg) was administrated to the subjects after lidocaine jelly instillation. The status of sedation was measured and divided according to five stages, as described in the Additional file 1. Cystoscopy was started when the stage was over three. After the procedure was finished, the midzolam antidote, flumazenil was administrated.

After the procedure, the patient was transferred to day care unit and was discharged when they displayed normal orientation of time and space with vital signs within the normal range.

Deep sedation with propofol

Patients received an injection of 0.2 mg glycopyrollate about 20 min before induction of deep sedation. Sedation was induced with propofol 2 mg/kg without muscle relaxation and was maintained using propofol 10 mg/kg/h. After induction, the anesthesiologist applied a face mask and assisted with ventilation with 100% O_2. After the procedure, the patient was transferred to day care unit and was discharged when they displayed normal orientation of time and space with vital signs within the normal range.

Cost calculation

Cost was described as medical insurance fee and real patient expense. In Korea, due to National Medical Insurance system, a patient may pay 20-100% of total medical insurance fee. Rate of exchange between Korea Won and the US dollar was 1120.6 won for 1 dollar.

Treatment satisfaction

The treatment satisfaction questionnaire included five subscales: "very satisfied", "satisfied", "average", "not satisfied", and "totally not satisfied". These subscales were divided into two groups: "Satisfactory" included "very satisfied" and "satisfied", and "Not satisfactory" included "average", "not satisfied", and "totally not satisfied".

Questionnaire about seeking another method

After the procedure, a questionnaire solicited responses about seeking other pain controlling method. The question asked was "Do you prefer another pain controlling method if it were effective although you could pay more?"

Statistical analyses

Data were analyzed using SAS version 9.1 (SAS Institute, Cary, NC, USA). The Kolmogorov-Smirnov test was used to verify the normality of distribution of continuous variables. Nonparametric tests of comparison were used for variables evaluated as not normally distributed. Median and minimal to maximal range were used as appropriate to describe statistics. Difference testing between groups was performed using Kruskal-Wallis test and Mann–Whitney test as appropriate.

Results

There was no significant difference among blood pressure, pulse rate, O2 saturation during the procedure including those 3 different methods. The differences of pre-operative and post-operative MMSEs including pre-

Table 1 Satisfaction and pain scores among the three groups

	Group 1	Group 2	Group 3	P value
Age	49.50 (26–70)	47.50 (15–70)	49.50 (29–72)	0.731
BMI	26.5 (19.8-31.2)	25.6 (21.4-28.3)	26.0 (22.6-29.4)	0.361
Time duration (min)	11.3 (8.6-30.5)	32.6 (29.6-40.5)	50.4 (45.3-75.4)	0.021
Duaration of procedure (min)	2.3 (1.5-3.3)	2.4 (1.3-3.4)	2.2 (1.0-3.2)	0.243
VAS	8.00 (6–10)*,†	5.00 (1–7)†,‡	0.00 (0–1)*,‡	<0.001
Satisfaction	1 (0–3)*,†	3 (1–5)†,‡	5 (4–5)*,‡	<0.001
Willing to undergo the procedure (VAS)	2 (0–4)*,†	5 (4–8)†,‡	7 (6–9)*,‡	<0.001

Group 1, Cystoscopy + IV analgesics, *Group 2*, Cystoscopy + midazolam, Group 3, Cystoscopy + propofol, *BMI* Body mass index, *VAS* Visual analog pain scale.
Time duration procuedural time + recovery time.
Data are expressed as median number with minimum to maximum number.
P values were analyzed by Kruskal-Wallis test.
*,†,‡:significant differences by Post hoc analysis.

operative and post-operative were not noted among the three groups. The time duration including procedural time and recovery time showed longer in group 2 and 3 than group1 (Table 1).

Group 1 experienced more pain and more dissatisfaction with the procedure than group 2 and group 3. VAS of group 1 was higher than that of group 2 and group 3 (P <0.001) (Table 1). Satisfaction scale of group 1 was lower than that of group 2 and group 3 (P <0.001) (Table 1). Comparison of group 2 and 3 revealed lower VAS in group 3 (P <0.001) and higher satisfaction rate in group 3 (P < 0.001) (Figures 1 and 2).

Total medical insurance fee for group 1, 2, and 3 was US102.63, US108.65, and US218.47, respectively (Table 2). For real patient expense, the cost in the same respective order was US57.94, US61.55, and US119.98 (Table 2). Detailed expenses are provided in Table 2.

Comparison of groups 2 and 3 revealed less pain and higher satisfaction rate in group 3 (P <0.001 for both). In group1, 17 (85%) patients wanted other treatment modalities, whereas in eight of group 2 patients (40%) and no group 3 patients wanted other treatment modalities. Group 1 revealed lower VAS score of willing to undergo the procedure again than group 2 and group 3 (<0.001).

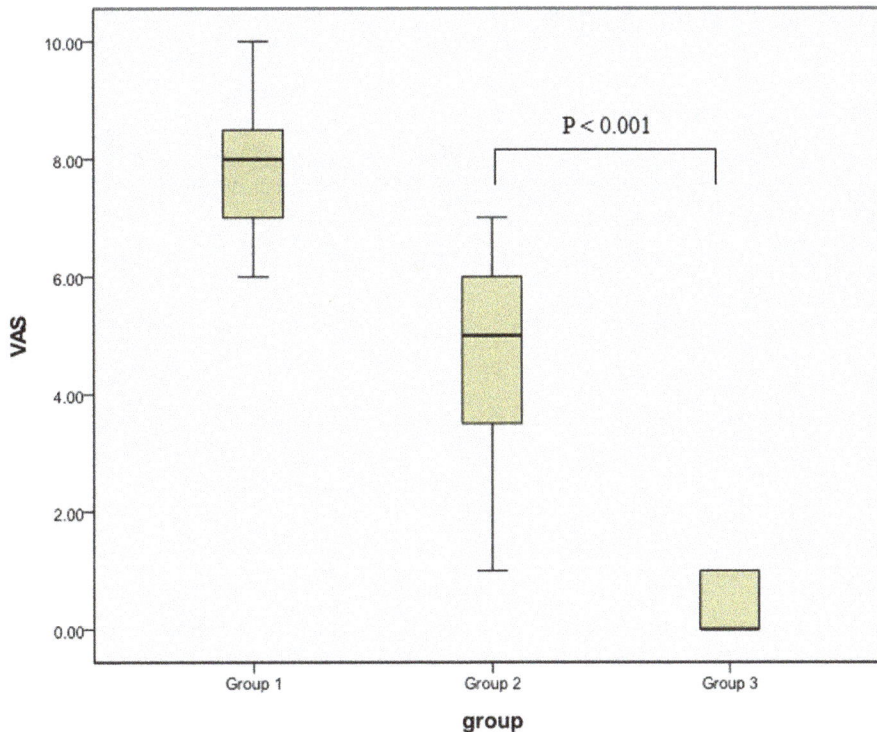

Figure 1 Comparison of VAS among group 1 (cystoscopy + IV analgesics), group 2 (cystoscopy + midazolam), and group 3 (cystoscopy + general anesthesia using propofol).

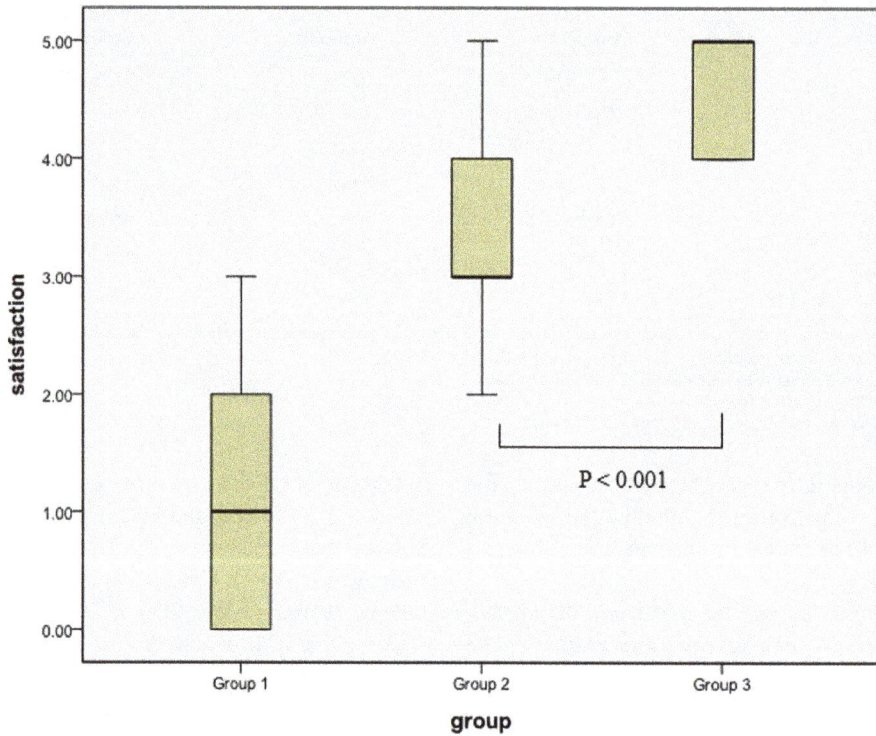

Figure 2 Comparison of satisfaction among group 1 (cystoscopy + IV analgesics), group 2 (cystoscopy + midazolam), and group 3 (cystoscopy + general anesthesia using propofol.

Table 2 Cost expenses among the three groups

	Group 1		Group 2		Group 3	
	Cost (won)	Patient expense (won)	Cost (won)	Patient expense (won)	Cost (won)	Patient expense (won)
Fee for procedure	75,647	45,388	75,647	45,388	75,647	45,388
Consultation fee	13,090	13,090	13,090	13,090	13,090	13,090
Normal saline 1 L	1,099	659	1,099	659	1,099	659
Intravenous injection fee	3,315	663	3,315	663	6,630	1,326
Day care unit					38000	38000
Aneshesia fee					92,950	18,590
Profopol					17,398	17,398
Midazolam			761	456		
Flumazenil			7,868	4,720		
IV NSAIDs	1,889	1,134				
Blood O2 saturation monitoring	5,490	1,098	5,490	1,098		
ECG monitoring	6,460	1,292	6,460	1,292		
Blood pressure monitoring	8,020	1,604	8,020	1,604		
Total costs (won)	115,010	64,928	121,750	68970	244,814	134,451
Total costs (US dollar)	102.63	57.94	108.65	61.55	218.47	119.98

Gourp 1 Cystoscopy + IV analgesics, *Group 2* Cystoscopy + midazolam, *Group 3* Cystoscopy + propofol, *ECG* electrocardiography, *NSAIDS* non-steroidal anti-inflammatory drugs.

Group 2 showed also lower VAS score of willing to undergo the procedure again than group 3 (<0.001) (Table 1).

Discussion

Cystscopy is the standard technique used to removal or exchange a ureteral stent. In addition to the large diameter of cystoscopies, which can induce pain, several conditions make this technique more difficult, especially in male patients, due to the longer urethra and prostatic enlargement.

Several retrograde methods without conventional cystoscopy have been developed [7-10]. Successful outcomes have been reported using retrograde ureteral stent removal or change under fluoroscopic guidance, but most patients in these studies were female, and only one study included male patients [10].

Ureteroscopy is one of the most common methods to treat urinary stones [11]. In many cases, ureteral stent insertion follows ureteroscopy [1]. Although cystoscopic ureteral stent removal is common, discomfort associated with the procedure is unclear. Our study is the first clinical trial to address this issue.

Local anesthesia has long been used in men undergoing rigid cystoscopy. Recent reports indicated that lidocaine gel has no effect on pain during cystoscopy [7-11]. The diverse efficacy of lidocaine gel may be because the absorption of topical lidocaine is slow and incomplete. Several groups have demonstrated that maximal lidocaine absorption requires 15 to 60 minutes [5,12].

To overcome this limited effect of lidocaine jelly, several methods have been introduced such as sleep induction using midazolam, pain killers, or listening to music [4,6,13]. Midazolam is a well-known sedative drug with amnesic properties. Previous studies have demonstrated that midazolam can yield anterograde amnesia without retrograde amnesia [14-17]. Midazolam produces the immediate onset of anterograde amnesia in patients, which could be useful in forgetting the painful events [14].

One of the prominent features of our study was that, for the first time, we adapted a propofol in cystoscopy or cysoscopic ureteral stent removal. Propofol is safe and effective during gastrointestinal endoscopy procedures [18,19]. Moreover, it has been associated with shorter recovery time, better sedation, and lack of a harmful effect on cardiopulmonary function. Our study showed that both the group with midazolam and propofol showed longer time duration but the differences were not large. Considering the nature of pilot study to use propofol, we had assistance of anesthetic department for safety. In the future, the procedures using propofol might be feasible in outpatient department.

In this study, the satisfaction was the greatest in the group with using propofol. Cystoscopic procedure with IV pain killers was not effective at all. Procedures using

midazolam yielded less pain and greater satisfaction than procedures with IV pain relievers. Patients treated with propofol reported the greatest satisfaction despite spending additional recovery time in the day care unit.

Moreover, the gap of real expense among the three groups was not large. This is might be due to a unique medical insurance system in Korea. The gap difference of cost should be validated in other countries with different medical systems.

The present study has several limitations. We did not assess the pain felt by patients during each step of the procedure. Moreover, the sample size was relatively small, and the study was not blinded for patients and physicians, which could result in some bias in data interpretation or reporting of satisfaction and pain levels. Second, the sample size was relatively small but owing to its nature of pilot study, the differences of main outcomes among each groups were definite.

Conclusions

Urologists have to pay more concern to cystscopic ureteral stent removal. With the traditional methods of lidocaine jelly and pain killers, patients have to suffer from pain and discomfort. Midazolam and propofol could be a options to control both. Considering the safety and the high prevalence of use of midazolam and propofol, urologists should not hesitate to adapt new methods in pain control during cystoscopic ureteral stent removal.

Competing interests
The authors declare that they have no competing interests.

Authors' contributions
JHK and YSS contributed with the conception and design of the study and drafted the manuscript, JHK, YSS, HC, DS, SWC, MKL, and SYP collected data and performed the analyses. All authors read and approved the final manuscript.

Acknowledgement
This work was supported by Soonchunhyang Univeristy Research Fund.

Author details
[1]Department of Urology, Soonchunhyang University Hospital, 657 Hannam-Dong, Yongsan-Gu, Seoul 140-743, Korea. [2]Department of Anesthesiology and Pain Medicine, Soonchunhyang University Hospital, Seoul, Korea. [3]Department of Urology, Korea University Hospital, Ansan, Korea. [4]Department of Surgery, Soonchunhyang University Hospital, Seoul, Korea.

References
1. Tang L, Gao X, Xu B, Hou J, Zhang Z, Xu C, Wang L, Sun Y: Placement of ureteral stent after uncomplicated ureteroscopy: do we really need it? *Urology* 2011, **78**:1248–1256.
2. Wetton CW, Gedroyc WM: Retrograde radiologic retrieval and replacement of double-J ureteric stents. *Clin Radiol* 1995, **50**:562–565.

3.   Park SW, Cha IH, Hong SJ, Yi JG, Jeon HJ, Park JH, Park SJ: **Fluoroscopy guided transurethral removal and exchange of ureteral stents in female patients: technical notes.** *J Vasc Interv Radiol* 2007, **18**:251–256.
4.   Demir E, Kilciler M, Bedir S, Erken U: **Patient tolerance during cystoscopy: a randomized study comparing lidocaine hydrochloride gel and dimethyl sulfoxide with lidocaine.** *J Endourol* 2008, **22**:1027–1029.
5.   Axelsson K, Jozwiak H, Lingårdh G, Schönebeck J, Widman B: **Blood concentration of lignocaine after application of 2% lignocaine gel in the urethra.** *Br J Urol* 1983, **55**:64–68.
6.   Song YS, Song ES, Kim KJ, Park YH, Ku JH: **Midazolam anesthesia during rigid and flexible cystoscopy.** *Urol Res* 2007, **35**:139–142.
7.   Birch BR, Ratan P, Morley R, Cumming J, Smart CJ, Jenkins JD: **Flexible cystoscopy in men: is topical anaesthesia with lignocaine gel worthwhile?** *Br J Urol* 1994, **73**:155–159.
8.   McFarlane N, Denstedt J, Ganapathy S, Razvi H: **Randomized trial of 10 mL and 20 mL of 2% intraurethral lidocaine gel and placebo in men undergoing flexible cystoscopy.** *J Endourol* 2001, **15**:541–544.
9.   Stein M, Lubetkin D, Taub HC, Skinner WK, Haberman J, Kreutzer ER: **The effects of intraurethral lidocaine anesthetic and patient anxiety on pain perception during cystoscopy.** *J Urol* 1994, **151**:1518–1521.
10. Chen YT, Hsiao PJ, Wong WY, Wang CC, Yang SS, Hsieh CH: **Randomized double-blind comparison of lidocaine gel and plain lubricating gel in relieving pain during flexible cystoscopy.** *J Endourol* 2005, **19**:163–166.
11. Kobayashi T, Nishizawa K, Mitsumori K, Ogura K: **Instillation of anesthetic gel is no longer necessary in the era of flexible cystoscopy: a crossover study.** *J Endourol* 2004, **18**:483–486.
12. Ouellette RD, Blute R Sr, Jaffee S, Bahde C: **Plasma concentration of lidocaine resulting from instillation of lidocaine jelly into genitourinary tract prior to cystoscopy.** *Urology* 1985, **25**:490–495.
13. Yeo JK, Cho DY, Oh MM, Park SS, Park MG: **Listening to music during cystoscopy decreases anxiety, pain, and dissatisfaction in patients: a pilot randomized controlled trial.** *J Endourol* 2013, **27**:459–462.
14. Dundee JW, Wilson DB: **Amnesic action of midazolam.** *Anaesthesia* 1980, **35**:459–461.
15. Koht A, Moss JI: **Does midazolam cause retrograde amnesia, and can Xumazenil reverse that amnesia?** *Anesth Analg* 1997, **85**:211–212.
16. Twersky RS, Hartung J, Berger BJ, McClain J, Beaton C: **Midazolam enhances anterograde but not retrograde amnesia in pediatric patients.** *Anesthesiology* 1993, **78**:51–55.
17. Bulach R, Myles PS, Russnak M: **Double-blind randomized controlled trial to determine extent of amnesia with midazolam given immediately before general anaesthesia.** *Br J Anaesth* 2005, **94**:300–305.
18. Qadeer MA, Vargo JJ, Khandwala F, Lopez R, Zuccaro G: **Propofol versus traditional sedative agents for gastrointestinal endoscopy: a meta-analysis.** *Clin Gastroenterol Hepatol* 2005, **11**:1049–1056.
19. Bo LL, Bai Y, Bian JJ, Wen PS, Li JB, Deng XM: **Propofol vs traditional sedative agents for endoscopic retrograde cholangiopancreatography: a meta-analysis.** *World J Gastroenterol* 2011, **17**:3538–3543.

Disease-specific outcomes of Radical Prostatectomies in Northern Norway; a case for the impact of perineural infiltration and postoperative PSA-doubling time

Sigve Andersen[1,2*†], Elin Richardsen[3,4†], Yngve Nordby[1,5], Nora Ness[3], Øystein Størkersen[6], Khalid Al-Shibli[7], Tom Donnem[1,2], Helena Bertilsson[8,9], Lill-Tove Busund[3,4], Anders Angelsen[8,9] and Roy M Bremnes[1,2]

Abstract

Background: Prostate cancer is the most common male malignancy and a mayor cause of mortality in the western world. The impact of clinicopathological variables on disease related outcomes have mainly been reported from a few large US series, most of them not reporting on perineural infiltration. We therefore wanted to investigate relevant cancer outcomes in patients undergoing radical prostatectomy in two Norwegian health regions with an emphasis on the impact of perineural infiltration (PNI) and prostate specific antigen- doubling time (PSA-DT).

Methods: We conducted a retrospective analysis of 535 prostatectomy patients at three hospitals between 1995 and 2005 estimating biochemical failure- (BFFS), clinical failure- (CFFS) and prostate cancer death-free survival (PCDFS) with the Kaplan-Meier method. We investigated clinicopathological factors influencing risk of events using cox proportional hazard regression.

Results: After a median follow-up of 89 months, 170 patients (32%) experienced biochemical failure (BF), 36 (7%) experienced clinical failure and 15 (3%) had died of prostate cancer. pT-Stage (p = 0.001), preoperative PSA (p = 0.047), Gleason Score (p = 0.032), non-apical positive surgical margins (PSM) (p = 0.003) and apical PSM (p = 0.031) were all independently associated to BFFS. Gleason score (p = 0.019), PNI (p = 0.012) and non-apical PSM (p = 0.002) were all independently associated to CFFS while only PNI (P = 0.047) and subgroups of Gleason score were independently associated to PCDFS. After BF, patients with a shorter PSA-DT had independent and significant worse event-free survivals than patients with PSA-DT > 15 months (PSA-DT = 3-9 months, CFFS HR = 6.44, p < 0.001, PCDFS HR = 13.7, p = 0.020; PSA-DT < 3 months, CFFS HR = 11.2, p < 0.001, PCDFS HR = 27.5, p = 0.006).

Conclusions: After prostatectomy, CFFS and PCDFS are variable, but both are strongly associated to Gleason score and PNI. In patients with BF, PSA-DT was most strongly associated to CF and PCD. Our study adds weight to the importance of PSA-DT and re-launches PNI as a strong prognosticator for clinically relevant endpoints.

* Correspondence: sigve.andersen@uit.no
[†]Equal contributors
[1]Institute of Clinical Medicine, The Arctic University of Norway, Tromso, Norway
[2]Department Oncology, University Hospital of North Norway, Tromso 9038, Norway
Full list of author information is available at the end of the article

Background

Prostate cancer (PC) is the most common male malignancy and the second most common cause of cancer mortality in Norway [1]. It is presently the most prevalent cancer and there has been an increasing incidence until 2007 where after a reduction was noted [1]. When PSA was widely introduced in Norway in the early 1990s, an increasing number of men were diagnosed and treated with curative intent (33% in 2001) [2]. Although declining, Norway has the highest mortality rate of all western countries [3,4]. There has been an increasing use of radical prostatectomy (RP), but a majority of patients diagnosed with PC will not have symptomatic disease or die of the disease as they have non-lethal P [5]. The reduced risk of prostate cancer specific mortality after a radical prostatectomy compared to watchful waiting has been estimated to range between 0-25% depending on tumor characteristics [6]. The only RCT evidence for a reduction in prostate cancer mortality is the SPCG-4 trial [7].

Disease-specific survival after RP has mainly been reported from a number of single institutions, but a few studies have reported on larger cohorts and three studies have described survival in nationwide cohorts in Europe [8-10]. Some of these larger studies lack sufficient follow-up, relevant prognostic parameters and clinically relevant end-points in the analysis.

Clinicopathological variables for predicting disease outcome after RP are numerous with Gleason grade and score, pTNM-stage, preoperative PSA and surgical margins as the most widely adopted ones [11,12]. User-friendly predictive tools like look-up tables, risk classifications and nomograms have been developed [11,13]. Some variables like lymphovascular invasion [14], tumor volume [15], pT2 subclassification [16] and tertiary Gleason grade [17] are conflicting or have insufficient supporting data yet.

For patients with biochemical failure (BF) there are several treatment options including continuous, intermittent or deferred androgen deprivation, salvage irradiation of the prostate bed and trial participation. To choose the optimal therapy for these patients it is crucial to understand the risk factors for a subsequent clinical failure or death of PC, especially since management strategy remains controversial [18-20]. After BF, PSA kinetics, or more specifically PSA-Doubling Time (PSA-DT), has emerged as a prognostic variable [21-25]. However, as a pretreatment marker, PSA-DT has not found its position [26,27].

The objective of the present study was to describe disease outcome data for patients operated in the PSA era in three urological centers in two major health regions in Norway, and to examine the impact of post-prostatectomy PSA-DT on clinical outcomes.

Methods
Patients

671 patients were retrospectively identified with RPs for adenocarcinoma of the prostate between 01.01.1995 to 31.12.2005 from the archives of the Departments of Pathology at St. Olav Hospital/Trondheim University Hospital (St. Olav) (n = 341), Nordlandssykehuset Bodo (NLSH) (n = 63) and the University Hospital of Northern Norway (UNN) (n = 267). Of these, 131 patients were excluded due to non-available tissue blocks for re-evaluation (St. Olav n = 112, NLSH n = 3, UNN n = 15), four patients were excluded due to other cancers (not superficial skin cancers) within 5 years of diagnosis (UNN n = 4), one patient was excluded due to previous radiotherapy to the pelvic region (NLSH) and one patient due to lack of follow-up data (St. Olav). Thus, 535 eligible patients had complete follow-up data and tissue blocks for re-evaluation. Preoperative clinical TNM staging was unevenly stated in the medical files and data are therefore not presented.

Definition of end-points and clinical variables

The preoperative PSA values were assessed right before surgery, except for those few patients who underwent transurethral resection of the prostate (TUR-P) prior to the RP. For these patients the PSA value before the TUR-P was used. PC was an incidental finding in these patients.

BF was defined as PSA ≥0.4 ng/ml in at least two consecutive postoperative blood samples according to Stephenson et al. [28]. Clinical failure (CF) was defined as verified symptomatic locally advanced progression after radical treatments and/or metastasis to bone, visceral organs or lymph nodes on CT, MR, bone scan or ultrasonography. Prostate cancer death (PCD) was defined as death with progressive and disseminated castration-resistant PC despite therapy. PSA-DT was calculated by the online available MSKCC-calculator (http://nomograms.mskcc.org/Prostate/PsaDoublingTime.aspx) which calculates a regression slope on the basis of all PSA values taken using natural log of 2 (0.693) divided by the slope of the relationship between the log of PSA and time of PSA measurement for each patient in months [24]. Up to four separate (at least 6 weeks apart) PSA measurements before supplementary treatment (endocrine therapy, radiotherapy or chemotherapy) were included. Optimal cut-off points for stratification of PSA-DT have been varying between reporters. We used cut-off values as the largest reported patient series to date from Johns Hopkins [21]. Hence, the four groups of patients with significantly differing prognosis for both CF and PCD were patients with PSA-DT < 3 months, 3–9 months, 9–15 months and >15 months.

Postoperative follow-up (FU) protocols were not completely uniform in the participating hospitals, but all FUs included PSA measurements and clinical examinations (including digital rectal examination in PSA recurrence) every three months for the first year, every six months for the second year and once yearly for the following years. Imaging with CT, MRI or radio nucleotide bone scans was done upon symptoms or rising PSA.

The follow-up of patients was done by examining the patient medical files at the operating centers and the patients' local hospital. Biochemical failure free survival (BFFS) was calculated from the date of surgery to the last FU date for BF, which was the last date of a measured PSA. Clinical failure free survival (CFFS) was calculated from the date of surgery to the last FU date for CF, which was the last date without symptoms or any evidence of metastasis. Prostate cancer death free survival (PCDFS) was calculated from the date of surgery to the date of death.

Tissues

All prostate specimens were re-evaluated regarding to histopathological variables and re-staged according to the 2010 revision of the TNM classification [29] independently by two experienced pathologists (E.R, L.T.B). A positive surgical margin (PSM) was defined as tumor extension to the inked surface of the resected specimen [30-32]. Tumor size was measured as the largest diameter of the index tumor and was used due to previous observations of excellent correlation to PC volume [15]. Median tumor size was 20 mm and was set as cut-off in further analyses. Perineural infiltration (PNI) was defined as tumor cells within the perineural space adjacent to a nerve *outside* of the prostate capsule. Lymphovascular infiltration (LVI) was defined as tumor cells found within lymphatic or blood vessels. Gleason grading was re-graded according to the 2005 International Society of Urological Pathology Modified Gleason System [33].

Statistical methods

Analyses for the patients with BF regarding the impact of PSA-DT on CFFS and PCDFS required the baseline date to be changed to date of BF as opposed to date of surgery for the other analyses.

The SPSS version 20 was used for the statistical analyses (Chicago, IL. USA). The non-parametric Spearman correlation coefficient (r) was used to calculate correlations between variables and only moderate or strong correlations (r > 0.3) are described. χ^2 statistics were utilized for distribution differences between groups. Plots of the event-free survivals were drawn using the Kaplan-Meier method, and the statistical significance between survival curves was assessed by the log-rank test. Univariate analyses for the various endpoints (Table 1) according to clinical and histopathological variables were done. Significant variables (bold text in Table 1) were entered in the multivariate analyses for all patients (Table 2). The backward Cox regression analysis was used with a probability for stepwise entry and removal at 0.05 and 0.10, respectively. A p-value < 0.05

was considered statistically significant for all analyses. For the patients with BF (Table 3), all significant variables from the univariate analyses for both CF and PCD, were entered in the multivariate analysis These were tumor size, the margin variables, PNI, LVI, pT stage, pN stage and Gleason score. Due to the low number of events for PCD (15 events) we used an enter model with manual inclusion and removal of variables to identify the three most significant variables (Gleason score, PNI and positive non-apical margin) before entering them into the models.

Ethics

This study was approved by the regional ethics committee, REK Nord, project application 2009/1393.

Results

Patient characteristics

Median age at surgery was 62 years (range 45–75), median follow-up of survivors was 89 months (range 6.3-188.3). 279 patients underwent a limited lymphadenectomy.

The pT2 group (n = 374) was sub-classified to pT2a (n = 139; 37%), pT2b (n = 34; 9%) and pT2c (n = 201; 54%). pT stage was correlated to PNI (r = 0.33, p < 0.001), T-Size (r = 0.30, p < 0.001) and positive non-apical margin (r = 0.373 p < 0.001).

Indications for lymph node dissection were not predetermined for the centers involved, but was done according to the surgeons preference which mostly was if Partin nomograms indicated >10% risk of N1 disease or Gleason ≥8, PSA ≥10 or suspected cT3. Three patients were found to have discrete metastasis in regional lymph nodes at re-evaluation (paraffin embedded tissue) of initial frozen-section-negative lymph nodes.

Preoperative PSA was available for 542 of 548 (99%) patients. Median value was 8.8 ng/ml (range 0.7-104.3). The variable was dichotomized with PSA = 10 ng/ml as chosen cut-off.

Distributions of Gleason scores are presented in Table 1. Patients with Gleason 4 + 5 (n = 26; 5%), Gleason 5 + 4 (n = 6; 1%) and Gleason 5 + 5 (n = 3, <1%) were pooled in the Gleason ≥9 group due to the low number of these patients. In patients with BF, Gleason score correlated inversely with PSA-DT (r = –0.37, p <0.001)

The maximum diameter of the index tumor (T-Size) had a median value of 20 mm (range 2–50). T-Size correlated significantly with pT stage (r = 0.30 p < 0.001). We explored the prognostic value of T-Size in the pT2 subgroup, but no significant association to event-free-survival was found in univariate analyses and the variable was consequently not entered into multivariate analysis.

PNI correlated to LVI (r = 0.393, p < 0.001), and pT stage (r = 0.33, p < 0.001 77 (14%) patients of the patients had both apical and non-apical PSM. There was a significant

Table 1 Patient characteristics and clinicopathological variables, and their prognostic value for the three endpoints in 535 prostate cancer patients (univariate analyses; log rank test)

Characteristic	Patients (n)	Patients (%)	BF (170 events)		CF (36 events)		PCD (15 events)	
			5-year EFS (%)	p	10-year EFS (%)	p	10-year EFS (%)	p
Age				0.55		0.085		0.600
≤ 65 years	357	67	76		92		97	
> 65 years	178	33	70		88		96	
pT-stage				<0.001		<0.001		0.027
pT2	374	70	83		96		98	
pT3a	114	21	60		86		98	
pT3b	47	9	43		73		89	
pN-stage				<0.001		<0.001		<0.001
NX	264	49	79		95		98	
N0	268	50	71		89		97	
N1	3	1	0		33		67	
Preop PSA				<0.001		0.085		0.061
PSA < 10	308	57	80		93		99	
PSA > 10	221	42	67		88		95	
Missing	6	1	-		-		-	
Gleason				<0.001		<0.001		0.001
3 + 3	183	34	83		98		99	
3 + 4	220	41	76		93		98	
4 + 3	80	15	69		84		95	
4 + 4	19	4	63		76		94	
≥9	33	6	34		67		87	
Tumor size				<0.001		0.019		0.098
0-20 mm	250	47	82		94		99	
>20 mm	285	53	67		88		96	
PNI				<0.001		<0.001		0.002
No	401	75	79		95		98	
Yes	134	25	60		81		93	
PSM				0.041		0.038		0.697
No	249	47	81		94		97	
Yes	286	53	69		89		97	
Non-apical PSM				<0.001		<0.001		0.029
No	381	71	81		95		98	
Yes	154	29	57		81		94	
Apical PSM				0.04		0.484		0.31
No	325	61	73		90		96	
Yes	210	39	77		92		98	
LVI				<0.001		<0.001		0.009
No	492	92	77		93		98	
Yes	43	8	46		71		88	

Table 1 Patient characteristics and clinicopathological variables, and their prognostic value for the three endpoints in 535 prostate cancer patients (univariate analyses; log rank test) *(Continued)*

Surgical proc				0.23	0.41	0.581
Retropubic	435	81	76	90	97	
Perineal	100	19	67	95	98	

Abbreviations: *BF* biochemical failure, *CF* Clinical failure, *EFS* event free survival in months, *LVI* lymphovascular infiltration, *PCD* prostate cancer death, *NR* not reached, *P* P value for log rank statistic for difference in event free survival, *PC* Prostate cancer, *PNI* Perineural infiltration, *Post op RT* postoperative radiotherapy, *Preop* preoperative, *PSA* Prostate specific antigen, *PSM* Positive surgical margin, *Surgical proc* surgical procedure. Significant p-values in bold (threshold p ≤ 0.05).

decline of PSMs for RPs performed during the latter part of the period (χ^2, $p < 0.001$). During the period 1995–2000 129/197 (66%) patients had PSM while in the period 2001–2005 162/351 (46%) patients had PSM. LVI correlated with PNI and to pT stage ($r = 0.33$, $p < 0.001$.

In pT3 patients, 109 of 161 (68%) patients had PSM while 182 of 387 (47%) pT2 patients had PSM. There was a significant association with operating center (χ^2, $p < 0.001$) with St. Olav having the lowest PSM rates.

In non-apical PSM, PSA correlated significantly with pT stage ($r = 0.373$, $p < 0.001$).

When stratifying for pT stage non-apical PSM had a significant impact in pT3a patients ($p = 0.001$), but not in pT2 ($p = 0.69$) or pT3b patients ($p = 0.075$).

Table 2 Multivariate analyses in models including significant univariate analyses for all patients (Cox regression, backward conditional)

Characteristic	BF (170 events)[†]			CF (36 events)			PCD (15 events)*		
	HR	CI95%	p	HR	CI95%	p	HR	CI95%	p
pT-stage			**0.001**	NS			NS		
pT2	1								
pT3a	1.70	1.14-2.54	**0.010**						
pT3b	2.40	1.45-3.97	**0.001**						
Preop PSA				NE			NS		
PSA < 10	1								
PSA > 10	1.39	1.01-1.91	**0.047**						
Gleason			**0.032**			**0.019**			0.087
3 + 3	1			1			1		
3 + 4	1.05	0.70-1.56	0.81	2.45	0.78-6.90	0.09	3.71	0.41-33.2	0.242
4 + 3	1.55	0.97-2.47	0.07	2.87	0.91-9.10	0.07	10.47	1.21-90.7	**0.033**
4 + 4	1.42	0.68-2.97	0.36	2.73	0.52-14.2	0.23	7.43	0.46-121	0.159
≥9	2.39	1.31-4.35	**0.004**	6.74	2.21-20.6	**0.001**	15.26	1.65-141	**0.016**
PNI			0.090			**0.012**			**0.047**
No	1			1			1		
Yes	1.35	0.95-1.92		2.48	1.23-5.04		3.17	1.02-9.87	
Non-apical PSM[±]			**0.003**			**0.002**	NS		
No	1			1					
Yes	1.70	1.20-2.40		3.22	1.56-6.64				
Apical PSM[±]			**0.031**	NE			NS		
No	1								
Yes	0.69	0.49-0.97							

Significant p-values in bold (threshold p ≤ 0.05).
Abbreviations: *BF* biochemical failure, *CF* Clinical failure, *LVI* lymphovascular infiltration, *NE* not entered, due to non-significance in the univariate analyses, *NS* not significant, the characteristic is removed by the backward conditional analysis due to insignificance, *PCD* prostate cancer death, *PNI* Perineural infiltration, *Post op RT* postoperative radiotherapy, *Preop* preoperative, *PSA* Prostate specific antigen, *PSM* Positive surgical margin.
[†]Tumor Size, pN-stage and LVI were removed by the backward conditional model due to insignificance in all models.
[±]Only the subgroups (apical/non-apical PSM) of PSM were entered.
*Due to the low number of events the model was carefully analyzed in advance with the inclusion and removal of variables in an enter analysis to find the most significant in advance before doing the final model with the three variables; Gleason score, perineural infiltration and positive non-apical margin.

Table 3 Multivariate analysis including significant univariate analyses for the 170 patients with biochemical failure (Cox regression, backward conditional)

	Patients		CF (36 events)[†]					PCD (15 events)*				
	N	(%)	5-year EFS (%)	HR	CI95%	p	Events (N)	10-year EFS (%)	HR	CI95%	p	Events (N)
PSA-DT						<0.001					0.029	
Missing	12	7	-	NE			3	-	NE			0
>15	71	42	98	1	Ref		5	93	1	Ref		1
9-14.9	27	16	77	3.28	0.9-11.9	0.09	5	86	4.60	0.41-52.0	0.22	2
3-8,9	46	27	69	6.44	2.26-18.3	**<0.001**	16	70	13.7	1.51-124	**0.020**	8
<3	14	8	59	11.2	3.35-37.7	**<0.001**	7	49	27.5	2.64-286	**0.006**	4
pN-stage						0.002					0.020	
NX	69	41		1	Ref		9		1	Ref		3
N0	98	57		1.38	0.61-3.13	0.45	24		1.20	0.31-4.59	0.80	11
N1	3	2		19.1	3.69-100	**<0.001**	2		32.5	2.61-405	**0.007**	1

Significant p-values in bold (threshold p ≤ 0.05).

Abbreviations: *BF* biochemical failure, *CF* Clinical failure, *NS* not significant, the characteristic is removed by the backward conditional analysis due to insignificance, *NE* not entered, *PCD* prostate cancer death, *PSA* Prostate specific antigen, *PSA-DT* PSA doubling time in months; [†]a positive non-apical margin, PNI, vasc inf, pT stage and Gleason were removed by the backward conditional model due to insignificance in all models. *Due to the low number of events the model was carefully analyzed in advance with the inclusion and removal of variables in an enter analysis to find the most significant in advance before doing the final model with the three variables; PSA-DT, Gleason score and pN-stage.

Events and PSA-DT

170 patients had BF during FU. Of these, 31 patients never reached postoperative PSA nadir < 0.4 ng/ml. When removing these patients (143 patients left) the median time to BF was 35 months (range 2.8-164). For CF patients the median time from BF to CF was 38.2 months (range 0–130.7). For PCD patients the median time from BF to PCD was 72.2 months (range 34.4-147). Kaplan-Meier curves illustrates event-free survivals are in Figure 1.

PSA data before salvage therapy was retrievable for 158 out of 170 patients with BF to calculate PSA-DT. Median PSA-DT was 13.6 months (range 0.4-332). Quartile cut-off values were 5.5, 13.4, and 23.9 months. We used the previously published cut-offs regarding PSA-DT [21] as these in our cohort reliably divided the patients into subgroups with differing hazard ratios for CF or PCD. PSA-DT correlated inversely with Gleason score (r = –0.37, p < 0.001) (Figure 2). Kaplan-Meier curves illustrating event-free survivals according to different PSA doubling times are in Figure 2.

For validation we did subgroup analyses stratifying for health regions. The results were highly significant in both Helse Nord (p < 0.001) and Helse Midt (p = 0.004).

Among the 36 (7%) patients with CF, 13 patients had symptomatic locally advanced progression, 18 had bone metastasis and 5 had regional lymph node metastasis. Median time to CF after RP was 64 months (range 15–159).

Concerning CF, 8/33 events (24%) were in patients with PSA-DT < 3 months and 23/33 events (70%) were in patients with PSA-DT less than 9 months. For PCD, 4/15 events were in patients with PSA-DT < 3 months and 12/15 events were in the patients with PSA-DT less than 9 months.

15 patients died of PC leaving 43/58 (74%) patients to have died of other causes at a mean time of 76 months after RP.

Impact of surgical center

Patients had their RP at one of three hospitals: UNN (n = 248, St.Olav (n = 228) and NLSB (n = 59). There was no statistical significant differences in risk of CF (p = 0.40) and PCD (p = 0.973) between the centers.

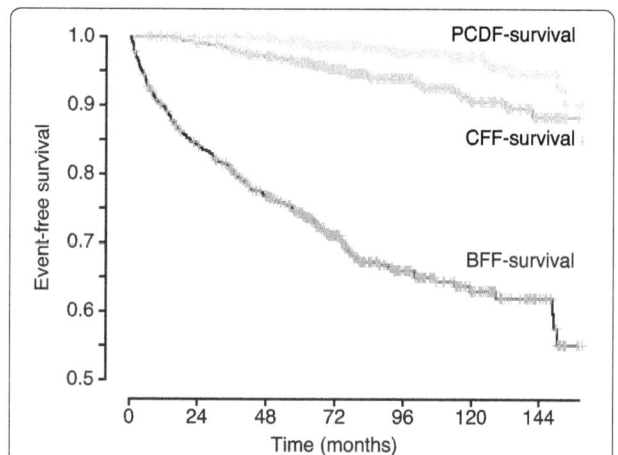

Figure 1 Overlapping Kaplan-Meier curves, each illustrating event-free survival for the whole cohort for the specific event. Note that the Y-axis has been modified with a proportion of 0.5 as the origin to better illustrate the differences. PCDF-survival = Prostate cancer death free-survival; CFF-survival = Clinical failure free-survival; BFF = Biochemical failure free-survival.

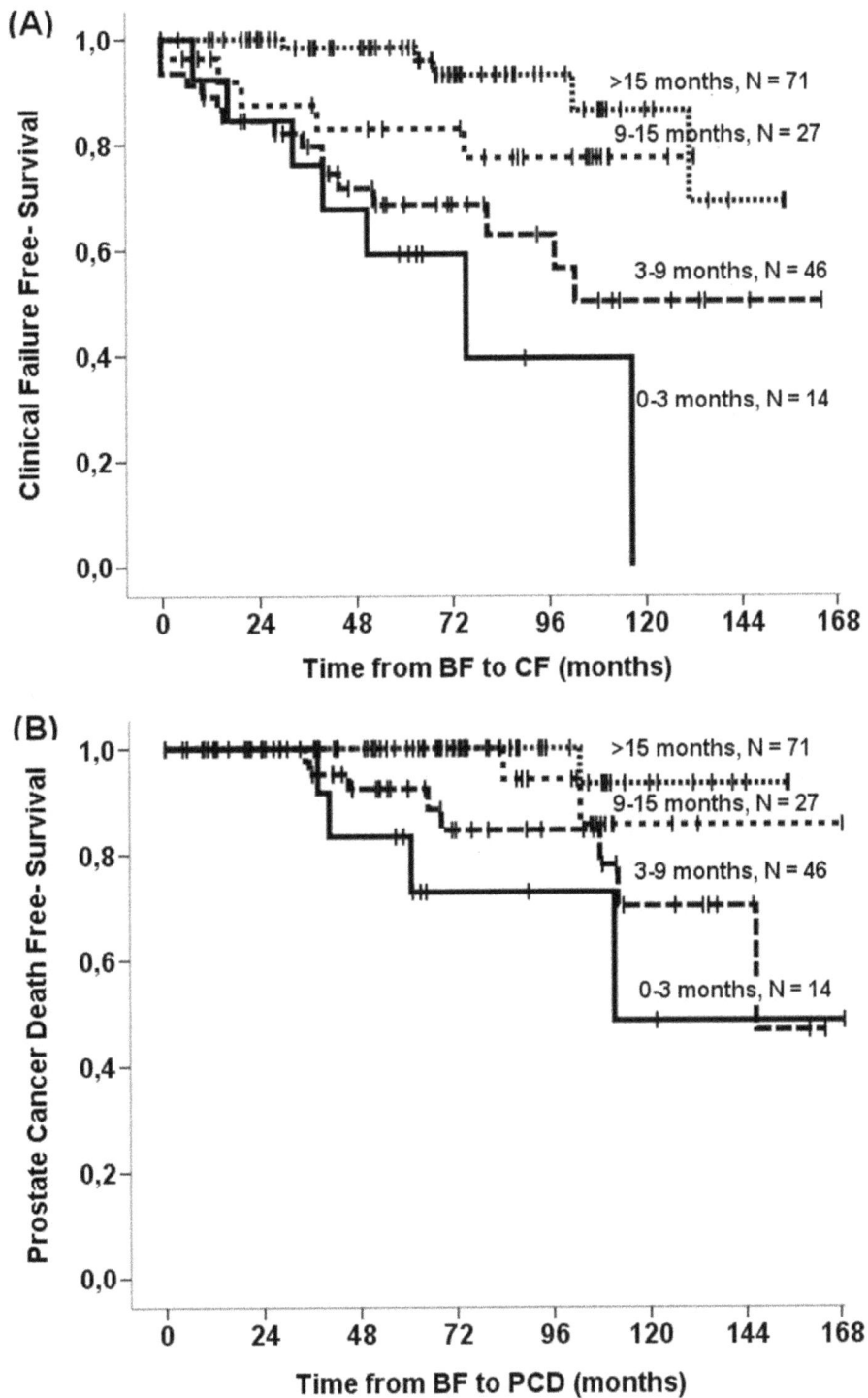

Figure 2 Kaplan-Meier curves of patients experiencing biochemical failure for (A) Clinical failure free-survival stratified by PSA-doubling time categories and (B) Prostate cancer death free-survival stratified by PSA-doubling time. See Table 3 for details regarding hazard levels and level of significance.

Discussion

This is the first large Scandinavian multicenter study presenting the impact of prognostic variable information regarding BF, CF and PCD in Scandinavia in the PSA era. We found post RP PSA-DT to be a strong predictor of CF and PCD, even outperforming Gleason score. In addition we found PNI to be an independently strong predictor of all event-free survivals. Otherwise we found the prognostic factors in this material to be mostly consistent to previously published larger series [34-36].

The strength of this paper is the unselected study population from Central and Northern Norway. It is reasonable to assess that more than 95% of men diagnosed with PC in this geographical area, were operated in hospitals that participated in this study. Moreover, the study has a relatively long FU, only patients in the PSA era were included, all tissues have been re-evaluated by two experienced pathologists, few patients had missing PSA-DT information, we have included relevant prognostic factors, and adjuvant treatment after RP was rare in the timeframe of this study. Weaknesses of the study are the retrospective design, the probable impact of salvage radiotherapy on the risk of time to events and events are low at longer follow-up times, contributing to low precision and large CIs (Tables 2 and 3). In addition, a number of tissue blocks were missing from one center, thereby reducing representativity.

Like other studies, we have found that the time from RP to CF and death of PC to be extensive, even in patients with a BF [21,37]. Prognostic factors to stratify patients for risk-adapted follow-up, treatment regimens or clinical trials are crucial since the majority of operated patients will not have BF. Furthermore an even greater majority will not experience symptoms of their disease and only a very few will die of PC. On the other hand, it will be important to identify those patients who otherwise will have symptoms from the recurrent disease or die. Another interesting observation is that the involved surgeons seem very capable to select patients for surgery with a long expected survival as only 8% patients died of other causes during follow up.

Our observation of post-prostatectomy PSA-DT as the strongest predictor of CF and PCD in patients with BF is consistent with numerous other studies recognizing the importance of PSA-DT as a predictor of CF [21,22,38] and PCD [37,39,40] after RP. We found the same pattern in both health regions, thereby internally validating these results. The importance of PSA-DT in patients treated with radiotherapy has also been reported [41]. In accordance with Antonarakis et al. we found patients in the two lowest PSA-DT categories (<3 months and 3–8,9 months) to have the worst prognosis with comparable Hazards ratios in the multivariable analysis. 64% of CF events and 80% of PCD deaths were in these two groups even though they collectively constituted only around 1/3 of the patients (35%). Although there was a correlation between Gleason Score and PSA-DT we saw the same trends of poor event-free survival when stratified for Gleason Score subgroups, but numbers were statistically insignificant due to the low number of patients in each subgroup. Our observation adds weight and validates the importance of PSA-DT for selecting BF-patients at high risk of developing clinically significant disease in the future.

At time of diagnosis, Gleason score has been shown to be a strong predictor of high risk PC [42], but also metastasis and PCD after RP [38,43]. Including all patients in the analyses we consistently found patients with a Gleason sum ≥9 to have the highest risk of BF (equal to pT3b), CF and PCD. This highlights a major impact of Gleason score in risk stratification following RP. Some have, however, suggested that Gleason score loses its value after including PSA-DT in the risk-stratification [44]. Analyzing patients with BF only, the PSA-DT removed Gleason score from the step-wise multivariate analyses due to its co-variation and prognostic strength. Antonarakis et al. found both Gleason score and PSA-DT to contribute to estimate metastasis free-survival [21] although PSA-DT was the strongest predictor.

Herein, extraprostatic PNI was in addition to Gleason score the only clinicopathological variable to predict both CF and PCD. Patients with an observed extraprostatic PNI had estimated HRs of CF and PCD at around 3. The ability of PNI to predict subsequent events has been controversial. Some have found PNI to independently predict BF [45-48] while others did not found PNI to be a predictive factor for any event [49-53]. D'Amico et al. reported PNI to be an independent predictor of BF, but only for low risk PC after evaluating biopsies [54]. Besides, the evaluation of its role as a prognostic factor has been hampered as it does not seem to be included as a histopathological variable in the large series of the world e.g. the Johns Hopkins database [55]. Most studies have only addressed the correlation between PNI and BF and not the more clinical relevant endpoints of CF and PCD. In the small, but interesting study by Aumayr et al. reported that a high amount of extraprostatic nerve infiltration correlated with tumor progression [45]. PNI found in preoperative biopsies, has also been found to be a predictor of metastasis and PCD in patients treated with dose-escalated radiotherapy [56]. Our finding of extraprostatic PNI as independently significant for prognosis with respect to CF and PCD, but not for BF, is in accordance with these findings.

PSM rates in our material are high (overall 53%) and among the highest that have seen published. In a large published single-center series from Mayo by Boorjian et al. in an almost identical period of time they found a PSM rate of 31.1% with an decreasing incidence over time [57]. The explanation could be the high incidence of pT3x cancers (30%) compared to 12% in the Mayo cohort and higher Gleason grades in our material, as these are independent predictors of PSM. In addition, as our centers during this timeframe were low-volume centers by international standards, this may have contributed to the high PSM rates [58]. Refinement of surgical technique and stage migration has been documented to improve the histopatological outcomes [59,60]. Margin location was relevant in our cohort, as non-apical PSM were associated with a poor BFFS and CFFS. Margin localization was not analyzed by Boorjian et al., but in a study from the same institution by Blute et al., they found PSM at the prostate base to be independently associated to outcome, as did Obek et al. [61,62]. A study by Godoy et al. found the base and anterior localization of PSM to be independently associated to an increased risk of BF compared to the other margin localizations. They specifically advocate that there is over-reporting of PSM from the apex and that an observation strategy is to be adopted for the large group of patients with a apical localization of PSM [63]. A Danish study also found non-apical PSM to be independently associated to BF, whereas apical margins were insignificantly associated to BF in multivariate analysis [64].

Conclusions

In conclusion, for the minority of patients with a subsequent BF we found a low PSA-DT to be the strongest prognosticator for CF and PCD, recognizing its superiority in risk-stratification in this subgroup. We also re-launch PNI in the pathological specimen as a possible strong predictor of CF and PCD following RP and a thorough evaluation in larger patient series is warranted.

As most patients, even after risk-stratification, will not experience a clinically significant relapse of the disease we need new prognostic markers to identify the relevant subgroups. We have included tissues from tumor and stroma of these thoroughly described and largely unselected patients in tissue micro array blocks. Hence, this forms an excellent platform for future molecular studies which will hopefully give us some of these answers.

Competing interests
The authors declare that they have no competing interests.

Authors' contributions
Collecting clinical data: SA, YN, NN, HB. Revising and collecting pathological data: ER, ØS, KA-S, L-TB. Drafting the manuscript: SA, ER, AA, RMB. Statistical analysis: SA, TD, YN. Design of study: SA, ER, TD, HB, L-TB, AA, RMB. All authors have read, revised and approved the final manuscript.

Acknowledgements
We would like to thank Dr. Cecilie Fiva for helping to collect tissues from Nordlandssykehuset Bodø, Dr. Raymond Mortensen for help to gather follow-up information from patients followed up at his clinic, the surgical department with Dr. Lars Hoem in Bodø for facilitating the collection of data from their region. At last we would like to thank all the medical doctors, secretaries and laboratory personnel at local hospitals who helped us to collect all the required data. The study was funded by the Norwegian Cancer Association, The Arctic University of Norway and the Northern Norway Regional Health Authority (Helse Nord RHF).

Author details
[1]Institute of Clinical Medicine, The Arctic University of Norway, Tromso, Norway. [2]Department Oncology, University Hospital of North Norway, Tromso 9038, Norway. [3]Institute of Medical Biology, The Arctic University of Norway, Tromso, Norway. [4]Department Pathology, University Hospital of North Norway, Tromso, Norway. [5]Department of Urology, University Hospital of North Norway, Tromso, Norway. [6]Department Pathology, St. Olavs Hospital, Trondheim University Hospital, Trondheim, Norway. [7]Department Pathology, Nordland Hospital, Bodoe, Norway. [8]Department of Urology, St. Olavs Hospital, Trondheim University Hospital, Trondheim, Norway. [9]Institute of Cancer research and Molecular Medicine, Norwegian University of Science and Technology, Trondheim, Norway.

References
1. Cancer registry of Norway: *Cancer in Norway 2010 - cancer incidence, mortality, survival and prevalence in Norway*. Oslo: Cancer registry of Norway; 2012. Ref Type: Report. www.kreftregisteret.no.
2. Kvale R, Skarre E, Tonne A, Kyrdalen AE, Norstein J, Angelsen A, Wahlqvist R, Fossa SD: Curative treatment of prostatic cancer in Norway in 1998 and 2001. *Tidsskr Nor Laegeforen* 2006, 126(7):912–916.
3. Center MM, Jemal A, Lortet-Tieulent J, Ward E, Ferlay J, Brawley O, Bray F: International variation in prostate cancer incidence and mortality rates. *Eur Urol* 2012, 61(6):1079–1092.
4. Kvale R, Moller B, Angelsen A, Dahl O, Fossa SD, Halvorsen OJ, Hoem L, Solberg A, Wahlqvist R, Bray F: Regional trends in prostate cancer incidence, treatment with curative intent and mortality in Norway 1980–2007. *Cancer Epidemiol* 2010, 34(4):359–367.
5. Wilt TJ, Brawer MK, Jones KM, Barry MJ, Aronson WJ, Fox S, Gingrich JR, Wei JT, Gilhooly P, Grob BM, Nsouli I, Iyer P, Cartagena R, Snider G, Roehrborn C, Sharifi R, Blank W, Pandya P, Andriole GL, Culkin D, Wheeler T: Radical prostatectomy versus observation for localized prostate cancer. *N Engl J Med* 2012, 367(3):203–213.
6. Vickers A, Bennette C, Steineck G, Adami HO, Johansson JE, Bill-Axelson A, Palmgren J, Garmo H, Holmberg L: Individualized estimation of the benefit of radical prostatectomy from the scandinavian prostate cancer group randomized trial. *Eur Urol* 2012, 62(2):204–209.
7. Bill-Axelson A, Holmberg L, Ruutu M, Garmo H, Stark JR, Busch C, Nordling S, Haggman M, Andersson SO, Bratell S, Spangberg A, Palmgren J, Steineck G, Adami HO, Johansson JE: Radical prostatectomy versus watchful waiting in early prostate cancer. *N Engl J Med* 2011, 364(18):1708–1717.
8. Roder MA, Brasso K, Christensen IJ, Johansen J, Langkilde NC, Hvarness H, Carlsson S, Jakobsen H, Borre M, Iversen P: Survival after radical prostatectomy for clinically localised prostate cancer: a population-based study. *BJU Int* 2014, 113(4):541–547.
9. Wehrberger C, Berger I, Willinger M, Madersbacher S: Radical prostatectomy in Austria from 1992 to 2009: an updated nationwide analysis of 33,580 cases. *J Urol* 2012, 187(5):1626–1631.
10. Etzioni R, Mucci L, Chen S, Johansson JE, Fall K, Adami HO: Increasing use of radical prostatectomy for nonlethal prostate cancer in Sweden. *Clin Cancer Res* 2012, 18(24):6742–6747.
11. Capitanio U, Briganti A, Gallina A, Suardi N, Karakiewicz PI, Montorsi F, Scattoni V: Predictive models before and after radical prostatectomy. *Prostate* 2010, 70(12):1371–1378.
12. Sutcliffe P, Hummel S, Simpson E, Young T, Rees A, Wilkinson A, Hamdy F, Clarke N, Staffurth J: Use of classical and novel biomarkers as prognostic risk factors for localised prostate cancer: a systematic review. *Health Technol Assess* 2009, 13(5):iii–xi–iiixiii.
13. Touijer K, Scardino PT: Nomograms for staging, prognosis, and predicting treatment outcomes. *Cancer* 2009, 115(13 Suppl):3107–3111.
14. Ng J, Mahmud A, Bass B, Brundage M: Prognostic significance of lymphovascular invasion in radical prostatectomy specimens. *BJU Int* 2012, 110(10):1507–1514.
15. Eichelberger LE, Koch MO, Daggy JK, Ulbright TM, Eble JN, Cheng L: Predicting tumor volume in radical prostatectomy specimens from patients with prostate cancer. *Am J Clin Pathol* 2003, 120(3):386–391.
16. Epstein JI: Prognostic significance of tumor volume in radical prostatectomy and needle biopsy specimens. *J Urol* 2011, 186(3):790–797.
17. Servoll E, Saeter T, Vlatkovic L, Lund T, Nesland J, Waaler G, Axcrona K, Beisland HO: Impact of a tertiary Gleason pattern 4 or 5 on clinical failure and mortality after radical prostatectomy for clinically localised prostate cancer. *BJU Int* 2012, 109(10):1489–1494.
18. Sandler HM, Eisenberger MA: Assessing and treating patients with increasing prostate specific antigen following radical prostatectomy. *J Urol* 2007, 178(3 Pt 2):S20–S24.
19. Moul JW, Banez LL, Freedland SJ: Rising PSA in nonmetastatic prostate cancer. *Oncology (Williston Park)* 2007, 21(12):1436–1445.
20. Bruce JY, Lang JM, McNeel DG, Liu G: Current controversies in the management of biochemical failure in prostate cancer. *Clin Adv Hematol Oncol* 2012, 10(11):716–722.
21. Antonarakis ES, Feng Z, Trock BJ, Humphreys EB, Carducci MA, Partin AW, Walsh PC, Eisenberger MA: The natural history of metastatic progression

in men with prostate-specific antigen recurrence after radical prostatectomy: long-term follow-up. *BJU Int* 2012, **109**(1):32–39.

22. Slovin SF, Wilton AS, Heller G, Scher HI: Time to detectable metastatic disease in patients with rising prostate-specific antigen values following surgery or radiation therapy. *Clin Cancer Res* 2005, **11**(24 Pt 1):8669–8673.

23. Okotie OT, Aronson WJ, Wieder JA, Liao Y, Dorey F, DeKERNION JB, Freedland SJ: Predictors of metastatic disease in men with biochemical failure following radical prostatectomy. *J Urol* 2004, **171**(6 Pt 1):2260–2264.

24. Pound CR, Partin AW, Eisenberger MA, Chan DW, Pearson JD, Walsh PC: Natural history of progression after PSA elevation following radical prostatectomy. *JAMA* 1999, **281**(17):1591–1597.

25. Freedland SJ, Humphreys EB, Mangold LA, Eisenberger M, Dorey FJ, Walsh PC, Partin AW: Death in patients with recurrent prostate cancer after radical prostatectomy: prostate-specific antigen doubling time subgroups and their associated contributions to all-cause mortality. *J Clin Oncol* 2007, **25**(13):1765–1771.

26. Ross AE, Loeb S, Landis P, Partin AW, Epstein JI, Kettermann A, Feng Z, Carter HB, Walsh PC: Prostate-specific antigen kinetics during follow-up are an unreliable trigger for intervention in a prostate cancer surveillance program. *J Clin Oncol* 2010, **28**(17):2810–2816.

27. O'Brien MF, Cronin AM, Fearn PA, Smith B, Stasi J, Guillonneau B, Scardino PT, Eastham JA, Vickers AJ, Lilja H: Pretreatment prostate-specific antigen (PSA) velocity and doubling time are associated with outcome but neither improves prediction of outcome beyond pretreatment PSA alone in patients treated with radical prostatectomy. *J Clin Oncol* 2009, **27**(22):3591–3597.

28. Stephenson AJ, Kattan MW, Eastham JA, Dotan ZA, Bianco FJ Jr, Lilja H, Scardino PT: Defining biochemical recurrence of prostate cancer after radical prostatectomy: a proposal for a standardized definition. *J Clin Oncol* 2006, **24**(24):3973–3978.

29. Cheng L, Montironi R, Bostwick DG, Lopez-Beltran A, Berney DM: Staging of prostate cancer. *Histopathology* 2012, **60**(1):87–117.

30. Kordan Y, Salem S, Chang SS, Clark PE, Cookson MS, Davis R, Herrell SD, Baumgartner R, Phillips S, Smith JA Jr, Barocas DA: Impact of positive apical surgical margins on likelihood of biochemical recurrence after radical prostatectomy. *J Urol* 2009, **182**(6):2695–2701.

31. Chang SS, Cookson MS: Impact of positive surgical margins after radical prostatectomy. *Urology* 2006, **68**(2):249–252.

32. Boorjian SA, Tollefson MK, Rangel LJ, Bergstralh EJ, Karnes RJ: Clinicopathological predictors of systemic progression and prostate cancer mortality in patients with a positive surgical margin at radical prostatectomy. *Prostate Cancer Prostatic Dis* 2012, **15**(1):56–62.

33. Epstein JI, Allsbrook WC Jr, Amin MB, Egevad LL: The 2005 International Society of Urological Pathology (ISUP) consensus conference on gleason grading of prostatic carcinoma. *Am J Surg Pathol* 2005, **29**(9):1228–1242.

34. Han M, Partin AW, Pound CR, Epstein JI, Walsh PC: Long-term biochemical disease-free and cancer-specific survival following anatomic radical retropubic prostatectomy. The 15-year Johns Hopkins experience. *Urol Clin North Am* 2001, **28**(3):555–565.

35. Tollefson MK, Blute ML, Rangel LJ, Bergstralh EJ, Boorjian SA, Karnes RJ: The effect of Gleason score on the predictive value of prostate-specific antigen doubling time. *BJU Int* 2010, **105**(10):1381–1385.

36. Eggener SE, Scardino PT, Walsh PC, Han M, Partin AW, Trock BJ, Feng Z, Wood DP, Eastham JA, Yossepowitch O, Rabah DM, Kattan MW, Yu C, Klein EA, Stephenson AJ: Predicting 15-year prostate cancer specific mortality after radical prostatectomy. *J Urol* 2011, **185**(3):869–875.

37. Freedland SJ, Humphreys EB, Mangold LA, Eisenberger M, Dorey FJ, Walsh PC, Partin AW: Risk of prostate cancer-specific mortality following biochemical recurrence after radical prostatectomy. *JAMA* 2005, **294**(4):433–439.

38. Okotie OT, Aronson WJ, Wieder JA, Liao Y, Dorey F, DeKERNION JB, Freedland SJ: Predictors of metastatic disease in men with biochemical failure following radical prostatectomy. *J Urol* 2004, **171**(6 Pt 1):2260–2264.

39. Trock BJ, Han M, Freedland SJ, Humphreys EB, DeWeese TL, Partin AW, Walsh PC: Prostate cancer-specific survival following salvage radiotherapy vs observation in men with biochemical recurrence after radical prostatectomy. *JAMA* 2008, **299**(23):2760–2769.

40. D'Amico AV, Moul J, Carroll PR, Sun L, Lubeck D, Chen MH: Prostate specific antigen doubling time as a surrogate end point for prostate cancer specific mortality following radical prostatectomy or radiation therapy. *J Urol* 2004, **172**(5 Pt 2):S42–S46.

41. Steigler A, Denham JW, Lamb DS, Spry NA, Joseph D, Matthews J, Atkinson C, Turner S, North J, Christie D, Tai KH, Wynne C: Risk stratification after

biochemical failure following curative treatment of locally advanced prostate cancer: data from the TROG 96.01 Trial. Prostate. *Cancer* 2012, 2012:814724.

42. Ploussard G, Epstein JI, Montironi R, Carroll PR, Wirth M, Grimm MO, Bjartell AS, Montorsi F, Freedland SJ, Erbersdobler A, van der Kwast TH: The contemporary concept of significant versus insignificant prostate cancer. *Eur Urol* 2011, **60**(2):291–303.

43. Roehl KA, Han M, Ramos CG, Antenor JA, Catalona WJ: Cancer progression and survival rates following anatomical radical retropubic prostatectomy in 3,478 consecutive patients: long-term results. *J Urol* 2004, **172**(3):910–914.

44. Tollefson MK, Slezak JM, Leibovich BC, Zincke H, Blute ML: Stratification of patient risk based on prostate-specific antigen doubling time after radical retropubic prostatectomy. *Mayo Clin Proc* 2007, **82**(4):422–427.

45. Aumayr K, Breitegger M, Mazal PR, Koller A, Marberger M, Susani M, Haitel A: Quantification of extraprostatic perineural spread and its prognostic value in pT3a pN0 M0 R0 prostate cancer patients. *Prostate* 2011, **71**(16):1790–1795.

46. Jeon HG, Bae J, Yi JS, Hwang IS, Lee SE, Lee E: Perineural invasion is a prognostic factor for biochemical failure after radical prostatectomy. *Int J Urol* 2009, **16**(8):682–686.

47. Tanaka N, Fujimoto K, Hirayama A, Torimoto K, Okajima E, Tanaka M, Miyake M, Shimada K, Konishi N, Hirao Y: Risk-stratified survival rates and predictors of biochemical recurrence after radical prostatectomy in a Nara, Japan, cohort study. *Int J Clin Oncol* 2011, **16**(5):553–559.

48. Ozcan F: Correlation of perineural invasion on radical prostatectomy specimens with other pathologic prognostic factors and PSA failure. *Eur Urol* 2001, **40**(3):308–312.

49. Lee JT, Lee S, Yun CJ, Jeon BJ, Kim JM, Ha HK, Lee W, Chung MK: Prediction of perineural invasion and its prognostic value in patients with prostate cancer. *Korean J Urol* 2010, **51**(11):745–751.

50. Masieri L, Lanciotti M, Nesi G, Lanzi F, Tosi N, Minervini A, Lapini A, Carini M, Serni S: Prognostic role of perineural invasion in 239 consecutive patients with pathologically organ-confined prostate cancer. *Urol Int* 2010, **85**(4):396–400.

51. Merrilees AD, Bethwaite PB, Russell GL, Robinson RG, Delahunt B: Parameters of perineural invasion in radical prostatectomy specimens lack prognostic significance. *Mod Pathol* 2008, **21**(9):1095–1100.

52. Jung JH, Lee JW, Arkoncel FR, Cho NH, Yusoff NA, Kim KJ, Song JM, Kim SJ, Rha KH: Significance of perineural invasion, lymphovascular invasion, and high-grade prostatic intraepithelial neoplasia in robot-assisted laparoscopic radical prostatectomy. *Ann Surg Oncol* 2011, **18**(13):3828–3832.

53. Freedland SJ, Csathy GS, Dorey F, Aronson WJ: Percent prostate needle biopsy tissue with cancer is more predictive of biochemical failure or adverse pathology after radical prostatectomy than prostate specific antigen or Gleason score. *J Urol* 2002, **167**(2 Pt 1):516–520.

54. D'Amico AV, Wu Y, Chen MH, Nash M, Renshaw AA, Richie JP: Perineural invasion as a predictor of biochemical outcome following radical prostatectomy for select men with clinically localized prostate cancer. *J Urol* 2001, **165**(1):126–129.

55. Partin AW, Pound CR, Clemens JQ, Epstein JI, Walsh PC: Serum PSA after anatomic radical prostatectomy. The Johns Hopkins experience after 10 years. *Urol Clin North Am* 1993, **20**(4):713–725.

56. Feng FY, Qian Y, Stenmark MH, Halverson S, Blas K, Vance S, Sandler HM, Hamstra DA: Perineural invasion predicts increased recurrence, metastasis, and death from prostate cancer following treatment with dose-escalated radiation therapy. *Int J Radiat Oncol Biol Phys* 2011, **81**(4):e361–e367.

57. Boorjian SA, Karnes RJ, Crispen PL, Carlson RE, Rangel LJ, Bergstralh EJ, Blute ML: The impact of positive surgical margins on mortality following radical prostatectomy during the prostate specific antigen era. *J Urol* 2010, **183**(3):1003–1009.

58. Urbanek C, Turpen R, Rosser CJ: Radical prostatectomy: hospital volumes and surgical volumes - does practice make perfect? *BMC Surg* 2009, **9**:10.

59. Berger AP, Volgger H, Rogatsch H, Strohmeyer D, Steiner H, Klocker H, Bartsch G, Horninger W: Screening with low PSA cutoff values results in low rates of positive surgical margins in radical prostatectomy specimens. *Prostate* 2002, **53**(3):241–245.

60. Eastham JA, Kattan MW, Riedel E, Begg CB, Wheeler TM, Gerigk C, Gonen M, Reuter V, Scardino PT: Variations among individual surgeons in the rate of positive surgical margins in radical prostatectomy specimens. *J Urol* 2003, **170**(6 Pt 1):2292–2295.

61. Blute ML, Bostwick DG, Bergstralh EJ, Slezak JM, Martin SK, Amling CL, Zincke H: **Anatomic site-specific positive margins in organ-confined prostate cancer and its impact on outcome after radical prostatectomy.** *Urology* 1997, **50**(5):733–739.
62. Obek C, Sadek S, Lai S, Civantos F, Rubinowicz D, Soloway MS: **Positive surgical margins with radical retropubic prostatectomy: anatomic site-specific pathologic analysis and impact on prognosis.** *Urology* 1999, **54**(4):682–688.
63. Godoy G, Tareen BU, Lepor H: **Site of positive surgical margins influences biochemical recurrence after radical prostatectomy.** *BJU Int* 2009, **104**(11):1610–1614.
64. Vrang ML, Roder MA, Vainer B, Christensen IJ, Gruschy L, Brasso K, Iversen P: **First Danish single-institution experience with radical prostatectomy: impact of surgical margins on biochemical outcome.** *Scand J Urol Nephrol* 2012, **46**(3):172–179.

Treatment of genital lesions with diode laser vaporization

Mário Maciel de Lima Jr[1][*], Mário Maciel de Lima[1] and Fabiana Granja[2]

Abstract

Background: Genital warts caused by human papillomavirus (HPV) infection are the most common sexually transmitted disease leading to anogential lesions. Although the laser therapy has been shown to be effective in a number of conditions, the use of laser diode vaporization in urological applications and the understanding on its effectiveness as a treatment for various urological conditions is limited. Therefore, the aim of this study was to evaluate the efficacy of diode laser vaporization as a treatment for genital lesions.

Methods: Patients presenting with genital lesions at the urology outpatient clinic at Coronel Mota Hospital, between March 2008 and October 2014, were enrolled into the study. Data collected included age, gender, duration of the lesion, site of the lesion and numbers of the lesions, length of follow-up, recurrence of lesions after treatment and whether there were any complications.

Results: A total of 92 patients were enrolled in the study; 92.4% (n = 85) male; mean age (± SD) 27.92 ± 8.272 years. The patients presented with a total of 296 lesions, with a median of 3 lesions each, including penis (n = 78), urethra (n = 4) lesions, and scrotum (n = 2) lesions. Lesions ranged in size from 0.1 to 0.5 cm^2, most commonly 0.3 cm^2 (n = 38; 41.3%), 0.4 cm^2 (n = 21; 22.8%) or 0.5 cm^2 (n = 20; 21.7%). Patients most commonly reported that they had their lesions for a duration of 12 (n = 29; 31.5%) or 6 months (n = 23; 25.0%). Eighteen patients (19.6%) had a recurrence after their 1st/conventional treatment. There were no incidences of post–operative infection or complications from the laser diode vaporization.

Conclusions: Laser diode vaporization can be considered as an alternative method for treating genital lesions in urology, with satisfactory results in terms of pain, aesthetic and minimal recurrence.

Keywords: Genital lesion, Laser treatment, Laser diode vaporization, Urology

Background

Genital lesions are a relatively common condition which may be caused either by sexually transmitted human papillomavirus (HPV) infection, as a result of non–infectious inflammatory diseases such as psoriasis and lichen planus, by a drug reaction and also as premalignant lesions that can progress to carcinoma. Regardless of origin, genital lesions are both a source of considerable discomfort and a cause of embarrassment and psychological repercussions. Genital lesions can often persist for prolonged periods, frequently a number of years and can re–occur after treatment.

Genital warts caused by HPV are the most common sexually transmitted disease and a major cause of anogential lesions. In addition to physical and psychological implications of HPV warts, there is also a substantial economic cost, estimated at $6 billion annually in the United States [1]. No specific antiviral therapies are available to cure HPV anogenital warts; treatment therefore relies on removal of warts or limiting spread through anti-proliferative or immunomodulation therapy [2]. However recurrence rates can be high due to the widespread infection or subclinical lesions that are not identified at the time of treatment. The variety of different treatment options for genital warts can be loosely grouped into three categories: topical agents, systemic agents, and surgical therapies [2].

* Correspondence: mmljr@uol.com.br
[1]Department of Urology, Coronel Mota Hospital, Rua Levindo Inácio de Oliveira, 1547, Paraviana, Boa Vista, RR CEP: 69307-272, Brazil
Full list of author information is available at the end of the article

One surgical therapy that is showing increasing use across dermatological conditions is diode laser therapy. Diode lasers are semiconductors that change electrical energy into light energy through the use of solid-state elements, such as aluminum and gallium. The light beam which is released by the diode laser falls within the visible and invisible range of near infrared waves (with wavelengths varying between 800 and 980 nm) and is able to vaporize soft tissue due to its high water content. These light beams are poorly absorbed by the hard tissue and therefore do not damage nearby hard tissue. By focussing the beam on the desired area for incision, a highly precise focal spot can be created. By adjusting the focus of the beam, the intensity of the laser light can be varied, which allows cauterization of small blood vessels and lymphatics to decrease post–operative swellings and sealing of nerve endings to reduce post-operative pain [3-5]. Studies suggest that side effects of diode laser therapy are generally mild [6-9]. However laser therapy can be expensive and is not widely available. Research to determine the efficacy of laser therapy for the treatment of different conditions is therefore important in order to justify investment in laser equipment and training in the use of laser therapy.

Laser therapy has been shown to be effective in a number of conditions, with probably the largest body of work conducted to examine the efficacy of laser surgery for the removal of different oral lesions such as simple soft tissue surgery (e.g. frenectomy, gingival contouring plasty) [3,10-12], vascular lesions (e.g. hemangiomas, telangiectasias) [4,5] and pigmented lesions [3]. Other areas where lasers have become a key option for treatment include cosmetic applications such as laser hair removal and laser tattoo removal, and various dermatological applications, including conditions such as syringoma, xanthelasma palpebrarum, recalcitrant warts, rhinophyma, epidermal nevi, condyloma and intraepithelial neoplasia and milia [13-19]. These studies have suggested a number of advantages of laser surgery over traditional scalpel surgical procedures, such as greater precision, a relatively bloodless surgical and postsurgical course, sterilization of the surgical area, minimal swelling and scarring, coagulation, vaporization, cutting, minimal or no suturing, and less or no postsurgical pain [12].

There have been few studies to date that have examined the efficacy of laser therapy as a destructive therapy for genital warts [20-23]. Because warts are vascular, laser therapy should result in instant coagulation and therefore provide bloodless removal of the lesion. The few studies of genital lesions conducted to date suggest clearance rates ranging between 23% and 52% for carbon dioxide and pulse dye laser therapy; however recurrence rates as high as 77% have also been reported [19,20,22].

However, the description of the use of laser diode vaporization in urological applications is still limited, and further work is required to fully understand the effectiveness of laser diode vaporization as a treatment for various urological conditions. The aim of this study was therefore to evaluate the efficacy of diode laser vaporization treatment in genital lesions.

Methods

Study population

This was a prospective study of patients presenting with genital lesions between March 2008 and October 2014. The study was conducted in the urology department outpatient clinic at Coronel Mota Hospital. Patients were eligible to be enrolled in the study if they presented with a genital lesion and were willing to provide informed written consent to the study. No other eligibility criteria were applied. The study was conducted under the ethical approval provided by ethical review board of Coronel Mota Hospital.

Data collection

Following consent, a full demographic and medical history was taken for each participant. Data collected included age, gender, duration of the lesion, site of the lesion and number of the lesions, length of follow-up, recurrence of lesions after treatment and whether there were any complications.

Diagnosis and treatment protocol

Upon presentation and written consent to participate in the study, patients underwent a physical examination to diagnose the lesion/s. No additional endoscopy was used at for diagnosis. Each patient then underwent laser diode vaporization of their lesion/s according to a standardized protocol. Firstly the warts lesion was prepared by sterilizing the area with povidone-iodine solution (10%) and infiltrating locally with 2% xylocaine hydrochloride without adrenalin. The laser light was then applied using either a circular or radial contact method. In all cases a Zap Laser, LLC® model Z2006AP was used, with a power density of 1.2 W/cm^2 CW (continue wave). Laser treatment was generally applied for 5–15 seconds for each lesion. For patients with a larger number of lesions, multiple treatment sessions were used. For example, for a patient with 10 lesions, a total of 4 treatment sessions were used.

Patient follow-up

After treatment, patients were seen at 7 days in order to check for early post-operative complications. They were then followed up at approximately 4 weeks intervals for 12 weeks. Any associated complications that occurred during this time, such as infection, scarring, hyperpigmentation, hypo- pigmentation or any other sequelae, were looked for and recorded if they occurred. Follow-up of patients continued at the end of the 12 weeks in order to collect data on potential longer term complications.

Results
Patient characteristics
A total of 92 patients were enrolled in the study, of which 7 (7.6%) were female and 85 (92.4%) were men (Table 1). All patients were treated with diode laser due to verrucoid lesions (<0.5 cm^2) in genital and skin. The mean age of the study cohort was 27.92 ± 8.272, ranging from 15 to 53 years. Together, the participants had a total of 296 lesions; this included one patient who had more than 10 lesions. Most commonly patients had three (n = 28; 30.4%), two (n = 18; 19.6%), four (n = 14; 15.2%), or five 5 (n = 15; 16.3%) lesions, with the median number of lesions being three. The lesions ranged in size from 0.1 to 0.5 cm^2, most commonly 0.3 cm^2 (n = 38; 41.3%), 0.4 cm^2 (n = 21; 22.8%) or 0.5 cm^2 (n = 20; 21.7%). A total of 78 patients had penis lesions, whilst four had external urethral meatus lesions, two had scrotum lesions, one had an anal mucosa lesion, and there were seven participants who had lesions on their face or neck (four with lesions on the neck, two with oral lesions and one with lesions on their face). A further four patients had a frenulectomy and therefore no lesions were reported for these patients.

Patients most commonly reported that they had had their lesions for a duration of 12 (n = 29; 31.5%) or 6 months (n = 23; 25.0%), with reported durations ranging from 1 to 36 months. A total of 18 patients (19.6%) had had a recurrence after their 1st/conventional treatment.

Treatment outcomes
Figure 1 shows examples from three cases of genital lesions before treatment, immediately post laser treatment and 15 days post laser treatment. Post-operative infection was not observed in any of the patients. Mild pain, oozing, oedema, and scales were observed during the first seven days after laser irradiation. Depending on the size of the lesions the healing process, which usually occurs by granulation tissue formation, took between 2–3 weeks. Patient follow up continued for between 2 months and 6 years (mean 33.90 ± 25.68 months) after the intensive follow-up period. No complications from the laser diode vaporization were observed, including no reported problems with urination or ejaculation and no strictures or scars.

Discussion
In our study we have evaluated the effect of diode laser vaporization for the treatment of genital warts. The treatment protocol used in our study is comparable to that used in the previous small studies examining pulsed dye laser therapy for the treatment of genital warts [22]. We found only a small incidence of recurrence after

Table 1 Patient characteristics

Characteristics	n (%)
Age (years)	
15–19	12 (13.0)
20–29	45 (48.9)
30–39	27 (29.3)
40–49	7 (7.6)
50–59	1 (1.1)
Gender	
Male	85 (92.4)
Female	7 (7.6)
Location of lesion	
Penis	78
Urethra	4
Scrotum	2
Anus	1
Face	1
Neck	4
Oral	2
Frenulectomy	4
Number of lesions	
1	8 (8.7)
2	18 (19.6)
3	28 (30.4)
4	14 (15.2)
5	15 (16.3)
6	2 (2.2)
7	1 (1.1)
8	1 (1.1)
>10	1 (1.1)
Size of largest lesion (cm^2)	
0.2	9 (9.8)
0.3	38 (41.3)
0.4	21 (22.8)
0.5	20 (21.7)
Duration of lesions (months)	
<6	15 (16.3)
6–11	27 (29.3)
12–23	30 (32.6)
24–35	14 (15.2)
36	2 (2.2)
Recurrent after 1st/conventional treatment	
Yes	18 (19.6)
No	70 (76.1)

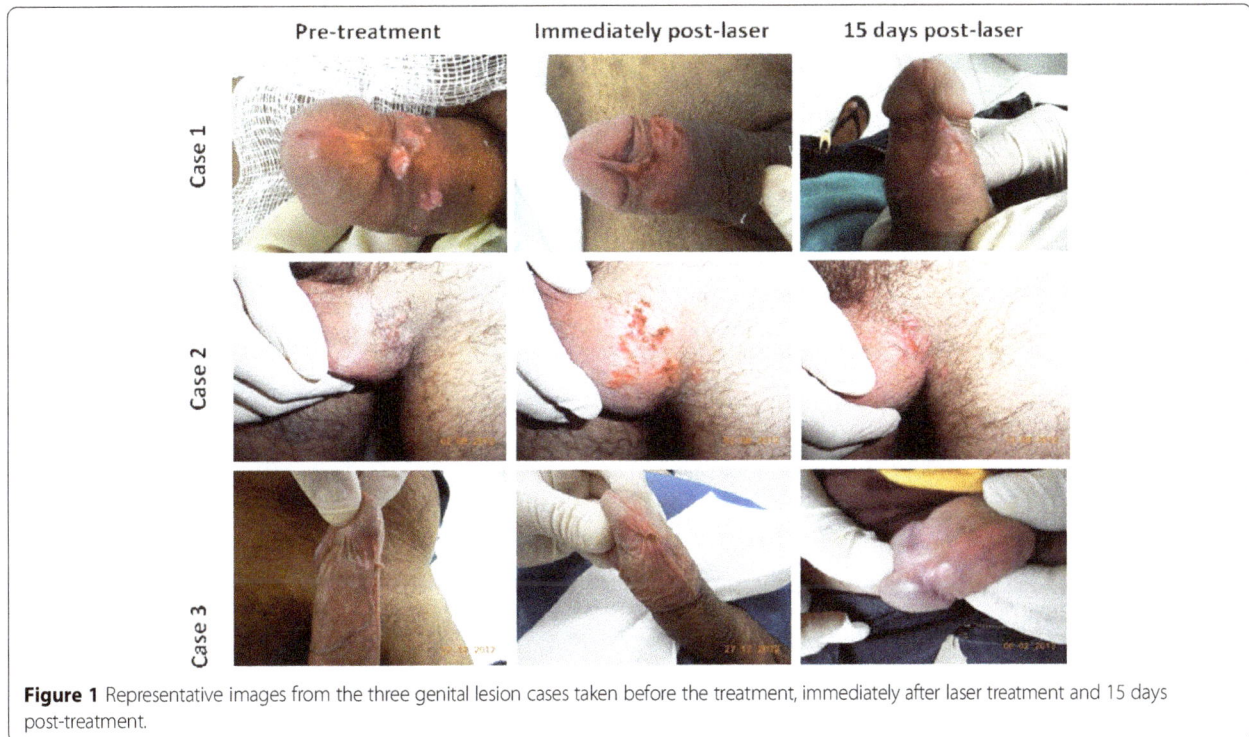

Figure 1 Representative images from the three genital lesion cases taken before the treatment, immediately after laser treatment and 15 days post-treatment.

laser diode treatment. Recurrence rates in previous studies have varied largely, with one study reporting a recurrence rate of 12.6% at one month post-laser therapy, whilst others have reported recurrence rates as high as 77% using carbon dioxide laser and pulsed dye laser [19,20,22]. Variation in reported recurrence rates may partially reflect the varying follow-up times within the individual studies. Some minimal discomfort and oedema was observed during the immediate period post–laser treatment, as expected and in line with findings in previous studies [24]. Notably, we also observed no long-term complications in any of the patients enrolled in the study, which is in line with previous reports of the excellent safety profile of laser therapy as a treatment for genital warts [9,19,22]. Importantly our study supports reports in the literature that laser treatment decreases post-operative pain by sealing nerve endings and reduces blood loss by cauterizing blood vessels [12].

We found no evidence of infection in any of the patients within our study. This may be expected since laser beams have a natural sterilization effect, causing the evaporation of bacteria, viruses and fungi within the immediate vicinity of the beam and therefore decreasing the possibility of local infection.

Conclusion

Our study suggests that laser diode vaporization provides a good option for the treatment of genital lesions.

Laser diode vaporization appears to provide a good clearance rate for the elimination of the verrucae, whilst at the same time having a low complication and side–effect profile, in terms of scarring and postoperative pain, and a low incidence of recurrence. Therefore laser diode vaporization can be considered as an alternative method for treating genital lesions in urology, with satisfactory results in terms of pain, aesthetic and minimal recurrence.

Consent

Written informed consent was obtained from the patient for the publication of this report and any accompanying images.

Competing interests
The authors declare that they have no competing interests.

Authors' contributions
MMLJ was the major contributor in writing the manuscript, and performed the surgery. MML analyzed and interpreted the patient data, and performed the surgery. FG analyzed and interpreted the patient data. All authors read and approved the final manuscript.

Acknowledgements
We acknowledge the assistance of Magna Bezerra Feitosa in collection of data. Additionally, this work was done with institutional support of Coronel Mota Hospital in Roraima, and there was no any external funding.

Author details
[1]Department of Urology, Coronel Mota Hospital, Rua Levindo Inácio de Oliveira, 1547, Paraviana, Boa Vista, RR CEP: 69307-272, Brazil. [2]Biodiversity Research Center, Federal University of Roraima (CBio/UFRR), Boa Vista, Brazil.

References

1. Division of STD Prevention. Prevention of Genital HPV Infection and Sequelae: Report of an External Consultants' Meeting. Atlanta, GA: Centers for Disease Control and Prevention; 1999.

2. Fathi R, Tsoukas MM. Genital warts and other HPV infections: Established and novel therapies. Clin Dermatol. 2013;32:229–306.

3. Desiate A, Cantore S, Tullo D, Profeta G, Grassi FR, Ballini A. 980 nm diode lasers in oral and facial practice: current state of the science and art. Int J Med Sci. 2009;6(6):358–64.

4. Genovese WJ, dos Santos MT, Faloppa F, de Souza Merli LA. The use of surgical diode laser in oral hemangioma: a case report. Photomed Laser Surg. 2010;28(1):147–51.

5. Saetti R, Silvestrini M, Cutrone C, Narne S. Treatment of congenital subglottic hemangiomas: our experience compared with reports in the literature. Arch Otolaryngol Head Neck Surg. 2008;134(8):848–51.

6. Campolmi P, Bonan P, Cannarozzo G, Bruscino N, Moretti S. Efficacy and safety evaluation of an innovative CO2 G laser/radiofrequency device in dermatology. J Eur Acad Dermatol Venereol. 2013;27:1481–90.

7. Tanzi EL, Alster TS. Comparison of a 1450-nm diode laser and a 1320-nm Nd:YAG laser in the treatment of atrophic facial scars: a prospective clinical and histologic study. Dermatol Surg. 2004;30((2 Pt 1)):152–7.

8. Park EJ, Youn SH, Cho EB, Lee GS, Hann SK, Kim KH, et al. Xanthelasma palpebrarum treatment with a 1,450-nm-diode laser. Dermatol Surg. 2011;37(6):791–6.

9. Carrozza PM, Merlani GM, Burg G, Hafner J. CO(2) laser surgery for extensive, cauliflower-like anogenital condylomata acuminata: retrospective long-term study on 19 HIV-positive and 45 HIV-negative men. Dermatology. 2002;205(3):v255–9.

10. Kafas P, Stavrianos C, Jerjes W, Upile T, Vourvachis M, Theodoridis M, et al. Upper-lip laser frenectomy without infiltrated anaesthesia in a paediatric patient: a case report. Cases J. 2009;2:7138.

11. Ishikawa I, Aoki A, Takasaki AA. Clinical application of erbium:YAG laser in periodontology. J Int Acad Periodontol. 2008;10(1):22–30.

12. Goharkhay K, Moritz A, Wilder-Smith P, Schoop U, Kluger W, Jakolitsch S, et al. Effects on oral soft tissue produced by a diode laser in vitro. Lasers Surg Med. 1999;25(5):401–6.

13. Oni G, Mahaffey PJ. Treatment of recalcitrant warts with the carbon dioxide laser using an excision technique. J Cosmet Laser Ther. 2011;13:231–6.

14. Pozo J, Castineiras I, Fernandez-Jorge B. Variants of milia successfully treated with CO(2) laser vaporization. J Cosmet Laser Ther. 2010;12(4):191–4.

15. Madan V, Ferguson JE, August PJ. Carbon dioxide laser treatment of rhinophyma: a review of 124 patients. Br J Dermatol. 2009;161(4):814–8.

16. Boyce S, Alster TS. CO2 laser treatment of epidermal nevi: long-term success. Dermatol Surg. 2002;28(7):611–4.

17. Cho SB, Kim HJ, Noh S, Lee SJ, Kim YK, Lee JH. Treatment of syringoma using an ablative 10,600-nm carbon dioxide fractional laser: a prospective analysis of 35 patients. Dermatol Surg. 2011;37(4):433–8.

18. Raulin C, Schoenermark MP, Werner S, Greve B. Xanthelasma palpebrarum: treatment with the ultrapulsed CO2 laser. Lasers Surg Med. 1999;24(4):122–7.

19. Aynaud O, Buffet M, Roman P, Plantier F, Dupin N. Study of persistence and recurrence rates in 106 patients with condyloma and intraepithelial neoplasia after CO2 laser treatment. Eur J Dermatol. 2008;18(2):153–8. 20.

20. Bellina JH. The use of the carbon dioxide laser in the management of condyloma acuminatum with eight-year follow-up. Am J Obstet Gynecol. 1983;147(4):375–8.

21. Taner ZM, Taskiran C, Onan AM, Gursoy R, Himmetoglu O. Therapeutic value of trichloroacetic acid in the treatment of isolated genital warts on the external female genitalia. J Reprod Med. 2007;52(6):521–5.

22. Tuncel A, Gorgu M, Ayhan M, Deren O, Erdogan B. Treatment of anogenital warts by pulsed dye laser. Dermatol Surg. 2002;28(4):350–2.

23. Garden JM, O'Banion MK, Shelnitz LS, Pinski KS, Bakus AD, Reichmann ME, et al. Papillomavirus in the vapor of carbon dioxide laser-treated verrucae. JAMA. 1988;259(8):1199–202.

24. Findakly JJI. Warts Treatment by 810 nm Diode Laser Irradiation: A New Approach. Iraqi J Laser. 2005;4:35–40.

Measuring the improvement in health-related quality of life using King's health questionnaire in non-obese and obese patients with lower urinary tract symptoms after alpha-adrenergic medication

Jae Heon Kim[1], Hoon Choi[2], Hwa Yeon Sun[1], Seung Whan Doo[1], Jong Hyun Yoon[1], Won Jae Yang[1], Byung Wook Yoo[3], Joyce Mary Kim[4], Soon-Sun Kwon[5], Eun Seop Song[6], Hong Jun Lee[7], Ik Sung Lim[8] and Yun Seob Song[1*]

Abstract

Background: The efficacy of medical treatment among obese men with lower urinary tract symptoms (LUTS) has been less clear, especially regarding the improvement of QoL. We aimed to investigate the difference in efficacy and consequent satisfaction of life quality after medical treatment of male LUTS according to obesity.

Methods: An 8-week prospective study was performed for a total of 140 patients >50 years old with International Prostate Symptom Scores (IPSS) > 12 points and prostate volume > 20 mL. Obesity was determined by either body mass index (BMI) or waist circumference (WC). Patients were divided into 2 groups according to BMI or WC. Patients received tamsulosin at a dose of 0.4 mg daily for 8 weeks. The changes from baseline in the IPSS, maximal urinary flow rate (Qmax), post-void residual volume, questionnaire of quality of life (QoL), and King's Health Questionnaire (KHQ) were analyzed.

Results: Of the 150 enrolled patients, 96 completed the study. Seventy-five patients (78.1%) had BMI $\geq$ 23 kg/m^2, and 24 (25.0%) had WC > 90 cm. Overall, the IPSS, IPSS QoL, and total KHQ showed significant improvement. Obese (BMI $\geq$ 23 kg/m^2) and non-obese (BMI < 23 kg/m^2) both showed improvement of the IPSS and IPSS QoL scores, but only the obese (BMI $\geq$ 23 kg/m^2) group showed improvement of the total KHQ score (P < 0.001 vs. P = 0.55). Only the obese (WC > 90 cm) group showed improvement of the IPSS and total KHQ scores (P < 0.001).

Conclusions: Our preliminary study showed the different efficacy of an alpha-blocker for improvement of LUTS and life quality according to obesity. Obese patients, defined by BMI or WC, showed the tendency toward a more favorable improvement of LUTS and life quality.

Keywords: Alpha-blocker, Prostatic hyperplasia, Body mass index, Waist circumference

* Correspondence: yssong@schmc.ac.kr
[1]Department of Urology, Soonchunhyang University College of Medicine, Seoul Hospital, 59, Daesagwan-ro, Yongsan-gu, Seoul 140-743, The Republic of Korea
Full list of author information is available at the end of the article

Background

Benign prostatic hyperplasia (BPH)/lower urinary tract symptoms (LUTS) is a common disease entity in older men and has a negative impact on quality of life (QoL) [1-3]. Obesity is also a common condition in older males and is related to LUTS [1,3]. As in Western countries, Korean men have a high prevalence of symptomatic BPH as they age, with a prevalence of 10.6%–31% in men > 50 years old [2,4]. Several studies have reported a significant relationship between LUTS and obesity [3,5,6]. Considering the objective evidence of a negative effect of both LUTS [7-13] and obesity [14] on QoL, LUTS plus obesity may result in a greater deterioration of QoL.

Among the alpha blockers, tamsulosin is one of the most commonly recommended because of its efficacy, safety, and tolerability [15]. The King's Health Questionnaire (KHQ) is a validated tool to measure the QoL in patients with LUTS [9]. Although the KHQ was developed originally for female urge incontinence, validity has been proven in studies that dealt with LUTS and health-related quality of life (HRQoL) in both sexes [9,16-19].

To date, efficacy of medical treatment among obese men with LUTS has been less clear, especially regarding the improvement of QoL within specific domains. Recently, Lee et al. [14] reported that alpha-blockers have a greater efficacy in improvement of LUTS when used in obese men. The main presumed hypothesis for this difference is that obese men have a greater level of sympathetic activity, which is suspected to be sensitive to alpha-blockers [20,21].

The main purpose of this preliminary study is to investigate the improvement of LUTS and QoL in different groups (obese and non-obese).

Methods

Study design

An eight-week prospective study was conducted between March 2010 and May 2011. The study was approved by the institutional review board of Soonchunhyang University Hospital.

At the initial visit, anthropometric parameters were evaluated, including weight, height, and waist circumference. Additional parameters measured included urinalysis, serum prostate-specific antigen [22], maximal urinary flow rate (Qmax), and post-void residual volume (PVR). Transrectal ultrasonography was also performed. At the initial and final visits, the International Prostate Symptom Score (IPSS) and KHQ were measured.

BMI was calculated as the body weight in kilograms divided by the square of the height in meters. After the first evaluation, eligible patients were treated with tamsulosin at a dose of 0.4 mg for 8 weeks. At each visit, adverse events were recorded.

Serum PSA tests were performed using the automated chemiluminescent microparticle immunoassay analyzer

Architect i2000 (Abbott Diagnostic Laboratories, Abbott Park, IL, USA). The prostate was measured in three dimensions by transrectal ultrasonography using an 8.0-MHz rectal probe (GE Healthcare, LOGIQ P6-PRO, Little Chalfont, UK), and prostate volume (PV) was estimated using a modification of the prolate ellipsoid formula and recorded in cm^3 (0.523 [length (cm) × width (cm) × height (cm)]).

Acquisition of questionnaire data was performed with face-to-face interviews conducted by one investigator with all study participants using a structured questionnaire. The severity of LUTS was measured using the IPSS, which is based on the American Urological Association [23] symptom index with one additional question on QoL, and is the most widely used objective assessment of LUTS.

The KHQ consists of 8 categories, including general health perceptions, impact on life, role limitations, physical/social limitation, personal relationships, emotions, sleep/energy, and incontinence severity measures. The KHQ has been validated in a Korean version [24].

Subjects

A total of 150 patients who visited the Department of Urology at Soonchunhyang University and provided informed consent were included in this study. Inclusion criteria were male ≥ 40 years of age, no history of prior treatment of BPH/LUTS, total IPSS ≥ 8, prostate volume > 20 mL as determined by transrectal ultrasound, no relevant medical history, and underlying comorbidities. Exclusion criteria were history of neurogenic bladder dysfunction, history of prostate or bladder cancer, treatment history of acute or chronic urinary retention within the previous 3 months, treatment history of acute or chronic prostatitis within the previous 3 months, PSA levels > 0.10 ng/mL, and history of urinary tract infection or bladder stones.

All patients were divided into 2 groups, non-obese (BMI < 23 kg/m^2) and obese (BMI ≥ 23 kg/m^2), according to the Asia-Pacific obesity criteria [25]. For additional analysis, we also categorized patients into 2 groups based on waist circumference (WC), normal waist (≤90 cm) and central obesity (>90 cm).

Power calculation

Sample size was not calculated because its being a preliminary study.

Statistical analysis

The primary outcome measurement was the degree of change of KHQ in the two groups, and secondary outcome measurement was the degree of change of IPSS in the two groups. All data are presented as mean ± SD. Statistical analysis was performed using SPSS (version 21.0; Chicago, IL, USA). Changes from baseline in total

IPSS, QoL scores, and KHQ scores were analyzed using Wilcoxon signed-rank test. A P value < 0.05 was considered significant.

Results

Of the 140 enrolled patients, 96 completed the study. Fifty four patients discontinued the trial. Of these, 22 were lost to follow-up, 14 refused to complete the final questionnaires, and 18 patients discontinued the medication because of low efficacy (9 patients) or adverse events (9 patients) (Figure 1).

The basic characteristics, including age, PSA, PV, Qmax, total IPSS, and KHQ questionnaire are described in Table 1. Between the obese group (BMI ≥ 23 kg/m^2) and non-obese group (BMI < 23 kg/m^2), no significant difference occurred among the variables. Between the central obesity group (WC > 90 cm) and non-central obesity group (WC ≤ 90 cm), no significant difference occurred among the variables except age.

After 8 weeks treatment with tamsulosin, overall improvement was seen in the total IPSS and IPSS QoL (P < 0.001) (Table 2). Total KHQ scores also improved after treatment (P < 0.001). Among the domains, general health, impact on life, role limitations, physical limitation, emotions, sleep/energy, and incontinence severity were improved or significantly improved. However, social limitation and personal relationships did not show improvement after treatment (Table 2).

In subgroup analysis, the non-obese group showed no improvement in total KHQ (P = 0.055) (Table 3). Among the KHQ domains, the obese group showed improvement only in general health (P = 0.025), impact on life (P = 0.020), and emotions (P = 0.047). The obese group showed improvement in total KHQ (P < 0.001) (Table 3). Among the KHQ domains, the obese group showed improvement in general health (P < 0.001), impact on life (P < 0.001), role limitations (P = 0.001), physical limitation (P < 0.001), and emotions (P < 0.001). The comparison of improvement of IPSS and KHQ revealed that obesity group showed significant greater improvement in total IPSS, physical limitation, and sleep/energy (Table 4).

In other subgroup analysis, the non-central obesity group showed no improvement in total IPSS, IPSS QoL, and total KHQ (Table 4). Among the KHQ domains, the non-central obesity group showed improvement only in general health (P = 0.020) and impact on life (P = 0.032). The central obesity group showed improvement in total IPSS, IPSS QoL, and total KHQ (Table 5). Among the KHQ domains, the central obesity group showed improvement in general health P < 0.001), impact on life (P < 0.001), role limitations (P < 0.001), physical limitation (P = 0.002), personal relationships (P = 0.029), emotions (P < 0.001), and sleep/energy (P = 0.024). The comparison of improvement of IPSS and KHQ revealed that central obesity group showed significant greater improvement in total IPSS, impact of life, and sleep/energy (Table 5).

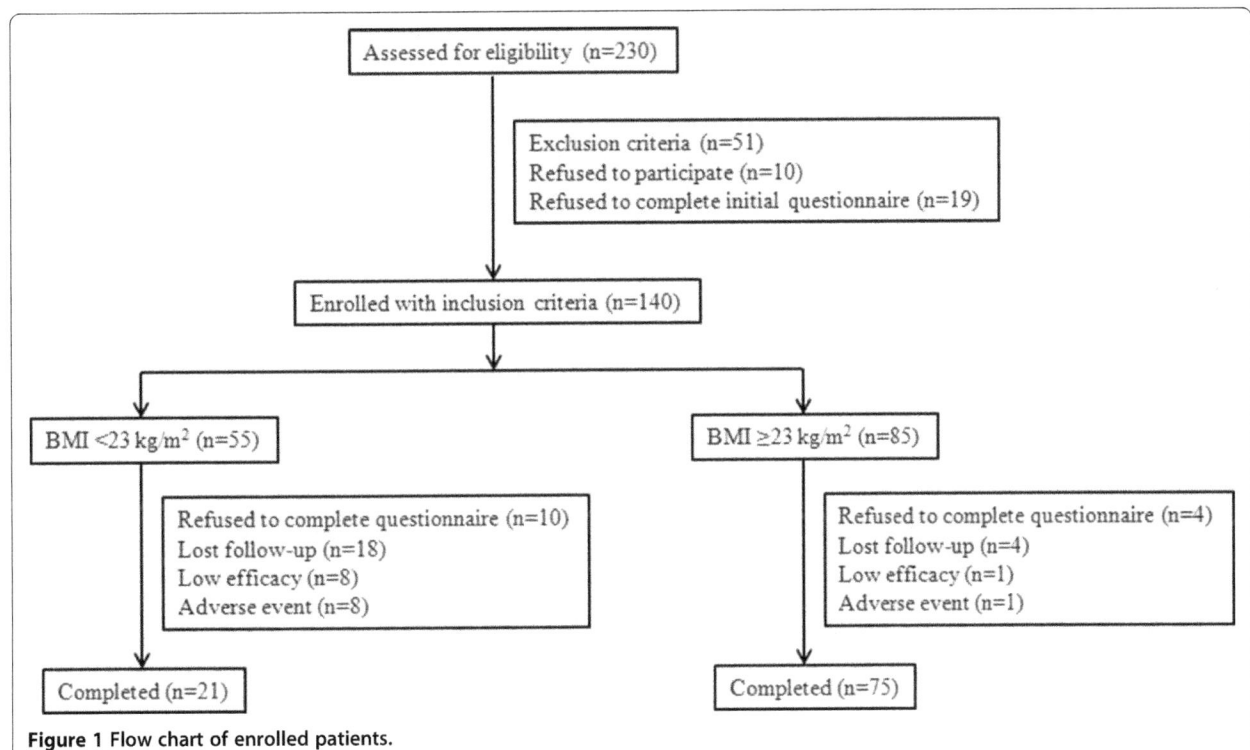

Figure 1 Flow chart of enrolled patients.

Table 1 Basic characteristics of participants

	BMI < 23	BMI ≥ 23	P value	WC ≤ 90	WC > 90	P value
No	21	75		72	24	
Age	61.25±9.80	61.48±7.09	0.982	60.58±7.60	64.20±7.54	0.045
PSA	2.12±	2.04±	0.231	2.13±	1.98±	0.312
PV	31.12±10.14	34.23±8.71	0.042	32.31±9.81	33.23±10.21	0.218
Qmax	12.32±2.21	13.25±1.75	0.134	11.46±1.89	13.33±2.34	0.185
IPSS questionnaire						
Total IPSS	14.90±7.58	13.41±6.79	0.388	15.00±7.57	13.31±6.74	0.308
IPSS QoL	3.47±1.21	3.54±1.22	0.830	3.56±1.40	3.51±1.15	0.864
KHQ questionnaire						
General health	41.66±18.25	47.66±23.67	0.286	47.91±26.49	45.83±21.39	0.698
Impact on life	53.91±30.65	58.60±30.40	0.534	58.27±28.20	57.35±31.22	0.898
Role limitations	25.29±33.45	28.77±31.98	0.664	33.20±37.91	26.28±30.10	0.364
Physical limitation	29.24±31.45	27.44±30.08	0.811	33.20±34.26	26.05±28.79	0.318
Social limitation	22.19±31.81	16.71±25.48	0.411	18.03±24.83	17.87±27.59	0.980
Personal relationships	21.71±37.96	25.39±32.24	0.724	24.90±35.34	24.55±32.84	0.972
Emotions	25.90±31.06	27.52±25.83	0.808	31.91±29.15	25.59±26.12	0.321
Sleep/Energy	26.08±29.49	21.02±26.64	0.454	18.67±24.13	23.28±28.22	0.475
Incontinence	14.14±27.47	9.85±14.73	0.343	16.50±21.31	8.89±16.76	0.076
Total KHQ	251.88±223.71	254.88±171.03	0.947	274.31±198.90	247.53±178.02	0.537

Adverse events were reported in 9 patients (6.0%) and included dizziness (3.3%), postural hypotension (1.3%), and gastric discomfort (1.3%).

Discussion

When obese patients with BPH have LUTS, a larger prostate is presumed to be one of the causes. The prostate grows faster in obese than in non-obese patients [26-28].

Many clinical studies have focused on prostate size or PSA in obese patients, but few studies have focused on the treatment outcome, including QoL, in obese patients. Although several studies have used the IPSS-QoL index to present the treatment outcome in obese patients

Table 2 Differences in IPSS and KHQ before and after treatment

	Mean difference	SD	95% CI		P value
IPSS					
IPSS questionnaire	3.521	6.764	2.150	4.891	< 0.001
QoL	1.011	1.487	.701	1.321	< 0.001
KHQ					
General health	13.281	25.380	8.139	18.424	< 0.001
Impact on life	18.417	32.513	11.829	25.004	< 0.001
Role limitations	10.302	26.954	4.841	15.764	< 0.001
Physical limitation	9.490	26.417	4.137	14.842	0.001
Social limitation	3.323	24.418	−1.625	8.271	0.186
Personal relationships	5.283	24.118	−1.365	11.931	0.117
Emotions	9.656	19.902	5.624	13.689	< 0.001
Sleep/Energy	4.632	22.549	.038	9.225	0.048
Incontinence	3.010	14.141	.145	5.876	0.040
Total KHQ	76.167	144.346	46.920	105.414	< 0.001

Table 3 Differences in IPSS and KHQ before and after treatment according to BMI

	BMI < 23			BMI ≥ 23		
	Mean difference	SD	P value	Mean difference	SD	P value
IPSS questionnaire						
Total IPSS	5.571	7.928	.004	2.947	6.341	< 0.001
QoL	1.105	1.243	.001	.986	1.552	< 0.001
KHQ questionnaire						
General health	10.714	20.266	.025	14.000	26.712	< 0.001
Impact on life	20.619	37.377	.020	17.800	31.269	< 0.001
Role limitations	9.381	27.006	.127	10.560	27.116	0.001
Physical limitation	3.190	34.945	.680	11.253	23.483	< 0.001
Social limitation	8.429	27.770	.180	1.893	23.400	0.486
Personal relationships	5.556	37.250	.666	5.227	21.101	0.108
Emotions	10.571	22.892	.047	9.400	19.146	< 0.001
Sleep/Energy	7.048	25.488	.220	3.946	21.785	.124
Incontinence	6.524	23.159	.211	2.027	10.357	.094
Total KHQ	79.762	179.641	.055	75.160	134.246	< 0.001

[14,29,30], the IPSS-QoL is not a disease-specific questionnaire. Rather, it represents the state of generalized HRQoL in men with LUTS.

The most prominent feature of our study was use of the KHQ questionnaire, a disease-specific HRQoL instrument for the evaluation of patients with LUTS, overactive bladder, and urinary incontinence [9,16-19]. The KHQ consists of nine domains. Seven of the domains include multiple questions including role limitations, physical limitations, social limitations, personal relationships, emotions, sleep/energy, and incontinence severity measures.

Our study revealed that comparison of improvement of IPSS QoL according to BMI and WC showed no significant difference. However, the comparison of improvement KHQ including impact on life, physical limitation, impact of life, and sleep/energy showed significant difference. Although improvement of total KHQ showed no significant difference, several domains of KHQ showed significant differences.

Although some controversies exist regarding the relationship between the severity of LUTS and obesity, obese patients usually have more severe LUTS than

Table 4 Differences in IPSS and KHQ before and after treatment according to waist circumference

	WC < 90			WC ≥ 90		
	Mean difference	SD	P value	Mean difference	SD	P value
IPSS questionnaire						
Total IPSS	2.667	7.191	.082	3.806	6.643	< 0.001
QoL	.957	1.637	.010	1.029	1.445	< 0.001
KHQ questionnaire						
General health	14.583	28.473	.020	12.847	24.464	< 0.001
Impact on life	15.292	32.742	.032	19.458	32.600	< 0.001
Role limitations	8.250	38.649	.307	10.986	22.053	< 0.001
Physical limitation	8.333	28.448	.165	9.875	25.904	0.002
Social limitation	.083	20.581	.984	4.403	25.610	0.149
Personal relationships	−4.714	21.084	.418	8.872	24.369	0.029
Emotions	3.667	18.253	.335	11.653	20.147	< 0.001
Sleep/Energy	−1.458	14.623	.630	6.690	24.404	0.024
Incontinence	3.000	12.487	.251	3.014	14.733	0.087
Total KHQ	52.333	165.817	.136	84.111	136.806	< 0.001

Table 5 Comparison of the differences in IPSS and KHQ according to BMI and waist circumference

	BMI < 23	BMI ≥ 23	P value	WC ≤ 90	WC > 90	P value
IPSS questionnaire						
ΔTotal IPSS	3.37±6.17	6.00±7.66	0.041	2.87±7.18	4.30±6.38	0.028
ΔIPSS QoL	0.96±1.52	1.00±1.22	0.830	0.79±1.79	1.02±1.34	0.231
KHQ questionnaire						
ΔGeneral health	10.71±20.26	14.00±26.71	0.286	14.58±28.47	12.84±24.46	0.321
ΔImpact on life	17.76±31.12	20.06±37.19	0.052	15.26±32.53	19.42±32.46	0.028
ΔRole limitations	10.61±27.10	9.48±27.05	0.564	8.30±38.54	11.06±22.11	0.356
ΔPhysical limitation	3.16±35.06	11.28±23.50	0.032	8.30±28.54	9.91±25.93	0.068
ΔSocial limitation	4.20±22.84	3.16±27.08	0.347	4.01±20.62	4.39±25.64	0.780
ΔPersonal relationships	5.71±27.96	5.39±22.24	0.561	5.09±22.05	4.71±28.32	0.814
ΔEmotions	9.47±19.19	10.57±22.87	0.706	10.91±18.41	11.76±20.14	0.415
ΔSleep/Energy	3.98±21.63	7.11±25.48	0.031	3.21±14.61	6.68±24.23	0.035
ΔIncontinence	19.69±24.66	18.35±24.96	0.381	18.43±24.99	19.72±24.64	0.451
ΔTotal KHQ	75.20±134.25	79.87±179.59	0.061	52.47±165.90	84.14±136.77	0.071

non-obese patients [29,30]. Possible reasons for this phenomenon are lower testosterone concentrations, lower serum globulin-binding protein levels, and greater prostate volumes in obese patients [31], as well as increased estrogen levels and increased free and total estradiol concentrations [32,33].

Our data demonstrate that the baseline total IPSS showed no significant difference between the obese and non-obese groups or central obesity and non-central obesity groups. This is mainly due to our lower IPSS inclusion criteria of more than 8 points total on the IPSS. We lowered the criteria for the IPSS because patients scoring higher on the IPSS could bias the results by showing more satisfaction with treatment.

Our data showed a more favorable treatment outcome in obese patients and those with central obesity. Although an improvement in the total IPSS was demonstrated in both obese and non-obese patients, the improvement in the total IPSS was only demonstrated in patients with central obesity. Improvement in total KHQ scores was demonstrated only in obese patients and patients with central obesity.

Greater estrogen levels in old age and obesity induce lower testosterone levels and may affect prostate cell growth [32]. Enlarged adipose tissue can secrete numerous hormones and proteins that influence fat metabolism [34,35], and leptin stimulates the cellular proliferation of BPH [36,37].

Besides an enlarged prostate, obese patients have increased sympathetic tone, which is suspected to be the main reason alpha blockers could have a greater impact in obese patients. Increased sympathetic tone can result in LUTS and subjective voiding complaints [19]. In particular, abdominal obesity increases the estrogen-to-

androgen ratio and may increase sympathetic nervous system activity, both of which are known to influence the development of BPH and the severity of LUTS [18]. In our study, obese patients showed improvement in 5 domains of the KHQ, but central obesity patients showed improvement in 7 domains of the KHQ. This result implies that obesity, especially central obesity, which is regarded as visceral obesity, could impact treatment outcomes. The main reason for this result is that obesity, and especially visceral adiposity, is closely related to sympathetic overactivity [38,39]. The whole body norepinephrine spillover rate is known to be quantitatively linked with waist circumference [17,31], and sympathetic nerve firing rates measured by microneurography have been reported to be 55% higher in men with visceral adiposity than in men with only subcutaneous obesity.

Sympathetic activity is increased in obese men and may be related to BPH/LUTS by a common link between norepinephrine and alpha-1 adrenoceptors [38,39]. Although general improvement of LUTS and KHQ were observed in this study, the obesity and central obesity groups showed more improvement in the IPSS and KHQ.

This study has several limitations. First, the study design has a relatively short follow-up period. However, 8 weeks is sufficient to judge the clinical outcome of alpha blockers. Moreover, the KHQ is a relatively long questionnaire and takes a long time to perform, which reduces patient compliance. Although the acquisition of questionnaire was performed by one special interviewer, a lot of patients showed negative response to the KHQ in our study. The most common reason for this negative response is that it takes quite a long time. This is why we did not perform an additional KHQ at 4 weeks. Second, this study has a relatively small size. However, considering the increasing prevalence of concomitant medical diseases, the availability of eligible patients is limited. This was a pilot; a preliminary study, and subsequent prospective study is needed.

Conclusions

Obese or central obesity patients with LUTS showed a better health-related quality of life than non-obese or non-centrally obese patients with LUTS after alpha-adrenergic medication. Therefore, alpha-adrenergic medication can be recommended to obese patients with LUTS preferentially for the improvement of quality of life.

Competing interest
The authors declare that they have no competing interest.

Authors' contributions
JHK and YSS contributed with the conception and design of the study and drafted the manuscript, JHK, HC, SHY, SWD, WJY, BWY, JHY and MJK collected data, SSK performed the statistical analyses, and ESS, HJL, ISL, YSS have contributed on the critical revision of this manuscript. All authors read and approved the final manuscript.

Acknowledgment
This research was supported by Research Program through the National Research Foundation of Korea (NRF) funded by the Ministry of Education, Science and Technology (2012-R1A1A2039317) and Soonchunhang University Research Fund.

Author details
[1]Department of Urology, Soonchunhyang University College of Medicine, Seoul Hospital, 59, Daesagwan-ro, Yongsan-gu, Seoul 140-743, The Republic of Korea. [2]Department of Urology, Korea University College of Medicine, Ansan Hospital, Ansan, Korea. [3]Department of Family Medicine, Soonchunhyang University School of Medicine, Seoul, Korea. [4]International Clinic Center, Soonchunhyang University Hospital, Seoul, Korea. [5]Biomedical Research Institute, Seoul National University Bundang Hospital, Seongnam, South Korea. [6]Department of Obstetrics and Gynecology, Inha University School of Medicine, Incheon, Korea. [7]Medical Research Institute, Chung-Ang University College of Medicine, Seoul, Korea. [8]Department of Industrial Management and Engineering, Namseoul University College of Engineering, Cheonan, Korea.

References

1. Lepor H: Phase III multicenter placebo-controlled study of tamsulosin in benign prostatic hyperplasia. Tamsulosin Investigator Group. *Urology* 1998, **51**:892–900.
2. Park YHC MK: The prevalence of clinical benign prostatic hyperplasia and lower urinary tract symptoms in South-East Korea: a community-based study. *J Pusan Natl Univ Hosp* 2001, **9**:141–157.
3. Giuliano F: Lower urinary tract symptoms and sexual dysfunction: a common approach. *BJU Int* 2008, **97**(Suppl 3):22–26.
4. Lee MWL MH: The prevalence of benign prostatic hyperplasia in self-referral populations over aged 50. *Korean J Urol* 1996, **37**:263–267.
5. Lee E, Lee C: Clinical comparison of selective and non-selective alpha 1A-adrenoreceptor antagonists in benign prostatic hyperplasia: studies on tamsulosin in a fixed dose and terazosin in increasing doses. *Br J Urol* 1997, **80**:606–611.
6. Giuliano F: Impact of medical treatments for benign prostatic hyperplasia on sexual function. *BJU Int* 2006, **97**(Suppl 2):34–38. discussion 44–35.
7. Na YJ, Guo YL, Gu FL: Clinical comparison of selective and non-selective alpha 1A-adrenoceptor antagonists for bladder outlet obstruction associated with benign prostatic hyperplasia: studies on tamsulosin and terazosin in Chinese patients. The Chinese Tamsulosin Study Group. *J Med* 1998, **29**:289–304.
8. McVary KT, Roehrborn CG, Avins AL, Barry MJ, Bruskewitz RC, Donnell RF, Foster HE Jr, Gonzalez CM, Kaplan SA, Penson DF, Ulchaker JC, Wei JT: Update on AUA guideline on the management of benign prostatic hyperplasia. *J Urol* 2011, **185**:1793–1803.
9. Watson V, Ryan M, Brown CT, Barnett G, Ellis BW, Emberton M: Eliciting preferences for drug treatment of lower urinary tract symptoms associated with benign prostatic hyperplasia. *J Urol* 2004, **172**(6 Pt 1):2321–2325.
10. Li NC, Chen S, Yang XH, Du LD, Wang JY, Na YQ: Efficacy of low-dose tamsulosin in chinese patients with symptomatic benign prostatic hyperplasia. *Clin Drug Investig* 2003, **23**:781–787.
11. Madersbacher S, Alivizatos G, Nordling J, Sanz CR, Emberton M, de la Rosette JJ: EAU 2004 guidelines on assessment, therapy and follow-up of men with lower urinary tract symptoms suggestive of benign prostatic obstruction (BPH guidelines). *Eur Urol* 2004, **46**:547–554.
12. Patrick DL, Martin ML, Bushnell DM, Yalcin I, Wagner TH, Buesching DP: Quality of life of women with urinary incontinence: further development of the incontinence quality of life instrument (I-QOL). *Urology* 1999, **53**:71–76.
13. Barry MJ, Williford WO, Chang Y, Machi M, Jones KM, Walker-Corkery E, Lepor H: Benign prostatic hyperplasia specific health status measures in clinical research: how much change in the American Urological Association symptom index and the benign prostatic hyperplasia impact index is perceptible to patients? *J Urol* 1995, **154**:1770–1774.
14. Lee SH, Oh CY, Park KK, Chung MS, Yoo SJ, Chung BH: Comparison of the clinical efficacy of medical treatment of symptomatic benign prostatic hyperplasia between normal and obese patients. *Asian J Androl* 2011, **13**:728–731.
15. Maldonado-Avila M, Manzanilla-Garcia HA, Sierra-Ramirez JA, Carrillo-Ruiz JD, Gonzalez-Valle JC, Rosas-Nava E, Guzman-Esquivel J, Labra-Salgado IR: A comparative study on the use of tamsulosin versus alfuzosin in spontaneous micturition recovery after transurethral catheter removal in patients with benign prostatic growth. *Int Urol Nephrol* 2014, **46**:687–690.
16. Okamura K, Usami T, Nagahama K, Maruyama S, Mizuta E: "Quality of life" assessment of urination in elderly Japanese men and women with some medical problems using International Prostate Symptom Score and King's Health Questionnaire. *Eur Urol* 2002, **41**:411–419.
17. Okamura K, Usami T, Nagahama K, Maruyama S, Mizuta E: The relationships among filling, voiding subscores from International Prostate Symptom Score and quality of life in Japanese elderly men and women. *Eur Urol* 2002, **42**:498–505.
18. Reese PR, Pleil AM, Okano GJ, Kelleher CJ: Multinational study of reliability and validity of the King's Health Questionnaire in patients with overactive bladder. *Qual Life Res* 2003, **12**:427–442.
19. Uemura S, Homma Y: Reliability and validity of King's Health Questionnaire in patients with symptoms of overactive bladder with urge incontinence in Japan. *Neurourol Urodyn* 2004, **23**:94–100.
20. Ahima RS, Stanley TL, Khor VK, Zanni MV, Grinspoon SK: Estrogen sulfotransferase is expressed in subcutaneous adipose tissue of obese humans in association with TNF-alpha and SOCS3. *J Clin Endocrinol Metab* 2011, **96**:E1153–E1158.
21. Hillebrand S, de Mutsert R, Christen T, Maan AC, Jukema JW, Lamb HJ, de Roos A, Rosendaal FR, den Heijer M, Swenne CA: Body fat, especially visceral fat, is associated with electrocardiographic measures of sympathetic activation. *Obesity (Silver Spring)* 2014, **22**:1553–1559.
22. Fedorchenko PM, Zhila VV, Sapsai VI, Volkov GP, Chernenko PS: [Postgraduate training and ways of improving it in a department of urology]. *Klin Khir* 1986, **10**:48–50.
23. Suzigan S, Drut R, Faria P, Argani P, De Marzo AM, Barbosa RN, Mello Denadai ER, Martins-Filho J, Martucci RC, Bauab T Jr: Xp11 translocation carcinoma of the kidney presenting with multilocular cystic renal cell carcinoma-like features. *Int J Surg Pathol* 2007, **15**:199–203.
24. Oh SJ, Ku JH: Comparison of three disease-specific quality-of-life questionnaires (Bristol Female Lower Urinary Tract Symptoms, Incontinence Quality of Life and King's Health Questionnaire) in women with stress urinary incontinence. *Scand J Urol Nephrol* 2007, **41**(1):66–71.
25. Kanazawa M, Yoshiike N, Osaka T, Numba Y, Zimmet P, Inoue S: Criteria and classification of obesity in Japan and Asia-Oceania. *World Rev Nutr Diet* 2005, **94**:1–12.

26. Hammarsten J, Hogstedt B: **Clinical, anthropometric, metabolic and insulin profile of men with fast annual growth rates of benign prostatic hyperplasia.** *Blood Press* 1999, **8**:29–36.

27. Hammarsten J, Hogstedt B, Holthuis N, Mellstrom D: **Components of the metabolic syndrome-risk factors for the development of benign prostatic hyperplasia.** *Prostate Cancer Prostatic Dis* 1998, **1**(3):157–162.

28. Ozden C, Ozdal OL, Urgancioglu G, Koyuncu H, Gokkaya S, Memis A: **The correlation between metabolic syndrome and prostatic growth in patients with benign prostatic hyperplasia.** *Eur Urol* 2007, **51**:199–203. discussion 204–196.

29. Mondul AM, Giovannucci E, Platz EA: **A prospective study of obesity, and the incidence and progression of lower urinary tract symptoms.** *J Urol* 2014, **191**:715–721.

30. Penson DF, Munro HM, Signorello LB, Blot WJ, Fowke JH, Urologic Diseases in America P: **Obesity, physical activity and lower urinary tract symptoms: results from the Southern Community Cohort Study.** *J Urol* 2011, **186**:2316–2322.

31. Lee S, Min HG, Choi SH, Kim YJ, Oh SW, Park Y, Kim SS: **Central obesity as a risk factor for prostatic hyperplasia.** *Obesity (Silver Spring)* 2006, **14**:172–179.

32. Matsuda T, Abe H, Suda K: **[Relation between benign prostatic hyperplasia and obesity and estrogen].** *Rinsho Byori* 2004, **52**:291–294.

33. Pasquali R, Casimirri F, Cantobelli S, Melchionda N, Morselli Labate AM, Fabbri R, Capelli M, Bortoluzzi L: **Effect of obesity and body fat distribution on sex hormones and insulin in men.** *Metab Clin Exp* 1991, **40**:101–104.

34. Considine RV, Sinha MK, Heiman ML, Kriauciunas A, Stephens TW, Nyce MR, Ohannesian JP, Marco CC, McKee LJ, Bauer TL, Caro JF: **Serum immunoreactive-leptin concentrations in normal-weight and obese humans.** *N Engl J Med* 1996, **334**:292–295.

35. Haque WA, Garg A: **Adipocyte biology and adipocytokines.** *Clin Lab Med* 2004, **24**:217–234.

36. Dahle SE, Chokkalingam AP, Gao YT, Deng J, Stanczyk FZ, Hsing AW: **Body size and serum levels of insulin and leptin in relation to the risk of benign prostatic hyperplasia.** *J Urol* 2002, **168**:599–604.

37. Hoon Kim J, Lee SY, Myung SC, Kim YS, Kim TH, Kim MK: **Clinical significance of the leptin and leptin receptor expressions in prostate tissues.** *Asian J Androl* 2008, **10**:923–928.

38. Alvarez GE, Beske SD, Ballard TP, Davy KP: **Sympathetic neural activation in visceral obesity.** *Circulation* 2002, **106**:2533–2536.

39. Eckel RH, Grundy SM, Zimmet PZ: **The metabolic syndrome.** *Lancet* 2005, **365**:1415–1428.

The role of diagnostic ureteroscopy in the era of computed tomography urography

Shay Golan[*], Andrei Nadu and David Lifshitz

Abstract

Background: To examine the contemporary role of ureteroscopy in the diagnosis of upper urinary tract urothelial carcinoma.

Methods: We retrospectively evaluated 116 diagnostic ureteroscopies, performed in our institution to rule out primary UTUC. Demographics, cytological findings and interpretation of preoperative imaging were obtained. Ureteroscopic diagnosis and histological results were recorded and the predictive values of diagnostic studies were determined. Follow-up data was reviewed to evaluate the oncological outcomes in patients treated endoscopically.

Results: The pre-ureteroscopic evaluation included CTU in 91 (78 %) patients. Positive and Negative predictive values of CTU were 76 and 80 %, respectively. Typical filling defect on CTU was demonstrated in 38 of 89 patients. UTUC has been ruled out in 9 patients (24 %) with suspicious filling defect on CTU. Endoscopic approach was implemented in 7 patients (18 %). During a median follow up period of 17 months (IQR, 9–25) none of the followed patients experienced disease progression.

Conclusions: Nephroureterectomy was spared from 42 % of patients who underwent diagnostic ureteroscopy for suspected UTUC, demonstrated on CTU. In about half of those patients tumor has been ruled out and the others were managed endoscopically. Therefore, diagnostic ureteroscopy is advised as a crucial step in confirming UTUC and treatment planning.

Keywords: Upper urinary tract urothelial carcinoma, Ureteroscopy, Computed tomography urography

Background

Upper urinary tract urothelial carcinoma (UTUC) is an uncommon malignancy, accounting for ~5 % of urothelial tumors [1]. The diagnosis of UTUC can be challenging, requiring a combination of radiographic, cytologic and endoscopic means. Time honored radiological tools such as intravenous urography and retrograde uretropyelograpy are currently replaced by modern computerized tomography urography (CTU) [2]. Diagnostic ureteroscopy is often performed following CTU. Flexible ureteroscopy allows exploration of the upper urinary tract and is beneficial when diagnostic uncertainty exists. It has the advantages of offering direct view of the tumor, ruling out other pathologies and achieving tissue diagnosis. Although nephroureterectomy is considered the gold standard

treatment of UTUC, endoscopic ablation and resection of the tumor can be successfully utilized in selected cases based on tumor size and histology, as determined during ureteroscopoy. In low grade low volume tumors endoscopic management provides cancer related and overall survival equivalent to that of nephroureterectomy [3]. Despite the above, the routine use of ureterosocpy following CTU is controversial. Ureteroscopy is an invasive procedure that may be associated with morbidity as well as a potential risk of tumor seeding [4, 5]. In the last edition of "Campbell's urology" the authors do not support a routine ureteroscopic confirmation of UTUC [6], while the European guidelines on UTUC (2015 version) advocate the use of diagnostic ureteroscopy with biopsy, especially in cases where additional information will impact treatment decisions. The purpose of this study was to evaluate the diagnostic value of ureteroscopy in patients who underwent workup for suspected UTUC and to assess the impact of ureteroscopy on the management of UTUC.

* Correspondence: shaygo1@yahoo.com
Institute of Urology, Rabin Medical Center, Petah Tikva, and Sackler Faculty of Medicine, Tel Aviv University, Tel Aviv, Israel

Methods

This study was approved by "Rabin Medical Center" ethics committee. Between 2003 and 2010, 1818 ureteroscopies, were performed at our institution, of which 116 (6.3 %) were diagnostic, aimed to rule out primary UTUC. The indications for diagnostic ureteroscopy included painless hematuria with positive urinary cytology and negative cystoscopy or imaging findings that may indicate UTUC. CTU was not performed in patients with chronic renal failure (eGFR < 30 mL/min/1.73 m^2) or severe contrast allergy. Although ultrasound is not accepted as a standard modality for UTUC investigation, we reported on ultrasound results when it was available (either performed as first imaging modality in the community or in cases of chronic renal failure or severe contrast allergy). The medical chart of each patient was reviewed to obtain demographics, cytological findings and the interpretation of preoperative imaging. Because of the retrospective design of this study our institutional ethics committee waived the need for written informed consent from participants.

Complete endoscopic examination of the ureter, renal pelvis and calyx has been performed in all patients. Ureteroscopy was performed following a retrograde study, using 8FR rigid ureteroscope (Wolf), advancing the instrument as much as possible. Renal inspection was performed using flexible ureteroscope (DUR-8 (ACMI) or in later years the Flex- X™ (Stortz)). Biopsy forceps or stone collection basket were used to obtain tissue from suspected lesion. Tumor grade and stage were assigned using the world health organization classification [7] and the 6th edition of the AJCC/UICC TNM staging system [8] by specialized pathologists at our institution. Patients with histologically confirmed UTUC were referred to nephroureterectomy usually within one month following the diagnostic procedure or, in selected cases, managed conservatively with endoscopic resection. Patients with low grade, <1 cm UTUC were eligible for endoscopic treatment. Holmium laser and a bugbee electrode were utilized for tumor resection and ablation.

Intra- and peri-operative complications were reviewed and staged according to Clavien-Dindo classification [9]. The first follow-up ureteroscopy was preformed 3 month after endoscopic tumor resection. Thereafter, patients were followed with ureteroscopy or CTU, alternately, every 3 months during the first two years. Patients with chronic kidney disease were referred to a nephrologist for consultation. Follow-up data was reviewed to include the oncological outcomes (disease recurrence and progression) of patients managed with nephron sparing endoscopic approach.

The diagnostic value (positive and negative predictive values) of urine cytology, ultrasound and CTU was determined. Positive cytology was defined as malignant cells or atypical cells, highly suggestive of urothelial carcinoma. Intraluminal Soft-tissue mass, demonstrated by ultrasound, or filling defect in contrast opacified collecting system, demonstrated by CTU, were considered positive for UTUC. The endoscopic appearance, supported by histologic examination, when available, served as the standard of reference.

Results

Clinical characteristics and diagnostic studies

The study cohort included 116 patients who underwent diagnostic ureteroscopy between November 2003 and December 2010. Demographics and clinical characteristics of the study patients are summarized in Table 1. Half (51 %) of the patients reported at least one episode of gross hematuria and 35 % had a history of lower urinary tract urothelial carcinoma. The preureteroscopic evaluation included urine cytology, ultrasound and CTU in 91 (78 %), 84 (72 %) and 89 (77 %) patients, accordingly. Results of all three studies were available in 47 patients (40.5 %). CTU was not performed in 22 patients with chronic renal failure and 3 patients with severe contrast allergy. Detailed description of the findings, according to the performed study is presented in Table 2. Visual diagnosis of UTUC was made in 47 patients (40 %), supported by histology in 38 of them (80 %). A reliable histological report could not be obtained in 9 patients due to insufficient amount of tissue or technical artifacts.

Of the 38 patients, 27 (71 %) had low grade disease and 11(29 %) had high grade disease on biopsy. In 24 cases tumor stage was determined. Ta, T1 and T2 were

Table 1 Demographic and clinical patient characteristics

Characteristic	N = 116
Age, years	
Median (IQR)	70.5
Mean (range)	68 (16–90)
Patient gender n, (%)	
Female	38 (33)
Male	78 (67)
Hematuria n, (%)	
Macroscopic	59 (51)
Microscopic[a]	88 (76)
History of LUTUC n, (%)	
None	75 (65)
Low grade	24 (21)
High grade	17 (14)

LUTUC Lower urinary tract urothelial carcinoma
[a] Defined as three or more red blood cells per high power microscopic filed on urinary sediment

Table 2 Results of preoperative evaluation - cytological, sonographic and radiographic findings

Method	
Urine Cytology (n, %)	
Atypia	26 (22)
Dysplasia	10 (9)
Normal	55 (48)
N/A	25 (21)
Ultra-Sound (n, %)	
Intra-luminal mass	9 (9)
Dilation	43 (37)
No finding	32 (27)
N/A	32 (27)
CTU (n, %)	
Filling defect	38 (33)
Wall thickening	14 (12)
Dilation	39 (33)
External mass	5 (4)
No finding	12 (10)
N/A	27 (22)

Table 3 Correlation of preoperative studies with the ureteroscopic results

Preoperative findings	Ureteroscopic results		
	Positive for UTUC	Negative for UTUC	Total
CTU			
Positive	29	9	38
Negative	10	41	51
Total	39	50	89
Ultrasound			
Positive	8	1	9
Negative	26	49	75
Total	34	50	84
Urine cytology			
Positive	17	19	36
Negative	23	32	55
Total	40	51	91

assigned in 21 (87 %), 2 (8 %) and 1 (5 %) cases, respectively.

All complications observed in this study were Clavien grade I or II. Intraoperative complications included contrast extravasation, observed during ureteroscopy, in 4 patients (3 %). All patients were managed with ureteral stent for one week with no clinical sequel. Febrile UTI and renal colic were observed after ureteroscopy in 7 (6 %) and 4 (3 %) patients, respectively. Conservative treatment was successfully applied in all cases.

Correlation with ureteroscopy findings
Positive urinary cytology, reported in 36 of 91 patients, included atypia in 26 and dysplasia in 10 patients. The calculated PPV and NPV for UTUC were 47 and 58 %, accordingly. Sonographic appearance of intraluminal mass in 9 patients (9 %), yielded PPV and NPV of 89 and 65 %. Typical filling defect, demonstrated during the excretory phase of CTU, was described in 38 of 89 patients. PPV and NPV of CTU were 76 and 80 %, respectively. Considering "wall thickening" as a positive result, increased the NPV to 90 % but decreased the PPV to 67 %. In 4/39 patients with confirmed UTUC no "filing defect" or "wall thickening" was demonstrated on CTU. Three of these patients had Ta low grade tumors in the ureter and one patient had carcinoma *in situ* of the renal pelvis. Table 3 summarizes the association between the results of preoperative studies and ureteroscopic diagnosis.

Filling defect on CTU – ureteroscopic results and therapeutic outcomes
UTUC had been confirmed during URS in 29 of 38 (76 %) patients with characteristic filling defect on CTU. 7 patients had high grade disease on biopsy, including: stage T1 in 4, T2 in 1 and non- determined stage in 2 patients. 20 patients had Ta low grade and in 2 patients neither stage nor grade could be determined. UTUC has been ruled out in 9 patients (24 %). Mucosa fold, small extraluminal mass and parapelvic hyperdense cyst and bullous mucosal edema of the renal pelvis were found in 4 patients and no findings, explaining the filling defects, were reported in the remaining 5 patients. No additional intervention was required in these cases.

Patients with UTUC were subjected to nephroureterectomy or endoscopic resection according to tumor characteristics (see above). Two patients, found to have metastatic disease, were referred to cisplatin based chemotherapy.

Overall, 20 patients underwent nephroureterectomy while nephron sparing endoscopic approach was implemented in 7 patients who underwent tumor resection with continues surveillance. One of these patients was lost to follow-up. During a median follow up period of 17 months (IQR, 9–25) none of the 6 followed patients experienced disease progression. Tumor recurrence was diagnosed and treated successfully in 2 patients, 5 and 14 months after initial resection (Fig. 1).

Discussion
CTU is currently the recommended imaging modality for evaluation of the upper urinary tract. With ongoing radiological improvements, the added value of diagnostic ureteroscopy is not always clear. We examined the

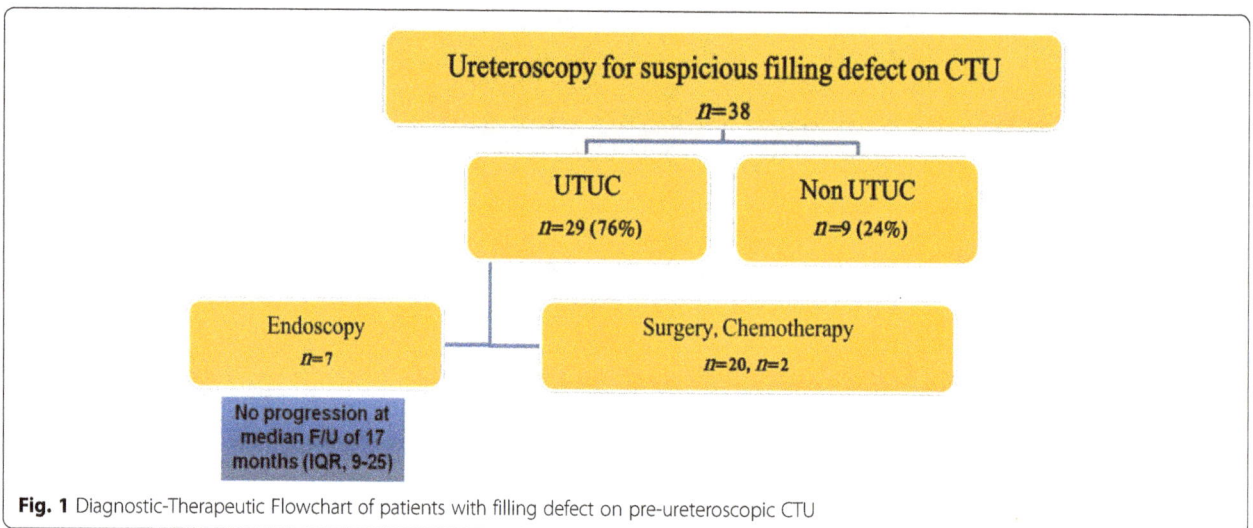

Fig. 1 Diagnostic-Therapeutic Flowchart of patients with filling defect on pre-ureteroscopic CTU

current role of ureteroscopy in the diagnosis of urothelial carcinoma. We found that nephroureterectomy was spared from 42 % (16/38) of patients who underwent ureteroscopy for presumptive UTUC, based on CTU. UTUC was ruled out in 9 patients and treated endoscopically in 7 patients. In the nephron sparing group we observed no disease progression during short term follow-up.

Although UTUC is relatively rare, its incidence has increased in the last decades [10, 11]. One possible explanation for this trend is increased use of CTU, a sensitive tool to detect upper urinary tract abnormalities [2]. The ability of CTU to demonstrate small tumors is well accepted but at the same time, growing use of CTU may increase the detection of benign findings. The positive predictive value (PPV) of CTU for the detection of UTUC is variable, depends on CTU technique and has been reported to be moderate (50-80 %) [12–15]. Intra- and extra-luminal conditions may simulate UTUC on CTU. Inflammatory changes, debris or blood clots may mimic intraluminal tumor. Indentation by extraluminal mass or vascular malformation may also cause false positive results [12]. In our study, the PPV of CTU was 80 %. Non-UTUC findings (mucosa fold, small extraluminal mass and parapelvic hyperdense cyst and bullous mucosal edema) were found during ureteroscopy in 4/9 cases and normal upper urinary tract was described in 5/9 cases. None of these patients had positive urinary cytology. Sadow *et al.* reported on extremely low PPV in small (≤5 mm) upper urinary tract filling defects on CTU [14]. All 17 cases of small filling defects in their study were found to be false positive. In accordance, the five completely normal ureteroscopies in our study were performed in patients with small filling defects on CTU.

The treatment options for confirmed UTUC include nephroureterectomy or, in selected patients, nephron sparing procedure. In the last two decades endoscopic management of UTUC has been extended from patients with imperative indications (chronic kidney disease, bilateral disease or solitary kidney) to selected patients with elective indications. In a review article, Cutress *et al.* reported that the long term renal preservation rate in patients treated endoscopically is 80 % [16]. This information is highly important when considering the potential cardiovascular and overall survival benefits of renal function preservation [17]. Recently published, long term retrospective studies showed that low grade UTUC can be managed endoscopically with cancer related and overall survival equivalent to that of nephroureterectomy [18–20]. Because tumor grade is a significant factor, determining the oncological outcomes of UTUC in patients treated endoscopically, ureteroscopic biopsy is of paramount importance. In our study, 7/38 patients with presumptive UTUC on CTU were treated endoscopically. All had biopsy confirming low grade UTUC less than 1 cm in size. Recurrence occurred in two patients and was amenable for repeat endoscopic resection. No progression was observed during a median follow-up time of 17 months. All complications observed in this study were Clavien grade I or II. Febrile UTI and renal colic were the only post operative complications, reported in 7 (6 %) patients and 4 (3 %) patients, respectively. All patients were successfully treated with antibiotics and analgesics. The potential adverse oncological effect that may be related to delayed nephroureterectomy was beyond the scope of our study, but was addressed in previous publications. No difference in 5 years metastasis-free, cancer specific or overall survival was found in patients who underwent diagnostic ureteroscopy prior to nephroureterectomy compared with patients who did not undergo ureteroscopy [21–23].

Our study is undoubtedly limited by its retrospective design and small size. By the reliance on imaging interpretation, CTU technique was not uniform and the results were subjected to inter observer bias. Despite that, the PPV of CTU in our study is in accordance with results of previous studies [12–15]. Another limitation is the relatively short follow up period of patients treated endoscopically. As mention above, high rate of renal preservation and favorable oncological outcomes were observed in long term studies when patients were carefully selected. This is also reflected by the European guidelines on UTUC, which recognize the option of endoscopic treatment in low grade low stage UTUC [24].

Conclusions

In this retrospective study, nephroureterectomy was spared from 42 % of patients with presumptive UTUC, demonstrated on CTU. In about half of those patients UTUC has been ruled out and the others were managed endoscopically. Although false positive seems to occur mainly in small filling defects on CTU, there is no room for diagnostic error when nephroureterectomy is being considered. Hence, our study favors ureteroscopy as a crucial step in confirming UTUC and treatment planning.

Abbreviations
UTUC: Upper tract urothelial carcinoma; CTU: Computerized tomography urography; PPV: Positive predictive value; NPV: Negative predictive value.

Competing interests
The authors declare that they have no competing interests.

Authors' contributions
SG has made substantial contributions to conception and design, acquisition of data and data analysis. He has drafted the manuscript and approved the submitted version. AN has made substantial contributions to study design and manuscript revising. He approved the submitted version. DL has made substantial contributions to conception and design, data analysis and interpretation. He has been involved in drafting and revising the manuscript and approved the submitted version. All authors read and approved the final manuscript.

Acknowledgements
No financial support was received for this study.

References
1. Siegel R, Naishadham D, Jemal A. Cancer statistics. CA Cancer J Clin. 2012;62(1):10–29.
2. Wang LJ, Wong YC, Huang CC, Wu CH, Hung SC, Chen HW. Multidetector computerized tomography urography is more accurate than excretory urography for diagnosing transitional cell carcinoma of the upper urinary tract in adults with hematuria. J Urol. 2010;183(1):48–55.
3. Gadzinski AJ, Roberts WW, Faerber GJ, Wolf Jr JS. Long-term outcomes of nephroureterectomy versus endoscopic management for upper tract urothelial carcinoma. J Urol. 2010;183(6):2148–53.
4. Grasso M, McCue P, Bagley DH. Multiple urothelial recurrences of renal cell carcinoma after initial diagnostic ureteroscopy. J Urol. 1992;147(5):1358–60.
5. Lim DJ, Shattuck MC, Cook WA. Pyelovenous lymphatic migration of transitional cell carcinoma following flexible ureterorenoscopy. J Urol. 1993;149(1):109–11.
6. Wein AJ, Kavoussi LR, Novick AC, Partin AW, Peters CA. Campbell-Walsh Urology, Vol two. 10th ed. 2011.
7. Epstein JI, Amin MB, Reuter VR, Mostofi FK. The World Health Organization/International Society of Urological Pathology consensus classification of urothelial (transitional cell) neoplasms of the urinary bladder. Bladder Consensus Conference Committee. Am J Surg Pathol. 1998;22(12):1435–48.
8. Greene GL, Page D, Fleming ID. AJCC Cancer Staging Manual. Genitourinary Sites: Renal Pelvis and Ureter. New York: Springer Verlag; 2002.
9. Dindo D, Demartines N, Clavien PA. Classification of surgical complications: a new proposal with evaluation in a cohort of 6336 patients and results of a survey. Ann Surg. 2004;240(2):205–13.
10. Eylert MF, Hounsome L, Verne J, Bahl A, Jefferies ER, Persad RA. Prognosis is deteriorating for upper tract urothelial cancer: data for England 1985–2010. BJU Int. 2013;112(2):E107–113.
11. Raman JD, Messer J, Sielatycki JA, Hollenbeak CS. Incidence and survival of patients with carcinoma of the ureter and renal pelvis in the USA, 1973–2005. BJU Int. 2011;107(7):1059–64.
12. Cowan NC, Turney BW, Taylor NJ, McCarthy CL, Crew JP. Multidetector computed tomography urography for diagnosing upper urinary tract urothelial tumour. BJU Int. 2007;99(6):1363–70.
13. Sudakoff GS, Dunn DP, Guralnick ML, Hellman RS, Eastwood D, See WA. Multidetector computerized tomography urography as the primary imaging modality for detecting urinary tract neoplasms in patients with asymptomatic hematuria. J Urol. 2008;179(3):862–7. discussion 867.
14. Sadow CA, Wheeler SC, Kim J, Ohno-Machado L, Silverman SG. Positive predictive value of CT urography in the evaluation of upper tract urothelial cancer. AJR Am J Roentgenol. 2010;195(5):W337–343.
15. Xu AD, Ng CS, Kamat A, Grossman HB, Dinney C, Sandler CM. Significance of upper urinary tract urothelial thickening and filling defect seen on MDCT urography in patients with a history of urothelial neoplasms. AJR Am J Roentgenol. 2010;195(4):959–65.
16. Cutress ML, Stewart GD, Zakikhani P, Phipps S, Thomas BG, Tolley DA. Ureteroscopic and percutaneous management of upper tract urothelial carcinoma (UTUC): systematic review. BJU Int. 2012;110(5):614–28.
17. Go AS, Chertow GM, Fan D, McCulloch CE, Hsu CY. Chronic kidney disease and the risks of death, cardiovascular events, and hospitalization. N Engl J Med. 2004;351(13):1296–305.
18. Grasso M, Fishman AI, Cohen J, Alexander B. Ureteroscopic and extirpative treatment of upper urinary tract urothelial carcinoma: a 15-year comprehensive review of 160 consecutive patients. BJU Int. 2012;110(11):1618–26.
19. Cutress ML, Stewart GD, Tudor EC, Egong EA, Wells-Cole S, Phipps S, et al. Endoscopic versus laparoscopic management of noninvasive upper tract urothelial carcinoma: 20-year single center experience. J Urol. 2013;189(6):2054–60.
20. Simhan J, Smaldone MC, Egleston BL, Canter D, Sterious SN, Corcoran AT, et al. Nephron sparing management versus radical nephroureterectomy for low or moderate grade, low stage upper tract urothelial carcinoma. BJU Int. 2014;114(2):216–20.
21. Hendin BN, Streem SB, Levin HS, Klein EA, Novick AC. Impact of diagnostic ureteroscopy on long-term survival in patients with upper tract transitional cell carcinoma. J Urol. 1999;161(3):783–5.
22. Boorjian S, Ng C, Munver R, Palese MA, Vaughan Jr ED, Sosa RE, et al. Impact of delay to nephroureterectomy for patients undergoing ureteroscopic biopsy and laser tumor ablation of upper tract transitional cell carcinoma. Urology. 2005;66(2):283–7.
23. Nison L, Roupret M, Bozzini G, Ouzzane A, Audenet F, Pignot G, et al. The oncologic impact of a delay between diagnosis and radical nephroureterectomy due to diagnostic ureteroscopy in upper urinary tract urothelial carcinomas: results from a large collaborative database. World J Urol. 2013;31(1):69–76.
24. Roupret M, Babjuk M, Comperat E, Zigeuner R, Sylvester R, Burger M, et al. European guidelines on upper tract urothelial carcinomas: 2013 update. Eur Urol. 2013;63(6):1059–71.

Clinical relevance of aortic calcification in urolithiasis patients

Toshikazu Tanaka[1], Shingo Hatakeyama[1]* iD, Hayato Yamamoto[1], Takuma Narita[1], Itsuto Hamano[1], Teppei Matsumoto[1], Osamu Soma[1], Yuki Tobisawa[1], Tohru Yoneyama[2], Takahiro Yoneyama[1], Yasuhiro Hashimoto[2], Takuya Koie[1], Ippei Takahashi[4], Shigeyuki Nakaji[4], Yuriko Terayama[3], Tomihisa Funyu[3] and Chikara Ohyama[1,2]

Abstract

Background: The aim of the present study is to investigate the clinical relevance of aortic calcification in urolithiasis patients.

Methods: Between January 2010 and September 2014, 1221 patients with urolithiasis were treated in Oyokyo Kidney Research Institute and Hirosaki University Hospital. Among these, 287 patients (Stone group) on whom adequate data were available were included in this retrospective study. We also selected 148 subjects with early stage (pT1N0M0) renal cell carcinoma from 607 renal cell carcinoma patients who underwent radical nephrectomy at Hirosaki University Hospital (Non-stone group) as control subjects. Validity of the Non-stone group was evaluated by comparison with pair-matched 296 volunteers from 1166 subjects who participated in the Iwaki Health Promotion Project in 2014. Thereafter, age, body mass index, aortic calcification index (ACI), renal function, serum uric acid concentrations, and comorbidities (diabetes, hypertension, or cardiovascular disease) were compared between the Non-stone and Stone groups. Independent factors for higher ACI and impaired renal function were assessed using multivariate logistic regression analysis.

Results: We confirmed relevance of Non-stone group patients as a control subject by comparing the pair-matched community-dwelling volunteers. Backgrounds of patients between the Non-stone and Stone groups were not significantly different except for the presence of hypertension in the Stone group. ACI was not significantly high in the Stone group compared with the Non-stone group. However, age-adjusted ACI was greater in the Stone group than the Non-stone group. Among urolithiasis patients, ACI was significantly higher in uric acid containing stone patients. The number of patients with stage 3B chronic kidney disease (CKD) was significantly higher in the Stone group than in the Non-stone group (12% vs. 4%, $P = 0.008$). Multivariate logistic regression analysis showed higher aortic calcification index (>13%), and being a stone former were independent factors for stage 3B CKD at the time of diagnosis.

Conclusion: Aortic calcification and being a stone former had harmful influence on renal function. This study was registered as a clinical trial: UMIN: UMIN000022962.

Keywords: Urolithiasis, Stone former, Aortic calcification, Chronic kidney disease, Renal function

* Correspondence: shingoh@hirosaki-u.ac.jp
[1]Department of Urology, Hirosaki University Graduate School of Medicine, 5 Zaifu-chou, Hirosaki 036-8562, Japan
Full list of author information is available at the end of the article

Background

Urolithiasis is a common urological disease, and its prevalence has been increasing in Japan similar to that in other developed countries [1]. In 2005, in Japan, the age-standardized annual incidences of the first episode of upper tract stones were reported to be 165.1/100,000 men and 65.1/100,000 women, which were 2-fold higher compared with that in 1965 [2]. During this period, life-style and dietary habits in Japan were more westernized, and the prevalence of obesity and metabolic syndrome (MetS) increased rapidly [3]. MetS refers to a cluster of risk factors, including high blood pressure, obesity, high cholesterol, type 2 diabetes, and atherosclerotic cardio-vascular disease [4]. Moreover, many epidemiological studies have suggested an association among urolithiasis, MetS, and chronic kidney disease (CKD) [5–7]. Because urolithiasis is considered as one of the consequences of MetS, we hypothesized that concurrent aortic calcifica-tion, complicated by arterial stiffness and atherosclerosis, may be responsible for developing CKD. Aortic calcifica-tion has recently been considered as a major complica-tion and an independent risk factor for CKD, coronary diseases, heart failure, and stroke [8–10]. Aortic calcifi-cation is widely used as an indicator of MetS-related disease [11], and it can be quantitatively measured by the aortic calcification index (ACI) using abdominal com-puted tomography (CT). We have previously reported the clinical relevance of ACI in hemodialysis patients, renal transplant recipients, and primary aldosteronism patients [12–14]. However, only a few studies have investigated aortic calcification and urolithiasis [15], and the implica-tion of aortic calcification in urolithiasis patients remains unclear. In the present study, we retrospectively assessed the distribution of aortic calcification, and in-fluence of aortic calcification on renal function in uro-lithiasis patients. This study was registered as a clinical trial: UMIN000022962.

Methods

Between January 2010 and September 2014, we treated 1221 stone patients with urolithiasis in Oyokyo Kidney Research Institute and Hirosaki University Hospital. We excluded the patients whose data including stone infor-mation and blood exam were inadequate. As a result, the remaining 287 patients (Stone group) who under-went pre-treatment abdominal CT and laboratory testing such as renal function, uric acid, lipid metabolism, and urinalysis were included in this retrospective study (Fig. 1a). The non-stone subjects comprised renal cell carcinoma (RCC) patients who had undergone radical nephrectomy at Hirosaki University Hospital between December 1986 and March 2015. Because pre-treatment abdominal CT and laboratory testing were necessary in those patients, we selected early stage RCC patients as a control group. Of 607 RCC patients, 148 early stage RCC patients (pT1N0M0) were selected as the non-stone control subjects (Non-stone group). Laboratory testing was performed before stone treatment or radical nephrectomy. The estimated glomerular filtration rate (eGFR) was calculated using the Modification of Diet in Renal Disease equation for Japanese patients [16].

To guarantee the validity of early stage RCC patients, we employed pair-matched 296 community-dwelling volunteers from 1166 subjects who participated in the Iwaki Health Promotion Project in 2014 [17]. The demographic data (age, sex, body mass index) and med-ical information (positive history of hypertension, car-diovascular disease, diabetes, and dyslipidemia) were obtained from self-questionnaires and interviews in this project. To select appropriate subjects, we used the propensity score matching strategy to compare renal function as described previously [18]. Propensity scores were calculated using logistic analysis, and the data used in the analyses included age, gender, body mass index, positive history of cardiovascular disease, hyper-tension, and diabetes. Based on the scores, two healthy subjects and one RCC patients with a score within 0.03 were selected as a pair (at a 2:1 ratio), and we com-pared renal function, serum uric acid concentration and lipid disorder between the volunteers and Non-stone group.

In the Non-stone and Stone groups, ACI was quantita-tively measured using abdominal CT images (TSX-301B, Toshiba Medical Systems Corp., Ohtawara, Japan, or CT750HD, GE Healthcare Japan, Tokyo, Japan) above the common iliac artery bifurcation by scanning 10 times at 10-mm intervals, as described previously [12]. ACI (%) expresses the calcification proportion in 12 sec-tors, and it is calculated as the average value of sections 1–10 (Fig. 1b).

After the validity evaluation of early stage RCC pa-tients for control subjects, we investigated the distribu-tion of ACI in urolithiasis patients. Patients' background including age, sex, body mass index, comorbidities (dia-betes, hypertension, or cardiovascular disease), renal func-tion, lipid metabolism, serum uric acid concentrations, voluntary urine protein, and ACI were compared between the Non-stone and Stone groups. Thereafter, the impact of stone disease on renal function were compared between the Non-stone and Stone groups.

Statistical analysis

The statistical analyses of the clinical data were per-formed using SPSS v. 22.0 (IBM Corporation, Armonk, NY, USA) and GraphPad Prism v. 5.03 (GraphPad Soft-ware, San Diego, CA, USA). Categorical variables were reported as percentages and compared using Fisher's exact test or Chi-square test. Quantitative data were

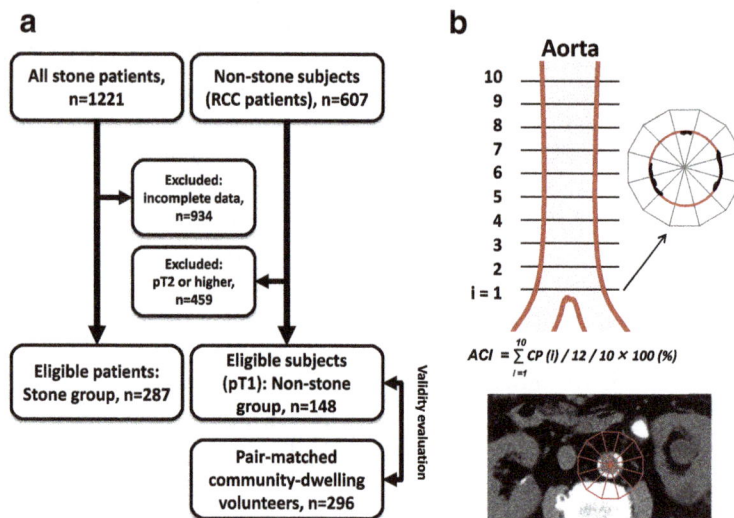

Fig. 1 Patient selection and measurement of aortic calcification index. Eligible stone patients and non-stone subjects were selected from our database in Oyokyo Kidney Research Institute and Hirosaki University Hospital. In the Stone group, 934 patients were excluded because of incomplete data. The non-stone subjects were selected from renal cell carcinoma (RCC) patients who underwent radical nephrectomy at Hirosaki University Hospital. Of those, we selected early-stage RCC patients (pT1N0M0) for the non-stone control subjects (Non-stone group). Validity of the Non-stone group was evaluated by comparison with pair-matched 296 community-dwelling volunteers from 1166 subjects who participated in the Iwaki Health Promotion Project in 2014 (**a**). Aortic calcification was quantitatively measured using pretreatment abdominal computed tomography images, scanned 10 times at 10-mm intervals above the abdominal aortic bifurcation. The calcification profile was calculated as the sum of calcification areas of 12 fractions in a single slice divided by 12. The sum of the calcification profile from 10 slices was divided by 10 and multiplied by 100 to obtain the percentage The typical computed tomography (CT) of stone patient is shown. The aortic calcification index (ACI) of this section is $10/12 \times 100 = 83.3\%$ (**b**)

expressed as medians with quartiles 1 and 3 (Q1-Q3). Differences between the groups were statistically compared using Student's t-test for data with normal distribution or Mann–Whitney U-test for data exhibiting a non-normal distribution. Differences among the three groups were statistically compared using Kruskal-Wallis test. When significant differences among the three groups were observed, we performed multiple comparisons. The correlation between two indices was analyzed using Spearman's correlation coefficient. Probability (P) values of <0.05 were considered to be statistically significant. The optimal cut-off value for stage 3B CKD was calculated using the following formula [19] :$(1 - \text{sensitivity})^2 + (1 - \text{specificity})^2$ with the receiver operating characteristic (ROC) curve.

Table 1 Clinical characteristic of community-dwelling volunteers and early stage renal cell carcinoma patients (Non-stone group)

	Volunteers	Non-stone group	P value
n	296	148	
Age (years)[a]	64 (56–72)	62 (54–72)	0.333
Gender (Male)[a], n=	176 (59%)	89 (60%)	0.919
Body mass index[a] (kg/m^2)	24 ± 4	24 ± 4	0.849
Comorbidities			
Hypertension[a], n=	85 (29%)	43 (29%)	1.000
Diabetes[a], n=	47 (16%)	31 (21%)	0.189
Cardiovascular disease[a], n=	42 (14%)	20 (14%)	0.886
eGFR (mL/min/1.73 m^2)	76 (66–85)	72 (61–87)	0.127
Stage 3B CKD, n=	12 (4%)	6 (4%)	1.000
Uric acid > 7.0 mg/dL, n=	34 (11%)	24 (16%)	0.180
Dyslipidemia (Total cholesterol >220, or Triglyceride >140 mg/dL), n=	21 (7%)	15 (10%)	0.401
Urine protein > 30 mg/dL, n=	N/A	22 (15%)	
Aortic calcification index (ACI)	N/A	6.7 (0.8-19.2)	

Median and interquartile range (Q1-Q3) was used for consecutive variables
[a], applied for propensity score-matching

Table 2 Patients' characteristics

	Non-stone group	Stone group	P value
n	148	292	
Age (years)	62 (54–72)	63 (54–72)	0.626
Sex (Male), n=	89 (60%)	169 (58%)	0.683
Body mass index (kg/m²)	24 ± 4	25 ± 4	0.171
Comorbidities			
Hypertension, n=	43 (29%)	142 (49%)	<0.001
Diabetes, n=	31 (21%)	72 (25%)	0.407
Cardiovascular disease, n=	20 (14%)	33 (11%)	0.536
eGFR (ml/min/1.73 m²)	72 (61–87)	76 (58–95)	0.250
Hyperuricemia (>7.0 mg/dL, n=	24 (16%)	45 (15%)	0.890
Dyslipidemia (total cholesterol >220, or triglyceride >140 mg/dL), n=	15 (10%)	31 (11%)	1.000
Voluntary urine protein > 30 mg/dL, n=	22 (15%)	57 (20%)	0.240
Type of stone			
Uric acid stone, n=		32 (11%)	
Non-uric acid stone, n=		216 (74%)	
Unknown, n=		44 (15%)	
Aortic calcification index (ACI)	6.7 (0.8–19.2)	7.1 (0.8–22.5)	0.856

Median and interquartile range (Q1, Q3) was used for consecutive variables

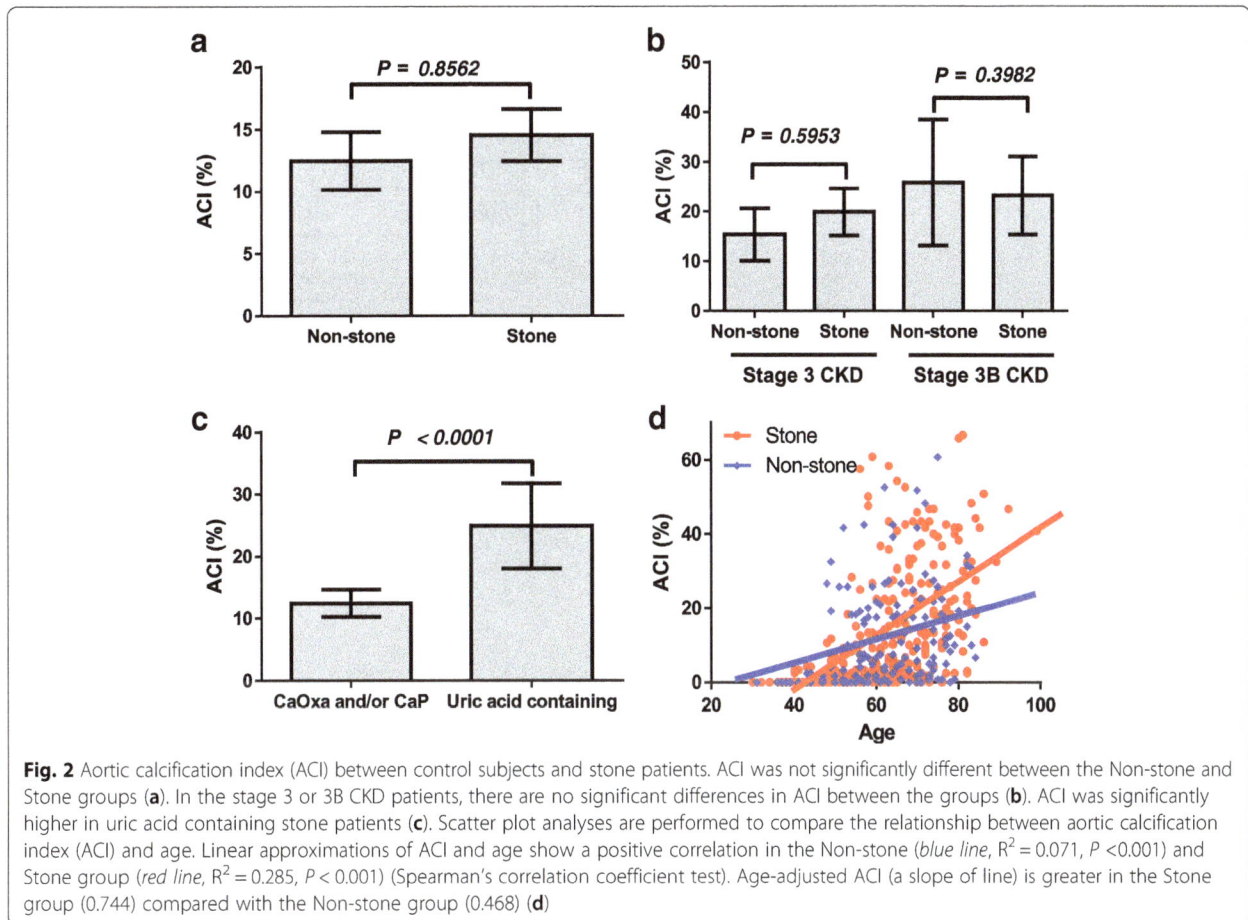

Fig. 2 Aortic calcification index (ACI) between control subjects and stone patients. ACI was not significantly different between the Non-stone and Stone groups (**a**). In the stage 3 or 3B CKD patients, there are no significant differences in ACI between the groups (**b**). ACI was significantly higher in uric acid containing stone patients (**c**). Scatter plot analyses are performed to compare the relationship between aortic calcification index (ACI) and age. Linear approximations of ACI and age show a positive correlation in the Non-stone (*blue line*, R^2 = 0.071, P <0.001) and Stone group (*red line*, R^2 = 0.285, P < 0.001) (Spearman's correlation coefficient test). Age-adjusted ACI (a slope of line) is greater in the Stone group (0.744) compared with the Non-stone group (0.468) (**d**)

Independent factors influencing stage 3B CKD at the time of diagnosis were identified by multivariate analyses using a logistic regression model. Odds ratios (ORs) with 95% confidence intervals (CIs) were calculated after concurrently adjusting for potential confounders. Data from healthy volunteers were not included in this multivariate model due to the absence of ACI and proteinuria information. We included nine variables in the logistic regression analysis because of the limited number of samples. Several independent variables that increased the postoperative renal impairment risk were included in the models: age (>65 years), sex (male), history of comorbidity (hypertension, type 2 diabetes, or cardiovascular disease), lipid metabolism abnormality (total cholesterol > 220 mg/dL or triglyceride > 140 mg/dL), serum uric acid concentration (>7.0 mg/dL), voluntary urine protein (>30 mg/dL), and ACI (>13.0%) at the time of diagnosis. Moreover, the predictive accuracy of the selected variables in the dataset was evaluated using the area under the curve (AUC) derived from the ROC curve.

Results

Comparison between community-dwelling volunteers and early stage RCC patients

We compared pair-matched 296 community-dwelling volunteers and 148 of early stage RCC patients. Median age, sex, body mass index, positive history of hypertension, diabetes, and cardiovascular disease were not significantly different. In addition, unadjusted parameters such as eGFR, the number of subjects with stage 3B CKD, hyperuricemia, and dyslipidemia were also not significantly different (Table 1). Based on these results, we regarded early stage RCC patients as appropriate candidate for control subjects.

Comparison between early stage RCC patients (Non-stone group) and stone patients (Stone group)

Thereafter, we compared the Non-stone and Stone groups. Component of stones were calcium oxalate ($n = 119$, 41.5%), calcium oxalate mixed stones ($n = 97$, 33.8%), uric acid containing stone ($n = 31$, 10.8%), cysteine ($n = 1$, 0.35%), and unknown ($n = 39$, 13.6%). Table 2 summarizes

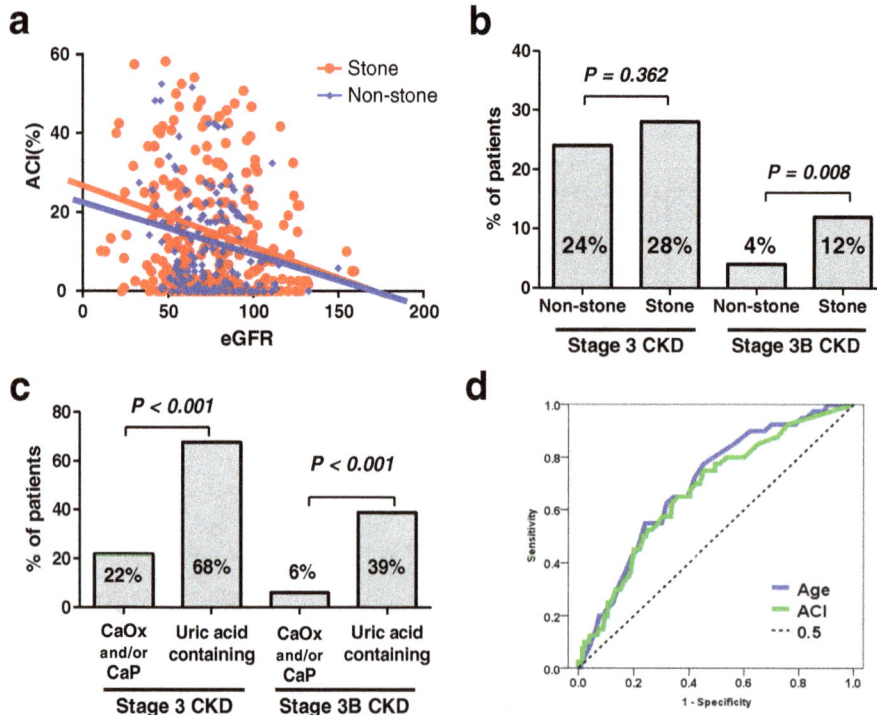

Fig. 3 Correlation eGFR and aortic calcification index (ACI), chronic kidney disease (CKD), and receiver operating characteristic curve (ROC) analysis for predictive accuracy of stage 3B chronic kidney disease. ACI and eGFR showed significant, but weak correlations in the Stone ($R^2 = 0.053$, $P < 0.001$) and Non-stone group ($R^2 = 0.032$, $P = 0.029$) (a). The number of patients with stage 3B CKD was significantly higher in the Stone group compared with the Non-stone group (12% vs. 4%, $P = 0.008$), although the number of patients with stage 3 CKD was not significantly different (b). The number of patients with stage 3 and 3B CKD was significantly higher in uric stone containing patients compared with calcium oxalate (CaOx) and/or calcium phosphate (CaP) stone patients (c). The optimal ACI cut-off value of age and ACI for stage 3B CKD was determined by analyzing ROC curves using the area under the curve (AUC) (d). An age of 65 years (AUC = 0.70; $P < 0.001$; 95% CI: 0.62–0.78, blue line) and ACI of 13.0% (AUC = 0.68; $P < 0.001$; 95% CI: 0.59–0.76, green line) were used as the cut-off values in this study

the patient characteristics. The number of patients with hypertension was significantly higher in the Stone group ($P = 0.001$). No significant differences were observed for any other parameter. ACI was not significantly different between the groups (Fig. 2a). In addition, there were no statistical significant differences in ACI in patients with stage 3 CKD or stage 3B CKD (Fig. 2b). Among urolithiasis patients, ACI was significantly higher in uric acid containing stone patients (Fig. 2c). Age and ACI showed positive correlations in the Stone group ($R^2 = 0.285$, $P < 0.001$) and Non-stone group ($R^2 = 0.071$, $P < 0.001$, Spearman's correlation coefficient test). Age-adjusted ACI (a slope of the line) was greater in the Stone group (0.744) than the Non-stone group (0.468) (Fig. 2d).

Although ACI and eGFR showed negative correlations (Fig. 3a), R^2 values showed weak correlation in both groups (Stone: $R^2 = 0.053$, $P < 0.001$, and Non-stone: $R^2 = 0.032$, $P = 0.029$). The number of patients with stage 3 CKD was not significantly different between the Non-stone and Stone groups (28% vs. 24%, $P = 0.362$). However, the number of patients with stage 3B CKD was significantly higher in the Stone group compared with the Non-stone group (12% vs. 4%, respectively, $P = 0.008$) (Fig. 3b). Similarly, patients with uric acid containing stone were higher in stage 3A/3B CKD (Fig. 3c, Table 3).

To investigate the implications of ACI in renal function, the optimal ACI cut-off value for age and ACI was determined by analyzing ROC curves. An age of 65 years (AUC = 0.70, $P < 0.001$, 95% CI: 0.62–0.78) and ACI of 13.0% (AUC = 0.68, $P < 0.001$, 95% CI: 0.59–0.76) were used as the cut-off values in this study (Fig. 3d).

Multivariate logistic regression analysis revealed that an age of >65 years, sex (male), presence of comorbidities, serum uric acid (>7.0 mg/dL) were selected as independent factors for higher ACI. Similarly, an age of >65 years, sex (male), hyperuricemia, voluntary urine protein > 30 mg/d, ACI >13.0%, and Stone group were selected as independent factors for stage 3B CKD at the time of diagnosis (Table 4). The three group comparisons among the community-dwelling volunteers, Non-stone and Stone groups were shown in Fig. 4.

Table 3 Relationship between stage of CKD and stone components

	Uric acid (%)	CaOx / CaP (%)	P value
Normal / CKD 1	0 (0%)	70 (32%)	<0.001
CKD 2	9 (41%)	99 (46%)	0.078
CKD 3A	9 (41%)	34 (16%)	0.068
CKD 3B	5 (19%)	10 (5%)	0.027
CKD 4	7 (29%)	3 (1%)	<0.001

CaOx calcium oxalate, *CaP* Calcium phosphate

Table 4 Multivariate logistic regression analyses of independent factors for higher ACI (>13%) and stage 3B CKD or higher (eGFR < 45 mL/min/1.73 m^2) at the time of diagnosis between the Non-stone and Stone groups

ACI	Factors	P value	OR	95% CI
Age	> 65 years	0.000	3.90	2.47-6.17
Sex	Male	0.013	1.76	1.13-2.76
Body mass index	> 25 kg/m^2	0.132	0.71	0.46-1.11
Comorbidities	Positive	0.049	1.60	1.00-2.55
Lipid metabolism abnormality	Positive	0.337	0.80	0.51-1.26
Serum uric acid	> 7.0 mg/dL	0.047	0.52	0.27-0.99
Urine protein	> 30 mg/dL	0.089	1.63	0.93-2.87
CKD stage	3B or higher	0.052	2.17	0.99-4.74
Stone formers	Positive	0.501	0.85	0.54-1.35
Stage 3B CKD	Factors	P value	OR	95% CI
Age	> 65 years	0.004	4.11	1.59-10.6
Sex	Male	0.030	2.56	1.09-5.99
Body mass index	> 25 kg/m^2	0.714	1.15	0.54-2.44
Comorbidities	Positive	0.606	1.26	0.52-3.03
Lipid metabolism abnormality	Positive	0.904	1.05	0.49-2.27
Serum uric acid	> 7.0 mg/dL	0.001	4.53	1.94-10.6
Urine protein	> 30 mg/dL	0.003	3.22	1.50-6.91
ACI	> 13.0%	0.047	2.28	1.01-5.17
Stone formers	Positive	0.005	4.00	1.52-10.5

Comorbidities included history of diabetes, hypertension, or cardiovascular disease
ACI aortic calcification index

Discussion

Aortic calcification is regarded as one of the consequences of systemic aortic degradation. Numerous studies have addressed the clinical importance of arterial calcification among CKD patients and cardiovascular high-risk patients [10–12, 14, 19–21]. Our previous study suggested that aortic calcification burden has a negative effect on postoperative renal function in renal transplant patients, [14] and the preoperative condition of aortic calcification has a significant impact on postoperative persistent hypertension after unilateral adrenalectomy in patients with aldosterone-producing adenomas. [13] However, only a few studies have demonstrated the impact of arterial calcification in urolithiasis patients. Yasui et al. [15] reported that aortic calcification scores were significantly different between stone and non-stone patients. They also suggested that a diet with high animal protein, cholesterol, and fat may cause urolithiasis and arteriosclerosis. Therefore, we hypothesized that aortic calcification may play an important role in renal function deterioration in urolithiasis patients. However, our results suggested that ACI was not significantly higher in urolithiasis patients with CKD, whereas the age-related aortic calcification is greater in urolithiasis

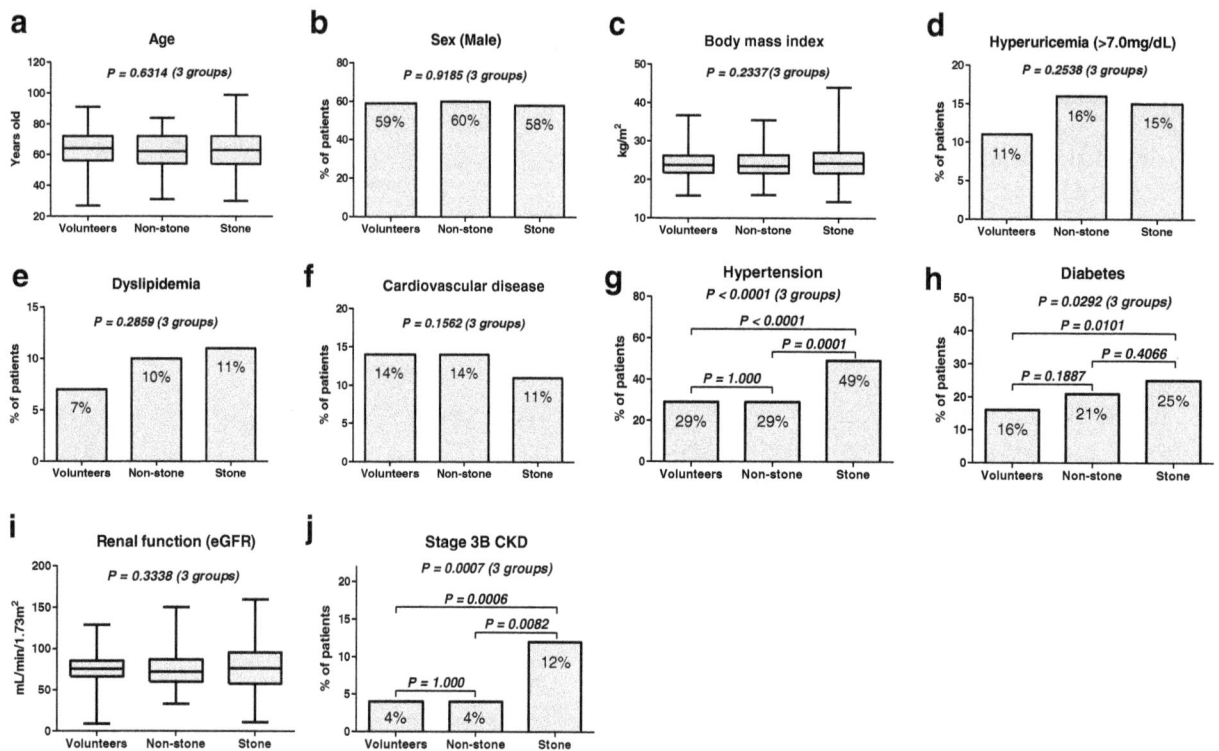

Fig. 4 The three group comparisons among the community-dwelling volunteers, Non-stone, and Stone groups. There were no significantly differences in age (**a**), sex (**b**), body mass index (**c**), hyperuricemia (**d**), dyslipidemia (**e**), positive history of cardiovascular disease (**f**) and eGFR (**i**), except for hypertension (**g**), diabetes (**h**), and prevalence of stage 3B CKD (**j**). It is remarkable that the prevalence of stage 3B CKD is significantly higher in the Stone group

patients. Although we could not prove the relationship between ACI and CKD in urolithiasis patients, the number of stage 3B CKD patients was significantly higher in the Stone group. The prevalence of stage 3B CKD in the community-dwelling volunteers, Non-stone, and Stone group showed 4%, 4%, and 12%, respectively (Fig. 4J). In addition, multivariate analysis identified ACI and being a stone former as potential factor for stage 3B CKD, which is similar to age, gender, hyperuricemia, and proteinuria. Our finding suggested that patients with poor renal function have more aortic calcification in stone formers as well as the control subjects. On the other hand, being a stone former was not selected as independent factors for higher ACI, whereas age, sex and hyperuricemia were associated with higher ACI. These results suggest a complicated relationship among vascular calcification, CKD and stone formation. Although precise mechanisms for urinary stone formation and aortic calcification remain unclear, higher age-adjusted ACI in urolithiasis patients suggested that MetS, including obesity, hypertension, impaired glucose metabolism, hyperuricemia, and atherogenic dyslipidemia, may play a key role in the vascular calcification and urolithiasis development, and resulted in premature vascular aging in stone formers.

Although mechanisms responsible for vascular calcification is still under investigation, it has been reported that vascular smooth muscle cells play a critical role in mediating vessel calcification by differentiating into osteoblast-like cells [22]. Calcifying vascular cells, which are a subpopulation of vascular smooth muscle cells, spontaneously form ossified nodules when cultured for a long time. These nodules express many bone-related molecules, including increased alkaline phosphatase activity, and osteocalcin, osteonectin, and osteopontin expressions [23]. Osteopontin is a glycoprotein secreted by macrophages, vascular smooth muscle cells, and endothelial cells and has been demonstrated to promote macrophage chemotaxis [24, 25]. It has been identified as a major matrix component of urinary calcium stones [26] and is strongly associated with urinary stone formation [27]. Recent studies have suggested that renal tubular inflammation, involving macrophages and osteopontin, plays a key role in renal calcium oxalate crystal formation [28]. Inflammation and osteopontin also play key roles in vascular calcification [25, 29] and inflammation, impaired calcium and phosphate homeostasis, and oxidative stress have been linked to vascular calcification in CKD patients. [30]. Furthermore, MetS has been considered as a chronic, low grade, systemic inflammatory disease [31]. Based on these results, vascular calcification and urinary stone formation might share similar mechanisms through inflammation, which is regarded as the key process underlying metabolic diseases. Further studies are necessary to address the detailed association between MetS, inflammation, oxidative stress, vascular calcification, urinary stone formation, and CKD.

Several limitations in this study need to be noted. The small sample size and retrospective design prevented definitive conclusions on the aortic calcification influence on renal function deterioration. We were unable to control selection bias and other unmeasurable confounding factors in both the stone and non-stone subjects even using matching methods. Although we used propensity matching methods to guarantee the validity of early stage RCC patients, adequacy of early stage RCC patients as a control subject remain unclear. We were also unable to include some other established factors that influence aortic calcification and renal function, such as cigarette smoking, information on blood pressure control, medications, and presence of hydronephrosis. We could not address the direct interaction between higher ACI and having urolithiasis because of cross-sectional study. In addition, we could not address the implication of uric acid stone on ACI and renal function due to the limited number of uric acid stone patients. Many statistics were also the limitation of the present study. Therefore, additional large-scale investigations are necessary to validate the ACI impact on renal function in urolithiasis patients.

Despite these limitations, the strength of this study is that it is the first report to assess the implication of aortic calcification in urolithiasis patients. Using this non-invasive modality, we could demonstrate an independent association between ACI and renal impairment in urolithiasis patients. In addition, a possible relation of ACI and hyperuricemia through MetS is suggested. Our findings may contribute for clinicians to take intensive care and educate urolithiasis patients with severe aortic calcification to prevent renal impairment progression.

Conclusion

In conclusion, aortic calcification and being a stone former had harmful influence on renal function. Premature vascular aging may be accelerated through MetS in stone formers. Further large-scale studies are needed to assess the clinical relevance of ACI on renal function in urolithiasis patients.

Abbreviations
ACI: Aortic calcification; AUC: Area under the curve; CaOx: Calcium oxalate; CaP: Calcium phosphate; CIs: Confidence intervals; CKD: Chronic kidney disease; CT: Computed tomography; eGFR: Estimated glomerular filtration rate; Mets: Metabolic syndrome; ORs: Odds ratios; Q1: First quartile; Q3: Third quartile; RCC: Renal cell carcinoma; ROC: Receiver operating characteristic

Acknowledgement
We thank Yuki Fujita and Mihoko Osanai for their invaluable help with the data collection.

Funding
This work was supported by a Grant-in-Aid for Scientific Research (No. 23791737, 24659708, and 22390301) from the Japan Society for the Promotion of Science.

Authors' contributions
Conceived and designed the experiments: SH Performed the experiments: TT, HY, TN, TM, OS, TY (Takahiro Yoneyama), YH Analyzed the data: YT (Yuriko Terayama), TY (Tohru Yoneyama) Contributed reagents/materials/analysis tools: YT (Yuki Tobisawa), TY (Tohru Yoneyama), IT, SN Wrote the manuscript: TT, SH, IH.Other: Supervision: CO, TK, TF. All authors read and approved the final manuscript.

Authors' information
TT: postgraduate student, SH: assistant professor, HY: assistant professor, TN: postgraduate student, IH: postgraduate student, TM: postgraduate student, OS: postgraduate student, YT: associate professor, TY: associate professor, TY: associate professor, YH: associate professor, TK: associate professor, IT: associate professor, SN: professor, YT: academic researcher, TF: administrative director, CO: professor and chairman.

Competing interests
The authors declare that they have no competing interests, and no financial conflict of interest.

Ethics approval and consent to participate
The study was performed in accordance with the ethical standards of the Declaration of Helsinki and was approved by the ethical committee of Hirosaki University Graduate School of Medicine (authorization number, 2015–184). For this type of retrospective study, formal patient consent is not required. The cross sectional data collection for the Iwaki Health Promotion Project was approved by the Ethics Committee of Hirosaki University School of Medicine (authorization number, 2014–015), and all subjects provided written informed consent before participating in the project.

Author details
[1]Department of Urology, Hirosaki University Graduate School of Medicine, 5 Zaifu-chou, Hirosaki 036-8562, Japan. [2]Department of Advanced Transplant and Regenerative Medicine, Hirosaki University Graduate School of Medicine, Hirosaki, Japan. [3]Department of Urology, Oyokyo Kidney Research Institute, Hirosaki, Japan. [4]Department of Social Medicine, Hirosaki University School of Medicine, Hirosaki, Japan.

References
1. Stamatelou KK, Francis ME, Jones CA, Nyberg LM, Curhan GC. Time trends in reported prevalence of kidney stones in the United States: 1976–1994. Kidney Int. 2003;63(5):1817–23.
2. Yasui T, Iguchi M, Suzuki S, Kohri K. Prevalence and epidemiological characteristics of urolithiasis in Japan: national trends between 1965 and 2005. Urology. 2008;71(2):209–13.
3. Yasui T, Okada A, Hamamoto S, Hirose M, Ando R, Kubota Y, Tozawa K, Hayashi Y, Gao B, Suzuki S, et al. The association between the incidence of urolithiasis and nutrition based on Japanese National Health and Nutrition Surveys. Urolithiasis. 2013;41(3):217–24.
4. Esposito K, Chiodini P, Colao A, Lenzi A, Giugliano D. Metabolic syndrome and risk of cancer: a systematic review and meta-analysis. Diabetes Care. 2012;35(11):2402–11.
5. Kawamoto R, Kohara K, Tabara Y, Miki T. An association between metabolic syndrome and the estimated glomerular filtration rate. Internal medicine (Tokyo, Japan). 2008;47(15):1399–406.
6. Rule AD, Krambeck AE, Lieske JC. Chronic kidney disease in kidney stone formers. Clin J Am Soc Nephrol . 2011;6(8):2069–75.
7. Thomas G, Sehgal AR, Kashyap SR, Srinivas TR, Kirwan JP, Navaneethan SD. Metabolic syndrome and kidney disease: a systematic review and meta-

8. Bahous SA, Blacher J, Safar ME. Aortic stiffness, kidney disease, and renal transplantation. Curr Hypertens Rep. 2009;11(2):98–103.

9. Walsh CR, Cupples LA, Levy D, Kiel DP, Hannan M, Wilson PW, O'Donnell CJ. Abdominal aortic calcific deposits are associated with increased risk for congestive heart failure: the Framingham Heart Study. Am Heart J. 2002;144(4):733–9.

10. Nakagami H, Osako MK, Morishita R. New concept of vascular calcification and metabolism. Curr Vasc Pharmacol. 2011;9(1):124–7.

11. Mizobuchi M, Towler D, Slatopolsky E. Vascular calcification: the killer of patients with chronic kidney disease. J Am Soc Nephrol. 2009;20(7):1453–64.

12. Tsushima M, Terayama Y, Momose A, Funyu T, Ohyama C, Hada R. Carotid intima media thickness and aortic calcification index closely relate to cerebro- and cardiovascular disorders in hemodialysis patients. Int J Urol. 2008;15(1):48–51.

13. Fujita N, Hatakeyama S, Yamamoto H, Tobisawa Y, Yoneyama T, Yoneyama T, Hashimoto Y, Koie T, Nigawara T, Ohyama C. Implication of aortic calcification on persistent hypertension after laparoscopic adrenalectomy in patients with primary aldosteronism. Int J Urol. 2016;23(5):412–7.

14. Imanishi K, Hatakeyama S, Yamamoto H, Okamoto A, Imai A, Yoneyama T, Hashimoto Y, Koie T, Fujita T, Murakami R, et al. Post-transplant renal function and cardiovascular events are closely associated with the aortic calcification index in renal transplant recipients. Transplant Proc. 2014;46(2):484–8.

15. Yasui T, Itoh Y, Bing G, Okada A, Tozawa K, Kohri K. Aortic calcification in urolithiasis patients. Scand J Urol Nephrol. 2007;41(5):419–21.

16. Imai E, Horio M, Iseki K, Yamagata K, Watanabe T, Hara S, Ura N, Kiyohara Y, Hirakata H, Moriyama T, et al. Prevalence of chronic kidney disease (CKD) in the Japanese general population predicted by the MDRD equation modified by a Japanese coefficient. Clin Exp Nephrol. 2007;11(2):156–63.

17. Satake R, Sugawara N, Sato K, Takahashi I, Nakaji S, Yasui-Furukori N, Fukuda S. Prevalence and Predictive Factors of Irritable Bowel Syndrome in a Community-dwelling Population in Japan. Intern Med. 2015;54(24):3105–12.

18. Hatakeyama S, Koie T, Narita T, Hosogoe S, Yamamoto H, Tobisawa Y, Yoneyama T, Yoneyama T, Hashimoto Y, Ohyama C. Renal Function Outcomes and Risk Factors for Risk Factors for Stage 3B Chronic Kidney Disease after Urinary Diversion in Patients with Muscle Invasive Bladder Cancer. PLoS One. 2016;11(2):e0149544.

19. Akobeng AK. Understanding diagnostic tests 3: Receiver operating characteristic curves. Acta Paediatr. 2007;96(5):644–7.

20. Li LC, Lee YT, Lee YW, Chou CA, Lee CT. Aortic arch calcification predicts the renal function progression in patients with stage 3 to 5 chronic kidney disease. Biomed Res Int. 2015;2015:131263.

21. Thomas IC, Ratigan AR, Rifkin DE, Ix JH, Criqui MH, Budoff MJ, Allison MA. The association of renal artery calcification with hypertension in community-living individuals: the multiethnic study of atherosclerosis. J Am Soc Hypertens. 2016;10(2):167–74.

22. Johnson RC, Leopold JA, Loscalzo J. Vascular calcification: pathobiological mechanisms and clinical implications. Circ Res. 2006;99(10):1044–59.

23. Watson KE, Bostrom K, Ravindranath R, Lam T, Norton B, Demer LL. TGF-beta 1 and 25-hydroxycholesterol stimulate osteoblast-like vascular cells to calcify. J Clin Invest. 1994;93(5):2106–13.

24. Sodek J, Ganss B, McKee MD. Osteopontin. Critical Reviews in Oral Biology and Medicine. 2000;11(3):279–303.

25. Gravallese EM. Osteopontin: a bridge between bone and the immune system. J Clin Invest. 2003;112(2):147–9.

26. Kohri K, Suzuki Y, Yoshida K, Yamamoto K, Amasaki N, Yamate T, Umekawa T, Iguchi M, Sinohara H, Kurita T. Molecular cloning and sequencing of cDNA encoding urinary stone protein, which is identical to osteopontin. Biochem Biophys Res Commun. 1992;184(2):859–64.

27. Kohri K, Nomura S, Kitamura Y, Nagata T, Yoshioka K, Iguchi M, Yamate T, Umekawa T, Suzuki Y, Sinohara H, et al. Structure and expression of the mRNA encoding urinary stone protein (osteopontin). J Biol Chem. 1993;268(20):15180–4.

28. Okada A, Yasui T, Hamamoto S, Hirose M, Kubota Y, Itoh Y, Tozawa K, Hayashi Y, Kohri K. Genome-wide analysis of genes related to kidney stone formation and elimination in the calcium oxalate nephrolithiasis model mouse: detection of stone-preventive factors and involvement of macrophage activity. J Bone Miner Res. 2009;24(5):908–24.

29. Buendia P, Montes de Oca A, Madueno JA, Merino A, Martin-Malo A, Aljama P, Ramirez R, Rodriguez M, Carracedo J. Endothelial microparticles mediate inflammation-induced vascular calcification. FASEB J. 2015;29(1):173–81.

30. Byon CH, Chen Y. Molecular Mechanisms of Vascular Calcification in Chronic Kidney Disease: The Link between Bone and the Vasculature. Curr Osteoporos Rep. 2015;13(4):206–15.

31. Nishimura S, Manabe I, Nagasaki M, Eto K, Yamashita H, Ohsugi M, Otsu M, Hara K, Ueki K, Sugiura S, et al. CD8+ effector T cells contribute to macrophage recruitment and adipose tissue inflammation in obesity. Nat Med. 2009;15(8):914–20.

Probiotics [LGG-BB12 or RC14-GR1] versus placebo as prophylaxis for urinary tract infection in persons with spinal cord injury [ProSCIUTTU]

Bonsan Bonne Lee[1,2], Swee-Ling Toh[2,3*], Suzanne Ryan[1], Judy M. Simpson[3], Kate Clezy[4], Laetitia Bossa[1,5], Scott A. Rice[5,9], Obaydullah Marial[2,6,7], Gerard Weber[6], Jasbeer Kaur[7], Claire Boswell-Ruys[1], Stephen Goodall[8], James Middleton[10,11], Mark Tudehope[7] and George Kotsiou[7]

Abstract

Background: Urinary tract infections [UTIs] are very common in people with Spinal Cord Injury [SCI]. UTIs are increasingly difficult and expensive to treat as the organisms that cause them become more antibiotic resistant. Among the SCI population, there is a high rate of multi-resistant organism [MRO] colonisation. Non-antibiotic prevention strategies are needed to prevent UTI without increasing resistance. Probiotics have been reported to be beneficial in preventing UTIs in post-menopausal women in several *in vivo* and *in vitro* studies. The main aim of this study is to determine whether probiotic therapy with combinations of Lactobacillus reuteri RC-14 + Lactobacillus rhamnosus GR-1 [RC14-GR1] and/or Lactobacillus rhamnosus GG + Bifidobacterium BB-12 [LGG-BB12] are effective in preventing UTI in people with SCI compared to placebo.

Method: This is a multi-site randomised double-blind double-dummy placebo-controlled factorial design study conducted in New South Wales, Australia. All participants have a neurogenic bladder as a result of spinal injury. Recruitment started in April 2011.
Participants are randomised to one of four arms, designed for factorial analysis of LGG-BB12 and/or RC14-GR1 v Placebo. This involves 24 weeks of daily oral treatment with RC14-GR1 + LGG-BB12, RC14-GR1 + placebo, LGG-BB12 + placebo or two placebo capsules. Randomisation is stratified by bladder management type and inpatient status. Participants are assessed at baseline, three months and six months for Short Form Health Survey [SF-36], microbiological swabs of rectum, nose and groin; urine culture and urinary catheters for subjects with indwelling catheters. A bowel questionnaire is administered at baseline and three months to assess effect of probiotics on bowel function.
The primary outcome is time from randomisation to occurrence of symptomatic UTI. The secondary outcomes are change of MRO status and bowel function, quality of life and cost-effectiveness of probiotics in persons with SCI. The primary outcome will be analysed using survival analysis of factorial groups, with Cox regression modelling to test the effect of each treatment while allowing for the other, assuming no interaction effect. Hazard ratios and Kaplan-Meier survival curves will be used to summarise results.

(Continued on next page)

* Correspondence: SweeLing.Toh@health.nsw.gov.au
[2]Department of Spinal and Rehabilitation Medicine, Prince of Wales Hospital, Sydney, Australia
[3]School of Public Health, University of Sydney, Sydney, Australia
Full list of author information is available at the end of the article

(Continued from previous page)

Discussion: If these probiotics are shown to be effective in preventing UTI and MRO colonisation, they would be a very attractive alternative for UTI prophylaxis and for combating the increasing rate of antibiotic resistance after SCI.

Keywords: Urinary prophylaxis, Multi-resistant organisms, Antibiotic resistance, Probiotics, Biofilm, Microbial community profiles

Background

Urinary tract infections [UTIs] are very common in people with a neurogenic bladder. People with a spinal cord injury [SCI] and people with the spinal demyelinating form of Multiple Sclerosis [MS] are highly susceptible to the development of neurogenic bladder dysfunction.

UTIs have a high societal cost and current prevention strategies do not work. People with neurogenic bladder are at significant risk from UTI with approximately two [2] UTI episodes per year on average for persons with SCI [1]. One of the major clinical challenges for SCI patients and clinicians is that when patients get a UTI, simple oral antibiotics frequently are ineffective due to the high numbers of multi-resistant-organism [s] [MROs] within SCI populations [about 40–50 % of SCI people] [1, 2]. This greatly amplifies the health, societal and economic consequences of disease and can even lead to life threatening clinical problems that can spread if not controlled through hospitals and the community. Health care costs associated with cross infection are estimated at US$18–30 billion yearly in the USA and UK combined. Australian costs are expected to be proportionate [3]. Furthermore, based on the existing SCI UTI prevention literature, we have demonstrated that current commonly used methods of non-antibiotic UTI prevention in SCI do not work [4]. The prevention of UTI, particularly the more difficult to treat MRO UTI, is therefore a clinical imperative for those people with SCI and neurogenic bladder. Non-antibiotic prevention is needed to prevent UTI without increasing the antimicrobial resistance burden [5].

Probiotics are defined as a preparation containing viable, defined micro-organisms in sufficient numbers, which alter the microflora [by implantation or colonization] in a compartment of the host and thus exert beneficial health effects in this host [6]. Reid postulated that probiotics could reduce antibiotic related superinfections, disrupt bacterial biofilms, and enhance generalised mucosal immunity in the gastrointestinal and genitourinary systems [7]. In a systematic review conducted by Falagas et al., it was concluded that several probiotics tested, e.g. Lactobacillus rhamnosus GR-1 and Lactobacillus fermentum RC-14, delivered either intravaginally or orally, were efficacious in restoring vaginal flora and in preventing recurrent UTIs in women [8]. In another trial, Manley et al. demonstrated clearance of vancomycin-related enterococci in stool after treatment with Lactobacillus rhamnosus GG [9].

There are currently no known trials of oral probiotics and its efficacy in prevention of UTIs in people with neurogenic bladders. Darouiche and others have conducted more invasive trials involving inoculating neurogenic bladders with benign strains of Escherichia coli and showed this approach was effective at lowering the rate of UTIs per year [10–12].

Study aims

Primary aim

To test the effectiveness of combination oral probiotic therapy Lactobacillus reuteri RC-14 + Lactobacillus rhamnosus GR-1 [RC14-GR1 capsules] and/or Lactobacillus rhamnosus GG + Bifidobacterium BB-12 [LGG-BB12 capsules] in preventing UTI in people with SCI compared to placebo.

Secondary aims

a) To examine whether probiotics may change or prevent colonisation or infection with MROs in persons with SCI.

b) To examine the effects of probiotics on bowel function in persons with SCI

c) Examination of indwelling and suprapubic catheters to determine:

i) How probiotic intervention affects microbial community composition in the urine and urinary catheter.

ii) Differences between microbial communities in individuals who are symptomatic versus asymptomatic for UTI.

d) To estimate the cost-effectiveness of probiotics in persons with SCI

A randomised controlled trial [RCT] was selected as the design most likely to provide a definitive conclusion to the primary aim.

Methods/design

This is a prospective multi-site randomised, double-blind, double-dummy, placebo-controlled factorial design trial conducted in the state of New South Wales [NSW] Australia, in order to test the effectiveness of two probiotic therapies in preventing UTI in people with SCI. Participants will be recruited from the NSW SCI community and all the specialist SCI units in NSW hospitals, including their regional and rural affiliations. These units are located at the Prince of Wales Hospital [POWH], Royal Rehabilitation Centre Sydney [RRCS] and Royal North Shore Hospital [RNSH].

Ethics approval

A multi-site ethics approval was obtained from the Human Research Ethics Committee [HREC] at each of the three SCI units in NSW, Australia. HREC Protocol no: 1008-282-CTN-GG [POWH SSA 1008-282 CTN, RR SSA 11/SSA03, RNSH SSA10/HAWKE/171].

The protocol for catheter sampling and culture independent technique of bacterial community identification was categorised as a low-risk study with separate ethics approval obtained from the HREC at each site [POWH HREC ref no. 11/036, RNSH HREC/10/HARBR/102 and SSA/10/HAWKE/171].

The trial was registered with the Australian New Zealand Clinical Trials Registry [ACTRN 12610000512022] on 21 June 2010. Informed consent will be provided prior to recruitment and participation. Participant recruitment commenced in April 2011.

Sample size

The trial uses a factorial design which allows the two probiotics to be compared with placebo simultaneously without inflating the sample size, on the assumption that they do not interact with each other. [Refer Table 1].

UTI prevention: In our previous RCT with the same study population [4], 45 % of participants had a symptomatic UTI within six months. To have 80 % power to detect [at 5 % two-sided significance level] a 30 % reduction in the treatment group requires a total sample size of 350. Allowing for a 5 % loss to follow-up a final sample size of 372 is required, 93 participants being randomly allocated to each of the four study groups.

MRO treatment: It is expected that approximately 40 % participants will be MRO-positive at enrolment. Assuming 5-10 % become MRO-negative in the control group, a 15–20 % reduction in MRO-positive colonisation rate with probiotics would be detectable as significant at the 5 % level, with 80 % power, with a sample size of 372.

Randomisation and blinding of assessors

A simple stratified [computer generated] randomisation protocol is used. JS is responsible for generating the allocation sequence. Randomisation is stratified by bladder management types [indwelling/suprapubic vs intermittent catheters vs condom drainage/reflex voiding] as well as inpatient/outpatient status. Randomisation occurs following participant's compliance check at Day 4. One central pharmacy is responsible for the assignment and distribution of the intervention for the entire study. All four treatment regimens will be indistinguishable by appearance and taste, and all participants receive the same quantity of tablets. All clinical staff, researchers and participants remain blind to treatment allocation throughout this process. An audit of randomisation, product allocation and dispensing stock will be performed at the completion of the study by MT, who is not affiliated with the final analysis and the clinical management of the study or study participants.

Participants

All participants are to be over 18 years of age and are required to provide written consent. All participants with known neurogenic bladder as a result of SCI who meet inclusion criteria and gave written consent are enrolled. BL, ST, SR, JK, LB, GW and CBR are responsible for enrolling participants.

Inclusion criteria:

1) Had a known neurogenic bladder;
2) Had a stable SCI or stable multiple sclerosis with a known spinal demyelinating lesion;
3) Had a stable bladder management technique [i.e. not receiving bladder management education for at least 4 weeks] and using a bladder management technique such as indwelling catheter, suprapubic catheter, clean intermittent self-catheterisation or reflex/condom drainage;
4) Agreed to fortnightly telephone consultation for themselves and their care team during the six month study period;
5) Agreed not to take any other probiotic in addition to the allocated intervention during the course of the study. This includes all oral or topical preparations of yoghurt and urinary antiseptics [e.g. methenamine hippurate (hiprex) or cranberry preparations].

Table 1 Study design for ProSCIUTTU

	LGG -BB12 (B) Active (186)	LGG -BB12 (b) Placebo (186)
GR1-RC14 (A) Active (186)	AB or Intervention A (93)	Ab or Intervention B (93)
GR1-RC14 (a) Placebo (186)	aB or Intervention C (93)	ab or Intervention D (93)

Exclusion criteria:

1. Receiving bladder management education within the last 4 weeks;
2. Being treated for, or symptomatic from a current infection or long-standing pressure sore;
3. Known to have a complex bladder disturbance requiring surgical intervention e.g. known cystoplasty, renal or bladder calculus, significant hydronephrosis, or current pyelonephritis;
4. Known to have chronic open wound/s or known long-standing osteomyelitis [greater than 6 weeks];
5. On long-term antibiotic therapy for any indication;
6. Known to have a history of adverse drug reaction to yoghurt products or a demonstrated intolerance to the probiotics used. Lactose intolerance was NOT an exclusion criterion;

7. Known to have severe renal or hepatic failure;
8. Requiring full [invasive] mechanical ventilation;
9. Receiving immunosuppressant medications or have an underlying immunosuppressive disease [for example HIV or end-stage/ progressive diabetes mellitus, multiple sclerosis or cerebrovascular disease];
10. Planning to have oral surgery during the intervention period;
11. Concurrently enrolled in another intervention study [observational studies or inclusion following completion of another study was allowed].

Each participant is enrolled for a six month study period, which includes 24 weeks of treatment [see Fig. 1]. Each participant randomised is required to take two tablets orally each day consisting of either RC14-GR1 + LGG-BB12

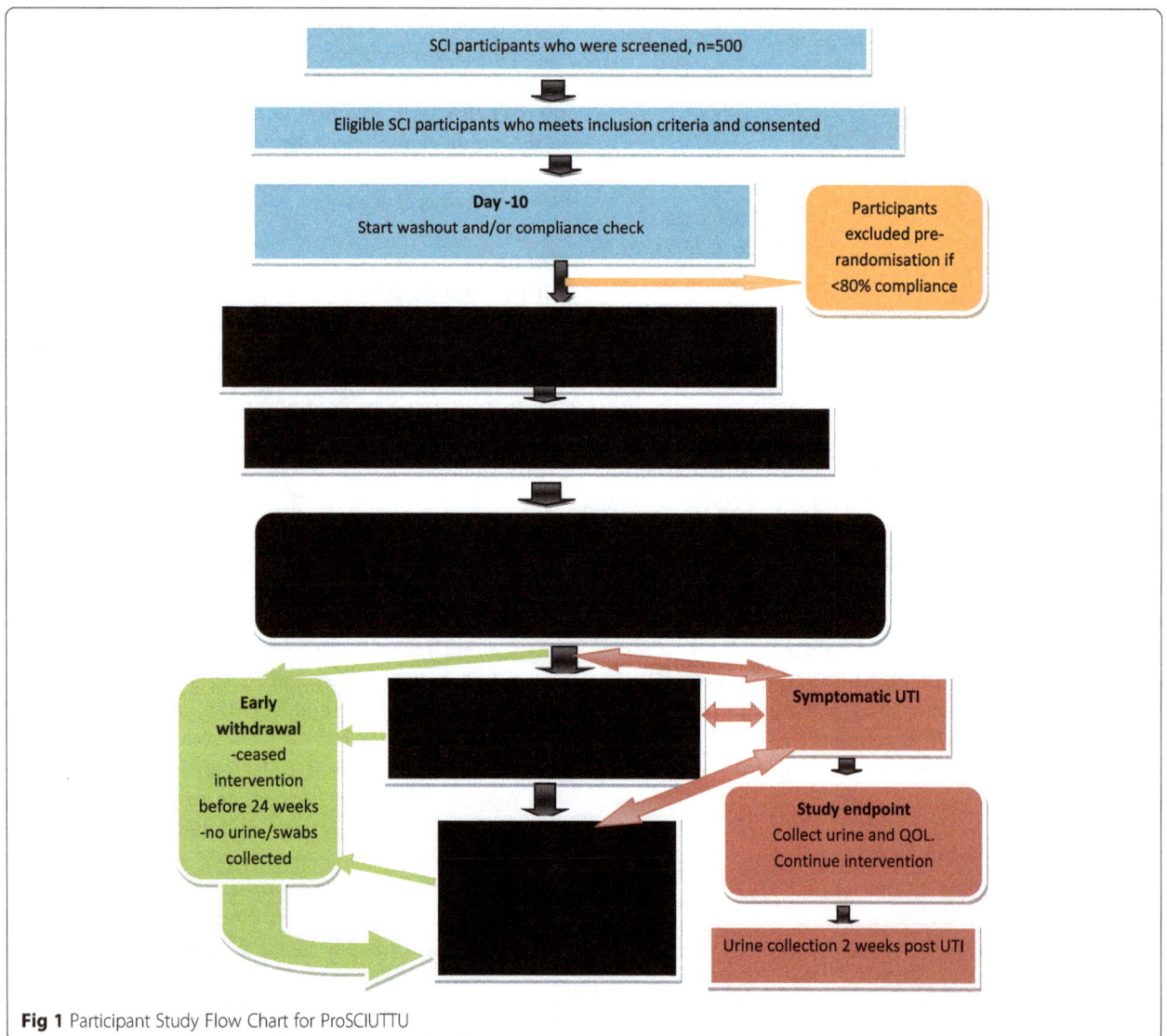

Fig 1 Participant Study Flow Chart for ProSCIUTTU

or RC14-GR1 + placebo or LGG-BB12 + placebo or 2 placebo tablets.

Active Interventions:

1. GR1-RC14. Concentration per capsule is 5.4×10^9 colony forming units.
2. LGG-BB12. Concentration per capsule is 7×10^9 colony forming units.

Participants will be assessed at Day 0, 3 months and 6 months, supported by fortnightly phone calls to determine health status and confirm intercurrent symptomatic UTI status. [Fig. 1] Following witnessed informed consent, evaluations conducted will be:

- Intervention issues and compliance.
- Quality of life assessment with the Short Form Health Survey [SF-36] – baseline and 6 months plus study endpoint if reached.
- Microbiological swabs of rectum, nose and groin, urine culture and collection of urinary catheters for participants with indwelling or suprapubic catheters – baseline, 3 months and 6 months. Urine cultures also performed if at study endpoint. Specific instructions for sampling were given by study co-ordinator to research assistants and community nurses performing the swabs to ensure consistency.
- Bowel questionnaire [13, 14] - baseline and 3 months.

Catheter-bioflora analysis

The indwelling urethral and suprapubic catheter biofilm is examined as a proxy for the urinary tract microbial community. Culture-independent techniques in profiling human microbes will be used to determine the composition of adherent microbes through the examination of the bacterial 16S rDNA gene by Terminal Restriction Fragment Length Polymorphism [TRFLP] [15] and via next-generation sequencing [16–19]

Samples are selected irrespective of interventional grouping.

Samples are also selected from groups with recurrent symptomatic UTI compared to no-UTI symptoms over the study follow-up period. All TRFLP and sequencing analysis will be conducted blinded by the use of a participant identification key that de-identifies the data.

TRFLP is done in collaboration with the Ramaciotti Centre for Genomics, University of New South Wales and sequencing through the Singapore Centre for Environmental Life Sciences Engineering at Nanyang Technological University, Singapore.

Study endpoints

1. The primary outcome measure is the time from randomisation to occurrence of "symptomatic UTI" [Fig. 2]. The date of the endpoint is the date participants develop symptoms consistent with a "symptomatic UTI" as per the algorithm, not the date participants start developing any symptoms. Table 2 outlines the definition of "symptomatic UTI" as primary endpoint for ProSCIUTTU. For participants who do not experience a "symptomatic UTI", the primary outcome is at six months. Participants who cease intervention early are followed up until the end of the study period.
2. The secondary endpoint is time to change of MRO colonisation status as determined by two successive cultures [See guidelines for MRO change or clearance in Additional file 1].

Data analysis

All analyses of outcomes will be by intention to treat, apart from safety outcomes which will be according to actual treatment received. Primary and MRO outcomes will be analysed using survival analysis. Cox regression modelling will be performed to test the effect of each treatment while allowing for the other, assuming no interaction effect. Hazard ratios and Kaplan-Meier survival curves will be used to summarise results. The extremely high prevalence of MRO in SCI will also allow us to explore whether probiotics can treat [or prevent] MRO colonisation in this group.

A survey was sent out to selected co-authors for determining the strength of association of several variables in regards to UTI in the SCI population [pre hoc review]. Only variables which have strong or moderate association will be included in the analysis.

Biofilms will be analysed using a combination of RNA based meta-community sequencing, TRFLP fingerprinting and culture based methods.

Trial data management

The data will be collected on trial specific case record forms. OM is responsible for designing and maintaining the trial database. Following each study visit, a study team member will ensure data is complete. Databases will be commissioned within the SCI units and will contain non-identifiable data. Re-identifiable data will be available for use only by the study team. Primary outcome measure endpoint determination will be verified by BL and ST. The two assessors will be blinded by each other's assessment. Discrepancies will be decided by a third investigator [KC].

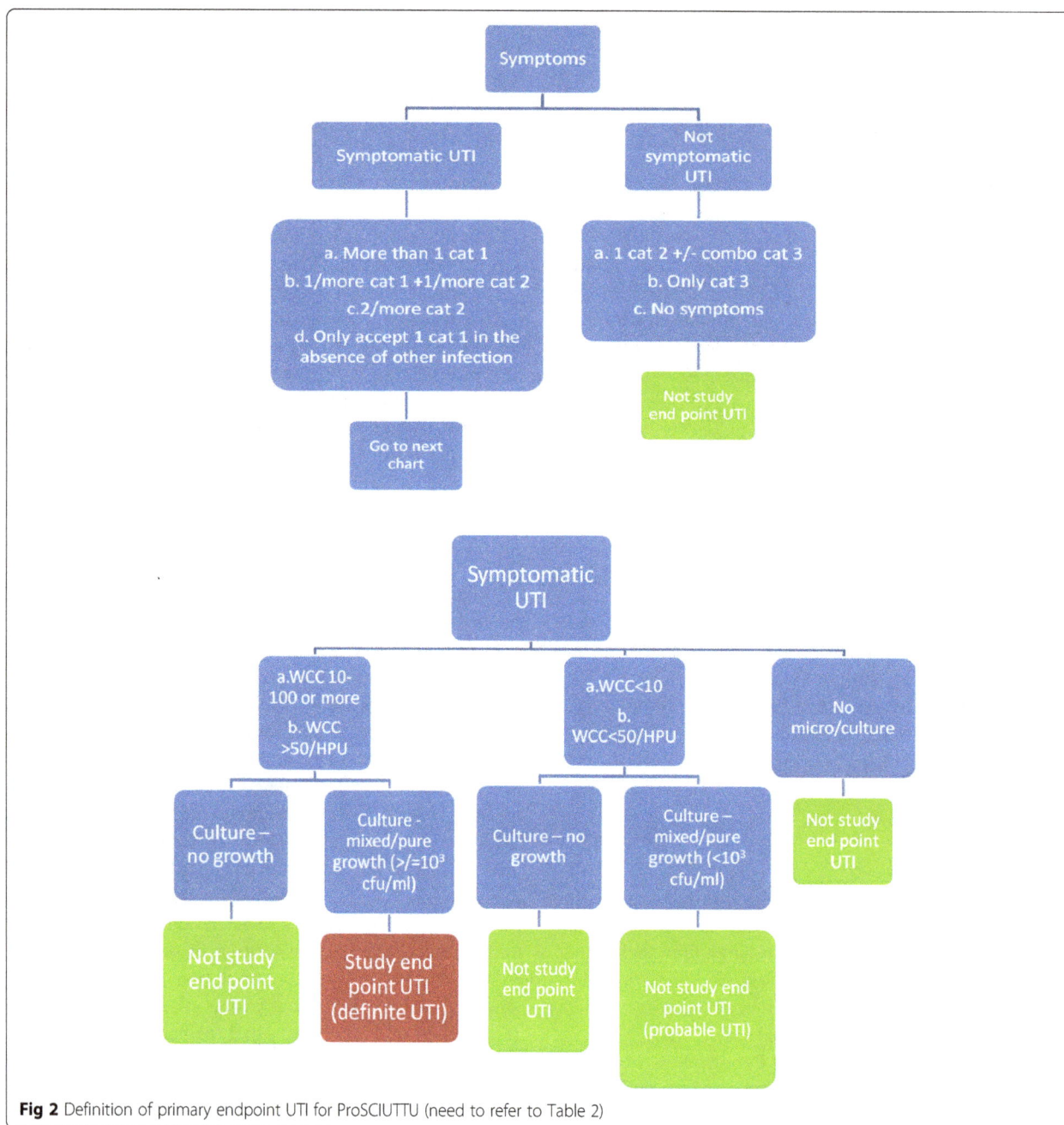

Fig 2 Definition of primary endpoint UTI for ProSCIUTTU (need to refer to Table 2)

Feasability, safety, efficacy

Efficacy

The primary study endpoint is symptomatic UTI with microbiological evidence of infection [refer to Fig. 2 and Table 2]. However, other secondary measures of interest include:

- Clinical infection.
- Hospital admissions and intensive care unit admissions related to infection.
- A diagnosis of laboratory infection defined by a positive blood culture.

- Clinical adverse events [grade 3–4] regardless of causality.
- All causes of mortality.
- Use of antibiotics.
- Change in of MRO colonisation/infection status as defined by two consecutive MRO swabs three months apart.
- Modifications of bladder management.
- SF-36
- A cost-effectiveness analysis will be undertaken using SF-6D utility weights derived from the SF-36. In addition to antibiotic use, the following

Table 2 Definition of "symptomatic UTI" as primary endpoint for ProSCIUTTU (need to refer to Fig. 2). Use the following table to assess "Category 1", or Two "Category 2" and any "Category 3" Symptoms: All symptoms should be asked in each category

"Category 1" Symptoms:*	"Category 2" Symptoms:*	"Category 3" Symptoms:
	Two or more	In themselves not enough to lead to treatment but recorded for International Spinal Cord Injury Urinary Tract Infection Datasets Compatibility
• Temperature:Greater than 38 ° C core Greater than 37.5 ° C per axilla • New or increasing symptoms of Autonomic Dysreflexia, as detected by any of the following signs: *Pulse < 50 or increased flushing or sweating or headache AND increased B.P Diastolic or Systolic > 25 % usual baseline.*	• Increased Frequency of Muscle Spasms or spasticity • Failure of usual control of urinary incontinence-*any of the following constitutes fulfillment of this category*-Bladder Spasm-Urinary frequency or need for increased catheterization-Urinary Retention-Urinary Urgency-Leaking around catheter site or per urethra if have suprapubic catheter • New Scrotal/Loin/Abdominal Discomfort unexplained by other pathology - *any of the following constitutes fulfillment of this category*-Abdominal Pain-Bladder/Suprapubic Pain-Loin/Back Pain-Scrotal Pain-Dysuria	*any of the following constitutes fulfillment of this category*-Anxiety/uneasiness-Feeling tired-Feeling sick-Arthralgias/Body Aches-Chills-Diaphoresis/sweating-Cloudy Urine-Foul smelling urine-Blood in urine *haematuria*-Catheter blockage

*Content adapted and modified from Box 1 of Spinal-injured neuropathic bladder antisepsis (SINBA) trial [4]

resource data will also be collected during the study:

– Use of isolation precautions: Single room; Personal Protective Equipment [PPE];
– Isolation ward;
– Terminal clean
– Infection control auditing

Safety monitoring

An independent Safety Monitoring Committee [SMC] is established. Clinicians or investigators responsible for the clinical care of study participants were not permitted to be members of the SMC. The SMC will monitor the trial and review safety data by treatment allocation. Safety monitoring will be carried out at various intervals through the trial depending on frequency of adverse events. The Committee will review laboratory data, Grade 3, Grade 4 and Grade 5 adverse events and serious adverse events [SAEs] and adverse events leading to cessation of study therapy [refer Table 3]. A summary of safety data will be undertaken when all recruited participants have completed 20 weeks on study.

The SMC Chairman had no formal affiliation with the trial and coordinated this process.

Project governance and administration support

The chief investigator Dr. Bon San Bonne Lee will be responsible for overall project management, but is assisted and advised by a project steering committee comprised of the collaborating researchers and administrative support from the administering institution [NeuRA]. The project steering committee will meet regularly and all agendas and minutes circulated to all stakeholders.

Table 3 Severity grade of adverse events

ESTIMATING SEVERITY GRADE				
PARAMETER	GRADE 1	GRADE 2	GRADE 3	GRADE 4
Clinical adverse event	Symptoms causing no or minimal interference with usual social & functional activities	Symptoms causing greater than minimal interference with usual social & functional activities	Symptoms causing inability to perform usual social & functional activities	Symptoms causing inability to perform basic self-care functions OR Medical or operative intervention indicated to prevent permanent impairment, persistent disability

Grades 1 and 2 Laboratory Abnormality or Clinical Event
Continue intervention at the discretion of the investigator
Grade 3 Laboratory Abnormality or Clinical Event
Grade 3 clinically significant laboratory abnormalities should be confirmed by repeat testing within three to five calendar days of receipt of results and before discontinuation, unless such a delay is not consistent with good medical practice
For grade 3 clinical events, continue if the event is considered to be unrelated to the intervention. For a grade 3 clinical event, or clinically significant laboratory abnormality confirmed by repeat testing, that is considered to be related to the intervention, both oral and bodywash interventions should be withheld until the toxicity returns to ≤ grade 2. When restarting following resolution of the adverse event, both interventions to be restarted simultaneously following discussion with the study monitor
Grade 4 Laboratory Abnormality or Clinical Event For grade 4 clinical event or clinically significant laboratory abnormality confirmed by repeat testing that is considered related to the intervention, the intervention should be permanently discontinued and subjects managed according to local practice. The subject should be followed as clinically indicated until the event resolves to baseline, or is otherwise explained, whichever occurs first. Study interventions may be continued without modification for non-clinically significant grade 4 laboratory abnormality (e.g. triglyceride elevation that is non-fasting or that can be medically managed) or clinical event considered unrelated to the study intervention

Abbreviations

BB12: bifidobacterium BB-12; GR1: lactobacillus rhamnosus GR-1; LGG: lactobacillus rhamnosus GG; MRO: multi-resistant organism; MS: multiple sclerosis; NHMRC: National Health and Medical Research Council of Australia; PPE: personal protective equipment; RC14: lactobacillus reuteri RC-14; RNA: ribonucleic acid; SAE: serious adverse event; SF-36: short form health survey; SCI: spinal cord injury; SMC: safety monitoring committee; TRFLP: terminal restriction fragment length polymorphism; UTI: urinary tract infection.

Competing interests

CHR Hansen has been paid commercial rates for providing the intervention product and placebo. The company had no input into the design of the trial. BL, JS, SG and JM have received competitive research funding support from the National Health and Medical Research Council of Australia [NHMRC]. They declare that they have no other financial or non-financial competing interests. The rest of the authors have no competing financial or non-financial interests.

Authors' contributions

The trial protocol has been developed by all authors over a series of teleconferences and workshops in Sydney, Australia in late 2009 and early 2010 from an original study design developed by BL and JS. LB and SAR were responsible for the protocol design and analysis of culture independent techniques of microbioflora identification. SR is the overall study project co-ordinator. SR is responsible for the study regulatory processes including designing the data collection forms, ethics and regulatory submissions as well as co-ordinating packaging of the investigational products. OM is responsible for designing and maintaining the trial database. JS is responsible for designing the biostatistical aspects of the trial and reviewing the statistical analysis. SG is responsible for designing the health economics aspects of the protocol and analysing the health economics data. GK is responsible in co-ordinating the microbiological sample analysis. MT is responsible for auditing the pharmacy compliance with protocol. BL, JK and GW are site investigators at the respective three spinal units. Recruitment is undertaken by BL, ST, SR, JK, GW, LB, CBR. Data collection is conducted by BL, SR, ST, OM, LB and CBR. ST, BL and KC are responsible for study endpoint determination. BL, SR and ST are responsible for initial manuscript preparation. All authors reviewed and were involved in writing up the final version of the manuscript prior to submission.

Acknowledgements

The authors would like to acknowledge Dr. Marcella Kwan and Ms. Elizabeth Rose, for their contributions as research assistants for the trial. The authors would like to thank Professor Ian Cameron for his role as the SMC Chairman. The authors would also like to thank Ms. Hanan Youssef and Ms. Alysia Wong for administrative support.

Funding

NHMRC is the organisation responsible for funding the supply of probiotics and matching placebo selected by the researchers for this study and budgeted within the NHMRC grant.

Author details

[1]Neuroscience Research Australia [NeuRA] and the University of New South Wales, Sydney, Australia. [2]Department of Spinal and Rehabilitation Medicine, Prince of Wales Hospital, Sydney, Australia. [3]School of Public Health, University of Sydney, Sydney, Australia. [4]Department of Infectious Diseases, Prince of Wales Hospital, Sydney, Australia. [5]Centre for Marine Bio-Innovation, University of New South Wales, Sydney, Australia. [6]Royal Rehabilitation Centre Sydney, Sydney, Australia. [7]Royal North Shore Hospital, Sydney, Australia. [8]Centre for Health Economics Research and Evaluation [CHERE], University of Technology Sydney, Sydney, Australia. [9]The Singapore Centre for Life Sciences Engineering and the School of Biological Sciences, Nanyang Technological University, Singapore, Singapore. [10]John Walsh Centre for Rehabilitation Research, Kolling Institute, Northern Sydney Local Health District, St Leonards, NSW 2065, Australia. [11]Sydney Medical School Northern, University of Sydney, Sydney, Australia.

References

1. Waites KB, Y-y C, DeVivo MJ, Canupp KC, Moser SA. Antimicrobial resistance in gram-negative bacteria isolated from the urinary tract in community-residing persons with spinal cord injury. Arch Phys Med Rehabil. 2000;81(6):764–9.
2. Mylotte JM, Kahler L, Graham R, Young L, Goodnough S. Prospective surveillance for antibiotic-resistant organisms in patients with spinal cord injury admitted to an acute rehabilitation unit. Am J Infect Control. 2000;28(4):291–7.
3. Pittet D. Infection control and quality health care in the new millenium. Am J Infect Control. 2005;33(5):258–67.
4. Lee B, Haran M, Hunt L, Simpson J, Marial O, Rutkowski S, et al. Spinal-injured neuropathic bladder antisepsis (SINBA) trial. Spinal Cord. 2007;45(8):542–50.
5. Murphy DP, Lampert V. Current implications of drug resistance in spinal cord injury. Am J Phys Med Rehabil. 2003;82(1):72–5.
6. Schrezenmeir J, de Vrese M. Probiotics, prebiotics, and synbiotics—approaching a definition. Am J Clin Nutr. 2001;73(2):361s–4.
7. Reid G. Probiotics to prevent the need for, and augment the use of, antibiotics. Can J Infect Dis Med Microbiol. 2006;17(5):291.
8. Falagas ME, Betsi GI, Tokas T, Athanasiou S. Probiotics for prevention of recurrent urinary tract infections in women. Drugs. 2006;66(9):1253–61.
9. Manley KJFM, Maynall BC, Power DA. Probiotic treatment of vancomycin-resistant enterococci : a randomised controlled trial. Med J Australia. 2007;186(9):454–7.
10. Darouiche RO, Donovan WH, Del Terzo M, Thornby JI, Rudy DC, Hull RA. Pilot trial of bacterial interference for preventing urinary tract infection. Urology. 2001;58(3):339–44.
11. Darouiche RO, Thornby JI, Stewart CC, Donovan WH, Hull RA. Bacterial interference for prevention of urinary tract infection: A prospective, randomized, placebo-controlled, double-blind pilot trial. Clin Infect Dis. 2005;41(10):1531–4.
12. Prasad A, Cevallos ME, Riosa S, Darouiche RO, Trautner BW. A bacterial interference strategy for prevention of UTI in persons practicing intermittent catheterization. Spinal Cord. 2009;47(7):565–9.
13. Krogh K, Perkash I, Stiens S, Biering-Sørensen F. International bowel function basic spinal cord injury data set. Spinal Cord. 2008;47(3):230–4.
14. Juul T, Bazzocchi G, Coggrave M, Johannesen I, Hansen R, Thiyagarajan C, et al. Reliability of the international spinal cord injury bowel function basic and extended data sets. Spinal Cord. 2011;49(8):886–91.
15. Liu W-T, Marsh TL, Cheng H, Forney LJ. Characterization of microbial diversity by determining terminal restriction fragment length polymorphisms of genes encoding 16S rRNA. Appl Environ Microbiol. 1997;63(11):4516–22.
16. Coolen MJ, Post E, Davis CC, Forney LJ. Characterization of microbial communities found in the human vagina by analysis of terminal restriction fragment length polymorphisms of 16S rRNA genes. Appl Environ Microbiol. 2005;71(12):8729–37.
17. Li F, Hullar MA, Lampe JW. Optimization of terminal restriction fragment polymorphism (TRFLP) analysis of human gut microbiota. J Microbiol Methods. 2007;68(2):303–11.
18. Khoruts A, Dicksved J, Jansson JK, Sadowsky MJ. Changes in the composition of the human fecal microbiome after bacteriotherapy for recurrent Clostridium difficile-associated diarrhea. J Clin Gastroenterol. 2010;44(5):354–60.
19. Fouts DE, Pieper R, Szpakowski S, Pohl H, Knoblach S, Suh M-J, et al. Integrated next-generation sequencing of 16S rDNA and metaproteomics differentiate the healthy urine microbiome from asymptomatic bacteriuria in neuropathic bladder associated with spinal cord injury. J Transl Med. 2012;10:174.

Genomic copy number variation association study in Caucasian patients with nonsyndromic cryptorchidism

Yanping Wang[1], Jin Li[3], Thomas F. Kolon[4], Alicia Olivant Fisher[1], T. Ernesto Figueroa[2], Ahmad H. BaniHani[2], Jennifer A. Hagerty[2], Ricardo Gonzalez[2,9], Paul H. Noh[2,10], Rosetta M. Chiavacci[3], Kisha R. Harden[3], Debra J. Abrams[3], Deborah Stabley[1], Cecilia E. Kim[3], Katia Sol-Church[1], Hakon Hakonarson[3,5,6], Marcella Devoto[5,6,7,8] and Julia Spencer Barthold[1,2]*

Abstract

Background: Copy number variation (CNV) is a potential contributing factor to many genetic diseases. Here we investigated the potential association of CNV with nonsyndromic cryptorchidism, the most common male congenital genitourinary defect, in a Caucasian population.

Methods: Genome wide genotyping were performed in 559 cases and 1772 controls (Group 1) using Illumina HumanHap550 v1, HumanHap550 v3 or Human610-Quad platforms and in 353 cases and 1149 controls (Group 2) using the Illumina Human OmniExpress 12v1 or Human OmniExpress 12v1-1. Signal intensity data including log R ratio (LRR) and B allele frequency (BAF) for each single nucleotide polymorphism (SNP) were used for CNV detection using PennCNV software. After sample quality control, gene- and CNV-based association tests were performed using cleaned data from Group 1 (493 cases and 1586 controls) and Group 2 (307 cases and 1102 controls) using ParseCNV software. Meta-analysis was performed using gene-based test results as input to identify significant genes, and CNVs in or around significant genes were identified in CNV-based association test results. Called CNVs passing quality control and signal intensity visualization examination were considered for validation using TaqMan CNV assays and QuantStudio® 3D Digital PCR System.

Results: The meta-analysis identified 373 genome wide significant ($p < 5 \times 10^{-4}$) genes/loci including 49 genes/loci with deletions and 324 with duplications. Among them, 17 genes with deletion and 1 gene with duplication were identified in CNV-based association results in both Group 1 and Group 2. Only 2 genes (*NUCB2* and *UPF2*) containing deletions passed CNV quality control in both groups and signal intensity visualization examination, but laboratory validation failed to verify these deletions.

Conclusions: Our data do not support that structural variation is a major cause of nonsyndromic cryptorchidism.

Keywords: Cryptorchidism, Genetics, CNV

* Correspondence: Julia.Barthold@nemours.org
[1]Nemours Biomedical Research, Nemours /Alfred I. duPont Hospital for Children, Wilmington, DE 19803, USA
[2]Division of Urology, Nemours/Alfred I. duPont Hospital for Children, Wilmington, DE 19803, USA
Full list of author information is available at the end of the article

Background

Nonsyndromic cryptorchidism, or isolated undescended testis, is one of the most common pediatric congenital anomalies, affecting 2-3 % of boys, and is associated with infertility and testicular malignancy later in life [1]. The etiology is largely unknown and likely multifactorial. Familial clustering suggests moderate genetic contribution to the disease [2].

A candidate approach to gene discovery has revealed some potential risk genes, but the results are inconsistent and population-specific [3–10]. Recently we performed a genome-wide association study (GWAS) in 912 nonsyndromic cryptorchidism cases and 2921 controls [11, 12] to identify common allelic variants across the genome associated with the disease. No variant reached genome-wide significance ($p \leq 7 \times 10^{-9}$) in full analysis, and one variant (rs55867206, near *SH3PXD2B*, $p = 2 \times 10^{-9}$) passed this threshold in a subgroup analysis of proximal testis position. Pathway analysis of suggestive association markers ($p \leq 10^{-3}$) using several bioinformatics tools identified overrepresentation of genes/functions linked to cytoskeleton-dependent processes, syndromic cryptorchidism and hypogonadotropic hypogonadism.

Over the past decade, evidence has shown that copy number variation (CNV) plays an important role in the occurrence of many diseases [13]. Analysis of CNVs using array comparative genomic hybridization found *VAMP7* duplication and *OTX1* deletion in individuals with congenital genitourinary defects [14, 15], with cryptorchidism as one of the primary traits. However, the association of CNVs with nonsyndromic cryptorchidism has not been explored. Through analysis of GWAS data [11, 12], we hypothesized that CNV is a significant cause of nonsyndromic cryptorchidism in Caucasian males.

Methods

Subjects and genotyping

Cases were self-reported Caucasian subjects with nonsyndromic cryptorchidism who underwent surgical repair at Nemours/Alfred I. DuPont Hospital for Children (Nemours) or The Children's Hospital of Philadelphia (CHOP). Subjects with multiple congenital anomalies or diagnosis of any syndrome, other genital anomalies (hypospadias, chordee or other penile anomalies) or abdominal wall defects were excluded from the study. Control subjects were recruited through the CHOP Health Care Network. They were self-reported Caucasian males who were at least 6 years old with no known history of testicular disease, penile anomaly, diagnosis of a syndrome or any additional medical disorder associated with cryptorchidism. Basic demographic and phenotypic data collected include age of diagnosis, race, ethnicity, laterality and the position of affected testes.

As described in detail in previous publications [11, 12], two groups of cases were genotyped at the Center for Applied Genomics at CHOP to match available control genotype data. In Group 1, 559 cases and 1772 controls were genotyped using the Illumina HumanHap550 v1, HumanHap550 v3 or Human610-Quad platforms that share over 535 K single nucleotide polymorphisms (SNPs) in common. In Group 2, 353 cases and 1149 controls were genotyped using the Illumina Human OmniExpress 12v1 or Human OmniExpress 12v1-1 platforms that share over 719 K SNPs. The global SNP and gene coverage of our SNP arrays are approximately 85 % and 80 %, respectively [16], and the average distance between probes is 4 kbp-5.5 kbp. At SNP genotype calling, cluster files (.egt) provided by Illumina were used as a common reference.

CNV detection and sample quality control

Due to differences in SNP coverage and less than 310 K intersection of SNPs between platforms used in the 2 case–control groups, CNV detection, sample quality control (QC), and association tests were performed separately in Groups 1 and 2. We used the PennCNV software package [17–20] to make CNV calls based on signal intensity data from genotyping arrays including log R ratio (LRR) and B allele frequency (BAF) for each SNP. Adjacent CNV calls were then automatically examined and merged using PennCNV software.

We used sample QC criteria from our prior genome-wide genotyping data analysis in PLINK [11, 12, 21–23]. Individuals were excluded from further analysis if one of below criteria were met: (1) discordance between reported sex and sex chromosome SNP data; (2) missing genotype rate >3 %; (3) potential duplicates or relatives (based on estimate of proportion of alleles shared identical by descent >0.1875); and (4) non-Caucasian ancestry based on multidimensional scaling (MDS) analysis using data from the Stanford Human Genome Diversity Project (HGDP) [24, 25]. We removed all samples that deviated from the means of the first or second MDS components by more than 3 standard deviations (SD). We also used a sample quality control function implemented in the ParseCNV software package [26, 27] and removed samples with (1) high intensity noise (measured by SDLRR (SD of LRR) > mean +3 SD); (2) extreme intensity waviness (measured by more than 3 SD of mean of GCWF (Guanine-Cytosine base pair wave factor)) and (3) high number of CNV counts per sample (measured by CNV count number > mean + 3 SD).

Gene based association analysis, meta-analysis and CNV based association analyses

Given that SNP overlap is low between the genotyping platforms used in Group 1 and 2, and the uncertainty of CNV boundary data from different platforms, we were unable to directly merge CNV from the two groups. Therefore, after removing individuals not passing samples QC, we performed gene-based association tests separately in Group 1 and 2 samples using the ParseCNV software package. We then performed meta-analyses of gene-based association results with METAL software [28, 29] using gene names as markers to identify significant genes ($p < 5X10^{-4}$, a conservative bar for CNV genome-wide significance suggested by ParseCNV). We also performed CNV-based association tests in cleaned Group 1 and 2 samples using ParseCNV software package. CNVs in or around significant genes from the gene-based meta-analyses were identified by searching the "gene" column in CNV-based association tests results. The CNVs were considered not passing CNV QC and removed if one of below criteria were met: average number of probes in CNV (AvgProbes) < 5, worst p-value in the span of CNV calls contributing to the significant CNV region (PenMaxP) > 0.5 and high frequency (Freq >0.5), nearly identical segmental duplications (SegDups) > 10, any locus frequently found in multiple studies such as T-cell receptor gene, human major histocompatibility complex gene etc. (Recurrent), the same inflated sample driving multiple CNV association signals (FreqInflated), the HMM confidence score in PennCNV calling (AvgConf) < 10, and allele A or B banding (ABFreq) in BAF low for duplications. Additionally, if more than three of below criteria were met, the CNV also was not considered for further analysis: CNV residing at centromere or telomere regions (TeloCentro), high or low GC content regions (AvgGC <30 or >60), CNV regions with high population frequency (PopFreq) >0.01, a large gap in probe coverage exists within CNV association signals (Sparse) >50 kbp, and average length of CNV <10 kbp [27].

CNV visualization, examination and laboratory validation
CNVs passing QC in both Groups 1 and 2 were examined by the plots of signal intensity (LRR/BAF) generated using the CNV visualization function implemented in the PennCNV package. Three CNVs passed CNV quality control in both groups and signal intensity visualization examination, and were chosen for further validation using TaqMan CNV probes located in the central region of each CNV (Hs04383175_cn, Hs06286795_cn and Hs06269635_cn), TaqMan CNV reference assay (human RNase P: 4403326) and QuantStudio® 3D Digital PCR System (Thermo Fisher Scientific, Waltham, MA USA) by the Nemours Biomolecular Core Laboratory, following the manufacturer's standard protocol.

Results
Based on sample quality control criteria, 66 cases and 186 controls were removed, leaving 493 cases and 1586 controls in Group 1. In Group 2, 46 cases and 47 controls were removed, leaving 307 cases and 1102 controls.

In Group 1, 7,376 deletions and 4,313 duplications were detected and 6,689 deletions and 6,635 duplications were detected in Group 2.

In gene-based association tests, 25 and 106 genes/loci with deletion, and 371 and 177 genes/loci with duplication reached genome-wide significance ($p < 5x10^{-4}$) in Group 1 and Group 2 (Additional file 1). After meta-analysis, 49 genes/loci with deletion and 331 genes/loci with duplication reached genome-wide significance (Additional file 2). For 49 genes with deletion, the direction of effect was consistent in the two groups. The direction of effect was inconsistent for 6 duplications and no direction was given in one duplication which was due to $p = 1$ for that gene in gene-based association test of Group 2, and they were removed from further consideration, leaving 324 genes/loci with duplication. Among these 373 significant genes/loci, 17 with deletion and 1 with duplication were identified in CNV-based association analysis in both Group 1 and Group 2 (Table 1). Five genes/loci (TCR gamma alternate reading frame protein (TARP), tonsoku-like DNA repair protein (TONSL), TONSL antisense RNA 1 (TONSL-AS1), nucleobindin 2 (NUCB2), and UPF2 regulator of nonsense transcripts homolog (yeast) (UPF2)) with deletion passed CNV quality control in both groups (Table 1). Signal intensity plots of CNVs in NUCB2 and UPF2 (Fig. 1: Array plot of Log R ratio and B allele frequency for NUCB2 and UPF2) suggested heterozygous deletions: the LRR decrease below 0 and the BAF cluster around either 0 or 1, but not near 0.5. Signal intensity plots of CNVs in TARP and TONSL/ TONSL-AS1 did not pass visualization examination (Additional file 3: Array plot of Log R ratio and B allele frequency for TARP and TONSL/TONSL-AS1) due to LRR close to 0, BAF cluster near 0.5, or both. Thus only CNVs in NUCB2 and UPF2 were further considered in our study.

The CNVs detected in NUCB2 are around 20 kbp and 6.7 kbp in Group 1 and Group 2, and they do not overlap. The Database of Genomic Variants (DGV) in The Hospital for Sick Children, a teaching hospital affiliated with the University of Toronto [30, 31] reported a 15 kbp deletion in 1 of 2026 individuals and a 719 bp deletion in 2 of 2504 individuals at the CNV region of Group 1 (chr11:17300844–17320797), and a 5 kbp deletion in 1 of 17421 individuals at the CNV region of Group 2 (chr11:17332461–17339127). Seven cases in Group 1 and 3 cases in Group 2 contained NUCB2 deletions based on this analysis. The CNVs detected in UPF2 were approximately 47.8 kbp and 13 kbp in Groups 1 and 2, respectively, and the 13 kbp segment is inside the 47.8 kbp segment. DGV reported a 47.8 kbp deletion in 2 of 17421 individuals in this CNV region detected in Group 1. Four cases in Group 1 and 9 cases in Group 2 contained UPF2 deletions. The CNV confidence scores of NUCB2 and UPF2 for each case generated

Table 1 Genes significant in meta-analysis and identified in CNV-based association tests

Gene Name	CNV Type	Group 1						Group 2					
		CNVR(hg19)	TagSNP	P value	Cases #	Control #	CNV QC Pass/Fail	CNVR(hg19)	TagSNP	P value	Cases #	Control #	CNV QC Pass/Fail
BBS5, KLHL41	Deletion	chr2:170354790–170368798	rs3769772	1.86E-11	30	11	PASS	chr2:170343083–170840224	rs2592804	0.217885025	1	0	FAIL
CDK19	Deletion	chr6:110972494–111696091	rs12198236	0.01327263	3	0	FAIL	chr6:111061814–111381468	rs9374202	0.010264833	3	0	PASS
SYNE1	Deletion	chr6:152938025–152969462	rs6940651	0.237247353	1	0	FAIL	chr6:152511420–152516441	rs7772542	2.04E-09	13	0	FAIL
TARP[a]	Deletion	chr7:38357194–38364605	rs11765884	3.74E-05	18	13	PASS	chr7:38341226–38341925	rs2736973	2.56E-07	29	26	PASS
TONSL-AS1, TONSL[a]	Deletion	chr8:144992103–146235564	rs11136344	0.027970085	7	7	PASS	chr8:145660543–145666578	rs2306384	5.04E-05	12	6	PASS
UPF2[a]	Deletion	chr10:12028228–12076043	rs7899260	0.00313275	4	0	PASS	chr10:12062959–12075960	rs7072007	8.15E-06	9	1	PASS
TET1	Deletion	chr10:70342775–70775081	rs7071780	0.05619918	2	0	FAIL	chr10:70410630–70432644	rs10762236	9.01E-11	15	0	PASS
MICU1	Deletion	chr10:74250792–74534174	rs7912170	0.237133237	1	0	FAIL	chr10:74304790–74433626	rs7909573	4.56E-08	11	0	PASS
ADK	Deletion	chr10:76092179–76099557	rs10824151	5.31E-06	14	5	FAIL	chr10:76372037–77001459	rs4746209	0.047420164	2	0	FAIL
NUCB2[a]	Deletion	chr11:17300844–17320797	rs12419530	4.08E-05	7	0	PASS	chr11:17332461–17339127	rs10466382	0.034028702	3	1	PASS
LARP4	Deletion	chr12:49846626–51537196	rs10876136	0.237133237	1	0	FAIL	chr12:50768339–50807570	rs7296212	2.21E-05	7	0	PASS
AQR	Deletion	chr15:34261920–35227613	rs16954263	0.237133237	1	0	FAIL	chr15:35233730–35252767	rs4513050	2.33E-09	17	3	FAIL
PIGL	Deletion	chr17:15043999–16221319	rs7210224	0.237133237	1	0	FAIL	chr17:16196056–16207526	rs11868284	2.21E-05	7	0	PASS
PAFAH1B1	Deletion	chr17:1811983–2578648	rs9674799	0.056145117	2	0	FAIL	chr17:2534710–2561169	rs11078288	0.000478637	5	0	PASS
SLC19A1	Deletion	chr21:46298869–47863025	rs2330183	0.138704428	2	1	FAIL	chr21:46945024–46953292	rs4819128	9.13E-06	10	2	PASS
FOLH1B	Duplication	chr11:89123768–89405190	rs7929532	0.237133237	1	0	FAIL	chr11:89374850–89405190	rs7112871	3.71E-35	54	2	FAIL

[a]Genes/loci passed CNV QC in both groups

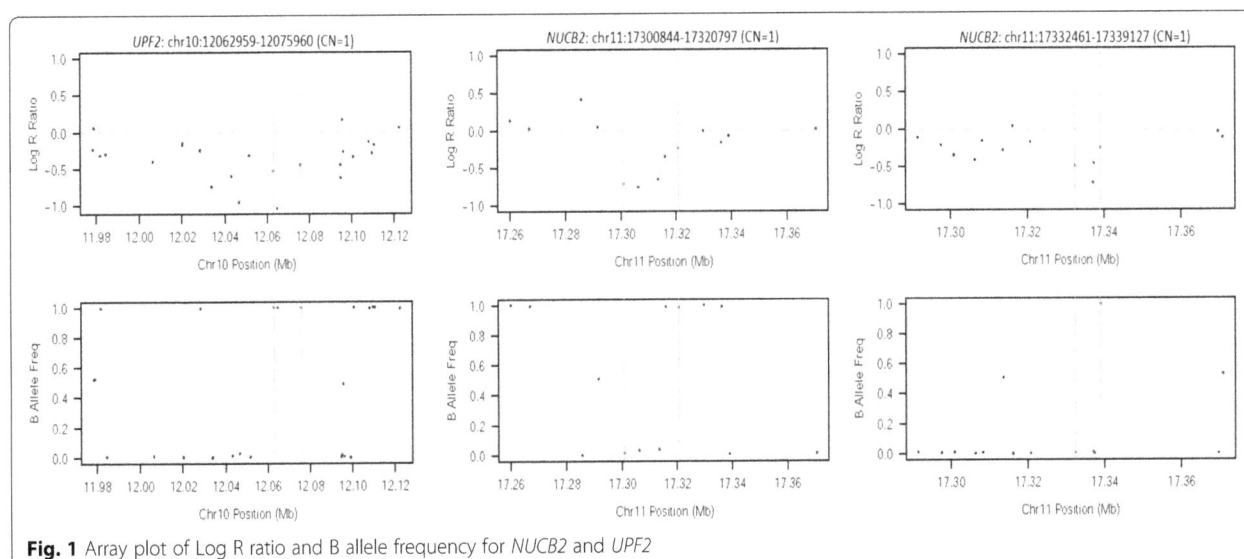

Fig. 1 Array plot of Log R ratio and B allele frequency for *NUCB2* and *UPF2*

during CNV calling by PennCNV are shown in Table 2. The score range was 12 to 55, which is considered borderline reliable for CNV detection.

We attempted to validate CNVs in *NUCB2* and *UPF2* in affected cases using TaqMan CNV assays and Quant-Studio® 3D Digital PCR System (Table 2). After validating the TaqMan CNV assays using 2 control DNAs without called CNVs in these regions, we tested 12 samples from Group 1 or 2 with called CNVs within these genes of interest (Table 2, noted in case IDs with underline). All 12 tested samples were diploid (Additional file 4), indicating that bioinformatically-called deletions were not validated by TaqMan CNV assays.

Discussion

Cryptorchidism is the most common male congenital genitourinary defect. While it is a manifestation of many congenital defect syndromes [32–34], the majority of cases are nonsyndromic and of unclear etiology. Our previous genome-wide association analyses of SNP data suggest that cryptorchidism is associated with significant genetic heterogeneity [11, 12]. In the present study, we performed genome-wide CNV association analysis to identify the potential association of structural variation with the occurrence of nonsyndromic cryptorchidism, and our results suggest that CNVs do not contribute to the genetic basis of the nonsyndromic form of the disease.

In a previous report, Jorgez and colleagues identified a 2p15 deletion encompassing *OTX1* in 6 subjects with genitourinary defects [15]. Three of these individuals had cryptorchidism and their genomic deletions also included *EHBP1* and *WDPC*. Other genitourinary anomalies of the three patients with cryptorchidism were variable including absent prepuce, micropenis, discontinuous raphe, penile cyst, hypoplastic scrotum, kidney stones or small testes. The three patients also had other defects including developmental delay, vision problems and dysmorphic facial features. Structural variations were also identified in studies of subjects with nonobstructive azoospermia or congenital genitourinary tract masculinization disorders from the same research group [14, 35]. In the study of nonobstructive azoospermia, 4

Table 2 Relevant validation information for genes (*UPF2* and *NUCB2*) passed CNV QC and signal intensity examination

Group	Gene Name	CNV (hg19)	Probe # in overlapping CNV region	CNV size (bp)	TaqMan CNV assays and location	Cases with deletion (CNV confidence score)
Group 1	*UPF2*	chr10:12028228–12076043	10	47815	Hs04383175_cn; Chr10:12063665	D10 (26)[a], D29 (55)[a], D34 (46), 1495 (27)
	NUCB2	chr11:17300844–17320797	5	19953	Hs06286795_cn; Chr11:17306162	D8 (24), D10 (28)[a], D24 (24), D29 (30)[a], D33 (26), D132 (27), D139 (30)
Group 2	*UPF2*	chr10:12062959–12075960	3	13001	Same as *UPF2* assay in group 1	7279 (15), 7334 (12)[a], 7338 (23), 7339 (16), 7341 (14), 7370 (26)[a], 7453 (16), 7475 (24), 7479 (17)
	NUCB2	chr11:17332461–17339127	4	6666	Hs06269635_cn; Chr11:17336218	7334 (17)[a], 7361 (14), 7370 (12)[a]

Case IDs with underline: samples tested by TaqMan CNV assays for validation
[a]samples with called deletions in both genes (*UPF2* and *NUCB2*)

patients with microduplications and 4 with microdeletions of *E2F1* were identified among 110 affected individuals, but not among 78 fertile controls [35]. Two of the 8 patients with CNVs had cryptorchidism. Two non-synonymous mutations of *E2F1* (Ala102Thr and Gly393-Ser) were also identified in three other patients, and one synonymous mutation (Leu415Leu) was identified in a patient with microduplication of *E2F1*. The patient with the Ala102Thr variant also had cryptorchidism. In the congenital genitourinary tract masculinization disorders study [14], copy number gains on Xq28 encompassing *VAMP7* were found in 4 of 296 patients. Two of them had idiopathic cryptorchidism, and the other two had hypospadias. They also found 1 case of hypospadias with *VAMP7* copy number gain in 28 distinct primary cultures of genital skin fibroblasts. All of the above three studies used array comparative genomic hybridization, a technology that enables efficient screening for CNVs, to discover the genomic variants. Other studies from Europe have also reported the microdeletions (2p14-p15, 2p15-16.1) in boys with cryptorchidism [36, 37]. However, all of these patients presented with other features besides cryptorchidism, including intellectual disability, developmental delay and/or dysmorphic features. In our study, subjects were excluded if there was evidence for other genital anomalies and/or other clinical features in addition to undescended testes.

Only autosomal CNVs were called and analyzed in our study, which may have led us to miss associated CNVs on the X or Y chromosome. The significant genes in our meta-analysis with CNVs that also passed QC in both groups and signal intensity visualization examination are *NUCB2* and *UPF2*, located at chromosome 11 and chromosome 10, respectively. However, these deletions were not validated by QuantStudio® 3D Digital PCR System with TaqMan CNV assays in our study samples, despite the signal intensity plots suggesting the presence of heterozygous deletions. The confidence score range of detected cases for these deletions is 12 to 55 (Table 2). The score numbers are lower in Group 2 cases with most of them less than 20. A confidence score of 10 has been suggested as a threshold to classify reliable CNV calls while the higher scores are more reliable and more likely to be replicated [38]. Most of our scores were less than the median score of 27.7 that was reported for deletions that could be replicated in the study of Ku et al. [38]. Due to different platforms with low overlapping SNP coverage that were used in genotyping Group 1 and Group 2 samples, we performed association tests separately in the two groups. Consequently, the whole study power was reduced compared to what it would have been if all samples had been genotyped on the same platform and some CNVs associated with disease may have been missed, even though we used meta-analysis to

combine the two data sets. The use of SNP genotyping array data for CNV analysis is a common and acceptable approach [39–42], but the global CNV coverage of our SNP arrays varies. Cooper GM et al. [43] reported approximately 40 % and 80 % CNV coverage for Illumina chips of HumanHap550 and Human 1 M. Besides HumanHap550, the other chips we used, Human610-Quad and Human OminiExpress, have fewer SNPs compared to the Human 1 M, and therefore likely have less than 80 % global CNV coverage. Cooper GM et al. also reported that only two-thirds of detected CNVs by SNP data from Human 1 M could be validated in independent experiments [43], indicating that using SNP array data for CNV analysis may result in false positives, as may be the case in the present analysis.

Conclusions

A sample size (800 cases and 2688 controls) greater than that of any other CNV analysis of nonsyndromic cryptorchidism failed to identify any associated variants, but weak effects at multiple genomic loci may still contribute to the etiology of this disease. It is also possible that CNVs are present but were not detected due to insufficient coverage by the SNP arrays we used and/or, the present analysis was underpowered to identify rare, strong effect CNVs that contribute to disease risk. Whole genome or exome sequencing, and comparative genomic hybridization are alternative approaches for discovery of disease-associated SNPs and CNVs, but beyond the scope of the present studies. It is possible that structural variation is more commonly associated with syndromic cryptorchidism, but our inability to validate the candidate CNVs in this analysis suggests that these variants are not a major cause of nonsyndromic cryptorchidism.

Additional files

Additional file 1: genome-wide significant genes/loci in gene-based association tests in each group. Listed all the genes/loci with genome-wide significance ($p < 5 \times 10^{-4}$) in gene-based association tests in each group and their *p*-values. (DOCX 55 kb)

Additional file 2: genome-wide signicant genes/loci in meta-analysis. Listed all the genes/loci with genome-wide significant *p*-values ($p < 5 \times 10^{-4}$) in meta-analyses of gene-based association results, and their *z*-scores, *p*-values and the direction of effect in the two groups. (DOCX 57 kb)

Additional file 3: Array plot of Log R ration and B allele frequency for *TARP* and *TONSL/TONSL-AS1*. Showed the signal intensity plots of 2 CNVs in *TARP* and 1 CNV in *TONSL/TONSL-AS1*. The array plots did not pass visualization examination due to LRR close to 0, BAF cluster near 0.5, or both. (DOCX 141 kb)

Additional file 4: CNVs validation using TaqMan CNV assays and QuantStudio® 3D Digital PCR System. Listed the samples tested for CNV validating and the results. (XLSX 10 kb)

Additional file 5: CNV calls for Group 1 cases passed sample QC. Each column in Additional file 5 represents CNV location, SNPs numbers contained within the CNV, the length of the CNV, copy number (cn) of the CNV call, sample id, the starting marker identifier and the ending marker identifier in the CNV, and confidence score in PennCNV calling. (XLSX 653 kb)

Additional file 6: CNV calls for Group 1 controls passed sample QC. Each column in Additional file 6 represents CNV location, SNPs numbers contained within the CNV, the length of the CNV, copy number (cn) of the CNV call, sample id, the starting marker identifier and the ending marker identifier in the CNV, and confidence score in PennCNV calling. (XLSX 1544 kb)

Additional file 7: CNV calls for Group 2 cases passed sample QC. Each column in Additional file 7 represents CNV location, SNPs numbers contained within the CNV, the length of the CNV, copy number (cn) of the CNV call, sample id, the starting marker identifier and the ending marker identifier in the CNV, and confidence score in PennCNV calling. (XLSX 534 kb)

Additional file 8: CNV calls for Group 2 controls passed sample QC. Each column in Additional file 8 represents CNV location, SNPs numbers contained within the CNV, the length of the CNV, copy number (cn) of the CNV call, sample id, the starting marker identifier and the ending marker identifier in the CNV, and confidence score in PennCNV calling. (XLSX 1952 kb)

Abbreviations

BAF: B allele frequency; CHOP: The Children's Hospital of Philadelphia; CNV: Copy number variation; DGV: Database of genomic variants; GCWF: Guanine-cytosine base pair wave factor; GWAS: Genome-wide association study; HGDP: Human genome diversity project; LRR: Log R ratio; MDS: Multidimensional scaling; NUCB2: Nucleobindin 2; QC: Quality control; SD: Standard deviation; SDLRR: Standard deviation of log R ratio; SNP: Single Nucleotide polymorphisms; UPF2: UPF2 regulator of nonsense transcripts homolog (yeast)

Acknowledgements

The authors would like to thank all our participants and their families for their gracious participation in this study.

Funding

Study design, data collection, data analysis and interpretation, and writing the manuscript were supported by R01HD060769 from the Eunice Kennedy Shriver National Institute for Child Health and Human Development (NICHD), and Nemours Biomedical Research Fund. Part of data analysis and interpretation, and manuscript publication were supported by an Institutional Development Award (IDeA) from the National Institute of General Medical Sciences (NIGMS) of the National Institutes of Health under grant numbers P20GM103464 and P30GM114736 Center for Pediatric Research (COBRE) and grant P20GM103446 (DE-INBRE). Part of data collection and analysis was supported by an Institute Development Fund to the Center for Applied Genomics at The Children's Hospital of Philadelphia.

Authors' contributions

YW: sample preparation, data analysis and draft of manuscript; JL: data analysis; TFK, AOF, TEF, AHB, JAH, RG, PHN, RMC, KRH, DJA, JSB: recruitment, sample collection and phenotyping; DS: CNV laboratory validation; CEK: genotyping; KSC, HH, MD, JSB: study design. All authors read and approved the final manuscript.

Competing interests

The authors declare that they have no competing interests.

Consent for publication

Not applicable.

Author details

[1]Nemours Biomedical Research, Nemours /Alfred I. duPont Hospital for Children, Wilmington, DE 19803, USA. [2]Division of Urology, Nemours/Alfred I. duPont Hospital for Children, Wilmington, DE 19803, USA. [3]Center for Applied Genomics, The Children's Hospital of Philadelphia, Philadelphia, PA 19104, USA. [4]Division of Urology, The Children's Hospital of Philadelphia, Philadelphia, PA 19104, USA. [5]Division of Genetics, The Children's Hospital of Philadelphia, Philadelphia, PA 19104, USA. [6]Department of Pediatrics, Perelman School of Medicine, University of Pennsylvania, Philadelphia, PA 19104, USA. [7]Department of Biostatistics and Epidemiology, Perelman School of Medicine, University of Pennsylvania, Philadelphia, PA 19104, USA. [8]Department of Molecular Medicine, Sapienza University, Rome, Italy. [9]Present address: Auf der Bult Kinder- und Jugendkrankenhaus, Hannover, Germany. [10]Present address: Division of Pediatric Urology, Cincinnati Children's Hospital Medical Center, Cincinnati, OH, USA.

References

1. Ashley RA, Barthold JS, Kolon TF. Cryptorchidism: pathogenesis, diagnosis, treatment and prognosis. Urol Clin North Am. 2010;37:183–93.
2. Schnack TH, Zdravkovic S, Myrup C, Westergaard T, Wohlfahrt J, Melbye M. Familial aggregation of cryptorchidism–a nationwide cohort study. Am J Epidemiol. 2008;167:1453–7.
3. Ferlin A, Zuccarello D, Zuccarello B, Chirico MR, Zanon GF, Foresta C. Genetic alterations associated with cryptorchidism. JAMA. 2008;300:2271–6.
4. Foresta C, Zuccarello D, Garolla A, Ferlin A. Role of hormones, genes, and environment in human cryptorchidism. Endocr Rev. 2008;29:560–80.
5. Bertini V, Bertelloni S, Valetto A, Lala R, Foresta C, Simi P. Homeobox HOXA10 gene analysis in cryptorchidism. J Pediatr Endocrinol Metab. 2004;17:41–5.
6. Galan JJ, Guarducci E, Nuti F, Gonzalez A, Ruiz M, Ruiz A, et al. Molecular analysis of estrogen receptor alpha gene AGATA haplotype and SNP12 in European populations: potential protective effect for cryptorchidism and lack of association with male infertility. Hum Reprod. 2007;22:444–9.
7. Kolon TF, Wiener JS, Lewitton M, Roth DR, Gonzales Jr ET, Lamb DJ. Analysis of homeobox gene HOXA10 mutations in cryptorchidism. J Urol. 1999;161:275–80.
8. Wang Y, Barthold J, Kanetsky PA, Casalunovo T, Pearson E, Manson J. Allelic variants in HOX genes in cryptorchidism. Birth Defects Res A Clin Mol Teratol. 2007;79:269–75.
9. Wang Y, Barthold J, Figueroa E, Gonzalez R, Noh PH, Wang M, et al. Analysis of five single nucleotide polymorphisms in the ESR1 gene in cryptorchidism. Birth Defects Res A Clin Mol Teratol. 2008;82:482–5.
10. Yoshida R, Fukami M, Sasagawa I, Hasegawa T, Kamatani N, Ogata T. Association of cryptorchidism with a specific haplotype of the estrogen receptor alpha gene: implication for the susceptibility to estrogenic environmental endocrine disruptors. J Clin Endocrinol Metab. 2005;90:4716–21.
11. Barthold JS, Wang Y, Kolon TF, Kollin C, Nordenskjöld A, Olivant Fisher A, et al. Phenotype specific association of the TGFBR3 locus with nonsyndromic cryptorchidism. J Urol. 2015;193:1637–45.
12. Barthold JS, Wang Y, Kolon TF, Kollin C, Nordenskjöld A, Olivant Fisher A, et al. Pathway analysis supports association of nonsyndromic cryptorchidism with genetic loci linked to cytoskeleton-dependent functions. Hum Reprod. 2015;30:2439–51.
13. Mikhail FM. Copy number variations and human genetic disease. Curr Opin Pediatr. 2014;26:646–52.
14. Tannour-Louet M, Han S, Louet JF, Zhang B, Romero K, Addai J, et al. Increased gene copy number of VAMP7 disrupts human male urogenital development through altered estrogen action. Nat Med. 2014;20:715–24.
15. Jorgez CJ, Rosenfeld JA, Wilken NR, Vangapandu HV, Sahin A, Pham D, et al. Genitourinary defects associated with genomic deletions in 2p15 encompassing OTX1. PLoS One. 2014; doi:10.1371/journal.pone.0107028
16. Li M, Li C, Guan W. Evaluation of coverage variation of SNP chips for genome-wide association studies. Eur J Hum Genet. 2008;16:635–43.
17. Wang K, Li M, Hadley D, Liu R, Glessner J, Grant SF, et al. PennCNV: an integrated hidden Markov model designed for high-resolution copy number variation detection in whole-genome SNP genotyping data. Genome Res. 2007;17:1665–74.
18. Wang K, Chen Z, Tadesse MG, Glessner J, Grant SF, Hakonarson H, et al. Modeling genetic inheritance of copy number variations. Nucleic Acids Res. 2008; doi:10.1093/nar/gkn641
19. Diskin SJ, Li M, Hou C, Yang S, Glessner J, Hakonarson H, et al. Adjustment of genomic waves in signal intensities from whole-genome SNP genotyping platforms. Nucleic Acids Res. 2008; doi:10.1093/nar/gkn556
20. PennCNV. http://penncnv.openbioinformatics.org/en/latest/. Accessed 9 Oct 2013.

21. Purcell S, Neale B, Todd-Brown K, Thomas L, Ferreira MA, Bender D, et al. PLINK: a tool set for whole-genome association and population-based linkage analyses. Am J Hum Genet. 2007;81:559–75.

22. PLINK v1.07. http://pngu.mgh.harvard.edu/purcell/plink/. Accessed 7 May 2011.

23. Anderson CA, Pettersson FH, Clarke GM, Cardon LR, Morris AP, Zondervan KT. Data quality control in genetic case–control association studies. Nat Protoc. 2010;5:1564–73.

24. Rosenberg NA. Standardized subsets of the HGDP-CEPH Human Genome Diversity Cell Line Panel, accounting for atypical and duplicated samples and pairs of close relatives. Ann Hum Genet. 2006;70:841–7.

25. Human Genome Diversity Project. http://www.hagsc.org/hgdp/files.html. Accessed 19 July 2013.

26. Glessner JT, Li J, Hakonarson H. ParseCNV integrative copy number variation association software with quality tracking. Nucleic Acids Res. 2013; doi:10.1093/nar/gks1346

27. ParseCNV. http://parsecnv.sourceforge.net/. Accessed 10 Nov 2014.

28. Willer CJ, Li Y, Abecasis GR. METAL: fast and efficient meta-analysis of genomewide association scans. Bioinformatics. 2010;26:2190–1.

29. METAL. http://csg.sph.umich.edu/abecasis/metal/. Accessed 2 Apr 2015.

30. MacDonald JR, Ziman R, Yuen RK, Feuk L, Scherer SW. The database of genomic variants: a curated collection of structural variation in the human genome. Nucleic Acids Res. 2014;42:D986–92. doi:10.1093/nar/gkt958.

31. Database of Genomic Variants. http://dgv.tcag.ca/dgv/app/home. Accessed 28 June 2015.

32. Neuhann TM, Müller D, Hackmann K, Holzinger S, Schrock E, Di Donato N. A further patient with van Maldergem syndrome. Eur J Med Genet. 2012;55:423–8.

33. Lipska BS, Brzeskwiniewicz M, Wierzba J, Morzuchi L, Piotrowski A, Limon J. 8.6 Mb interstitial deletion of chromosome 4q13.3q21.23 in a boy with cognitive impairment, short stature, hearing loss, skeletal abnormalities and facial dysmorphism. Genet Couns. 2011;22:353–63.

34. Fei X, Qi M, Zhao Y, Li-Ling J. Identification and characterization of a complex pure mosaic of small supernumerary marker chromosomes involving 11p11.12 → q12.1 and 19p12 → q12 regions in a child featuring multiple congenital anomalies. Am J Med Genet A. 2011;155A:3116–21.

35. Jorgez CJ, Wilken N, Addai JB, Newberg J, Vangapandu HV, Pastuszak AW, et al. Genomic and genetic variation in E2F transcription factor-1 in men with nonobstructive azoospermia. Fertil Steril. 2015;103:44–52.

36. Hancarova M, Vejvalkova S, Trkova M, Drabova J, Dleskova A, Vlckova M, et al. Identification of a patient with intellectual disability and de novo 3.7 Mb deletion supports the existence of a novel microdeletion syndrome in 2p14-p15. Gene. 2013;516:158–61.

37. Piccione M, Piro E, Serraino F, Cavani S, Ciccone R, Malacarne M, et al. Interstitial deletion of chromosome 2p15-16.1: report of two patients and critical review of current genotype-phenotype correlation. Eur J Med Genet. 2012;55:238–44.

38. Ku CS, Pawitan Y, Sim X, Ong RT, Seielstad M, Lee EJ, et al. Genomic copy number variations in three Southeast Asian populations. Hum Mutat. 2010;31:851–7.

39. Dajani R, Li J, Wei Z, Glessner JT, Chang X, Cardinale CJ, et al. CNV Analysis Associates AKNAD1 with Type-2 Diabetes in Jordan Subpopulations. Sci Rep. 2015;5:13391.

40. Li J, Fung I, Glessner JT, Pandey R, Wei Z, Bakay M, et al. Copy Number Variations in CTNNA3 and RBFOX1 Associate with Pediatric Food Allergy. J Immunol. 2015;195:1599–607.

41. Peiffer DA, Le JM, Steemers FJ, Chang W, Jenniges T, Garcia F, et al. High-resolution genomic profiling of chromosomal aberrations using Infinium whole-genome genotyping. Genome Res. 2006;16:1136–48.

42. Komura D, Shen F, Ishikawa S, Fitch KR, Chen W, Zhang J, et al. Genome-wide detection of human copy number variations using high-density DNA oligonucleotide arrays. Genome Res. 2006;16:1575–84.

43. Cooper GM, Zerr T, Kidd JM, Eichler EE, Nickerson DA. Systematic assessment of copy number variant detection via genome-wide SNP genotyping. Nat Genet. 2008;40:1199–203.

Developing a preoperative predictive model for ureteral length for ureteral stent insertion

Takashi Kawahara[1,3]* , Kentaro Sakamaki[2], Hiroki Ito[1,3], Shinnosuke Kuroda[3], Hideyuki Terao[3], Kazuhide Makiyama[1], Hiroji Uemura[1], Masahiro Yao[1], Hiroshi Miyamoto[4] and Junichi Matsuzaki[3]

Abstract

Background: Ureteral stenting has been a fundamental part of various urological procedures. Selecting a ureteral stent of optimal length is important for decreasing the incidence of stent migration and complications. The aim of the present study was to develop and internally validate a model for predicting the ureteral length for ureteral stent insertion.

Methods: This study included a total of 127 patients whose ureters had previously been assessed by both intravenous urography (IVU) and CT scan. The actual ureteral length was determined by direct measurement using a 5-Fr ureteral catheter. Multiple linear regression analysis with backward selection was used to model the relationship between the factors analyzed and actual ureteral length. Bootstrapping was used to internally validate the predictive model.

Results: Patients all of whom had stone disease included 76 men (59.8%) and 51 women (40.2%), with the median and mean (± SD) ages of 60 and 58.7 (±14.2) years. In these patients, 53 (41.7%) right and 74 (58.3%) left ureters were analyzed. The median and mean (± SD) actual ureteral lengths were 24.0 and 23.3 (±2.0) cm, respectively. Using the bootstrap methods for internal validation, the correlation coefficient ($R2$) was 0.57 ± 0.07.

Conclusion: We have developed a predictive model, for the first time, which predicts ureteral length using the following five preoperative characteristics: age, side, sex, IVU measurement, and CT calculation. This predictive model can be used to reliably predict ureteral length based on clinical and radiological factors and may thus be a useful tool to help determining the optimal length of ureteral stent.

Keywords: Ureteral length, Ureteral catheter, Predictive model, Ureter, Ureteral stent

Background

Since the first description by Zimskind et al. in 1967 [1], ureteral stenting has been a fundamental part of various urological procedures for the treatment of obstructing ureteral calculi, ureteral stricture, ureteropelvic junction obstruction, retroperitoneal tumor and fibrosis, and the procedures that were developed after open or endoscopic ureteral surgery [2]. Placement of a stent that is too long often causes complications, such as frequent or urgent urination, incontinence, hematuria, and bladder or flank pain, which have a negative impact on quality of life of patients [3–9]. Conversely, a short ureteral stent increases the risk of migration, resulting in complications that require retraction and replacement [10, 11]. Thus, choosing a stent of optimal length is important for reducing the incidence of stent migration and other complications [10, 12–14]. In our previous study, 4% of the ureteral stents were found to be too short and 19.5% were too long [15].

Actual ureteral stent measurement is the most accurate method to measure the ureteral length. However, actual stent measurement requires additional radiation exposure around 5.2 s and operation time of 0.2 min

* Correspondence: takashi_tk2001@yahoo.co.jp
[1]Department of Urology, Yokohama City University, Graduate School of Medicine, 3-9 Fukuura, Kanazawa-ku, Yokohama, Kanagawa 2360004, Japan
[3]Department of Urology, Ohguchi Higashi General Hospital, Yokohama, Japan
Full list of author information is available at the end of the article

[15]. Moreover, in some hospitals, assorted lengths of ureteral stents are not stocked. Therefore, preoperative prediction of ureteral length is often needed. We previously reported the usefulness of direct measurement with a ureteral catheter in predicting the actual ureteral length [15]. In another study, we showed the reliability of multiple modalities for approximating the ureteral length in the same group of patients [16]. The length from renal vein to ureteral orifice measured by CT scan (axial CT distance: ACTD) showed a stronger association than any other variables tested, including body height (BH) and intravenous urography (IVU) measurement [17]. Accurately predicting the ureteral length is necessary for determining the optimal stent length [10, 12].

The aim of the present study was to develop and internally validate a preoperative predictive model for predicting the actual ureteral length (AUL).

Methods

Patients

We measured the ureteral length in 362 patients by direct measurement, as described below, at Ohguchi Higashi General Hospital (Yokohama, Japan) from 2010 to 2014. In these patients, a total of 127 ureters had previously been assessed by both IVU and CT scan, preoperatively. This study was approved by the Review Board of Kanagawa Prefecture Medical Association (Approved number: H25-3169) and written informed consent was obtained from the patients for their data to be used for research purpose.

Measurement of actual ureteral length

The AUL, which was defined as the length between the ureteropelvic junction (UPJ; detected by fluoroscopy after retrograde pyelography) and the ureteral orifice (detected by cystoscopy), was determined by direct measurement using a 5-Fr ureteral catheter (TigerTail®, BARD, Murray Hill, NJ, USA), as we previously described [15]. In order to avoid overly straightening of the ureter, which might decrease its length, we measured the AUL, using a ureteral catheter without the guidewire.

Preoperative factors

The correlations between the actual ureteral length and the following variables were assessed: (1) BH, (2) age, (3) sex, (4) side, (5) IVUa (the linear distance from the UPJ to the uretero-vesicle junction [UVJ] by IVU), (6) IVUb (the linear distance from the mid-kidney to the UVJ by IVU), (7) IVUc (the ureteral trace was measured by tracing the ureter from the ureteropelvic junction to the ureterovesical junction and measuring the length of the trace with a flexible ruler which was in the form of a string by IVU), and (8) the distance from the level of the renal vein to the ureteral trace by non-contrast ACTD. ACTD was the distance from the renal vein level to the urinary orifice level. It was defined as the number of CT slices multiplied by the distance between each slice using axial CT. The upper slice was defined as the level of the renal vein, and the lower slice was defined as the level of UVJ.

Statistical analysis

Variables were selected by backward selection. Multiple linear regression analysis with backward selection was used to model the relationship between the factors analyzed and actual ureteral length. The selection criterion of $p < 0.1$ was used for elimination of a variable. Some variables were initially excluded from the model because of multicollinearity. Before multiple linear regression, we exclude IVUc, because of the strong association between IVUa and IVUc (r = 0.924). Decisions with respect to the coding of the predictive model variables were made before variable selection. A bootstrapping method was a nonparametric data generating method in which new datasets were repeatedly generated from an original dataset. Using the bootstrap methods for internal validation, the coefficient of determination (variance explained, R2) was assessed. Statistical analyses were performed using SAS 9.3 (SAS Institute Inc., Cary, NC, USA).

Results

A total of 127 patients all with stone disease, including 76 men (59.8%) and 51 women (40.2%), were enrolled in this study. The median and mean ($\pm$ SD) ages were 60 and 58.7 ($\pm$14.2) years (range: 28 - 86), respectively (Table 1). Fifty-three (41.7%) were right ureters (41.7%) and 74 (58.3%) were left ureters (58.3%). The median and mean ($\pm$ SD) AULs were 24.0 and 23.3 ($\pm$2.0) cm (range: 16.0 – 27.5). Left side ureter are significantly

Table 1 Patients' characteristics

Variables	Number (%) or median (mean ± SD)	Range (min., max.)
Ureteral Length (cm)	24 (23.3 ± 2.0)	16.0 - 27.5
Age	60 (58.7 ± 14.2)	28 - 86
Side		
Right	53 (41.7%)	
Left	74 (58.3%)	
Sex		
Male	76 (59.8%)	
Female	51 (40.2%)	
Body Height (cm)	163 (161.7 ± 9.7)	128 - 180
IVUa (cm)	24.0 (23.9 ± 2.8)	14.0 - 30.0
IVUb (cm)	26.0 (25.7 ± 2.7)	15.0 - 32.0
IVUc (cm)	20.5 (24.8 ± 2.7)	15.0 - 31.0
ACTD (cm)	22.4 (22.9 ± 2.7)	16.1 - 22.4

IVU intravenous urography, *ACTD* axial CT distance

longer than right side $(23.7 \pm 1.69$ versus 22.7 ± 2.2, $P = 0.007$) Ureteral length in male was not longer than in female $(23.4 \pm 1.86$ versus 23.1 ± 2.15, $P = 0.350$). On the other hand, multiple linear regression showed that sex was an independent factor (Table 2). The results of multiple linear regression are presented in Table 2. This predictive model contained five characteristics, including age, side, sex, IVUa, and ACTD. The total score of the predictive model was derived from the sum of the individual scores of each predictive variable (Fig. 1). The predicting ureteral length was written as follow formula; Ureteral Length = 10.1 + 0.27 x ACTD (cm) - 0.016 x Age + 0.302 x IVUa (cm) + 0.504 x side (Right:0, Left:1) + 0.716 x Sex (Male:0, Female:1). Using the bootstrap method, the explained variance (R2) was 0.57 ± 0.07 (range; 0.291 to 0.805).

Discussion

We previously reported the effectiveness of loop-type ureteral stent that decreased the prevalence of stent-related symptoms, compared with double pigtail ureteral stents. Significantly lower scores for almost all of stent-related symptoms, other than nocturia, were seen with loop-type ureteral stents than in double pigtail stents [18]. On the other hand, even when using with loop-type ureteral stent, the stent-related symptoms were not prevented with over-long ureteral stent position (unpublished data). We previously demonstrated the relationship between the AUL and the ureteral stent position using direct ureteral length measurements in 226 patients with loop-type ureteral stents [15]. The migration rate and overlong rate were correlated with the ureteral length, when the proximal end of the stent was in the renal pelvis. The appropriate length of ureteral stent was the same or up to 1 cm shorter than the measured ureteral length. In that study 89.0% of loop-type ureteral stents with the same length of the ureter were appropriately positioned, whereas 11.0% seemed to be overlong than AUL. When loop-type ureteral stents were 1 cm shorter than AUL were placed, 88.6% were in appropriate positions, 8.6% were too long, and 2.9% had migrated into the ureter. In addition, loop-type ureteral stents that were more than 2 cm shorter than the measured ureteral length increased the incidence of migration to more than 10% [15]. Direct measurement

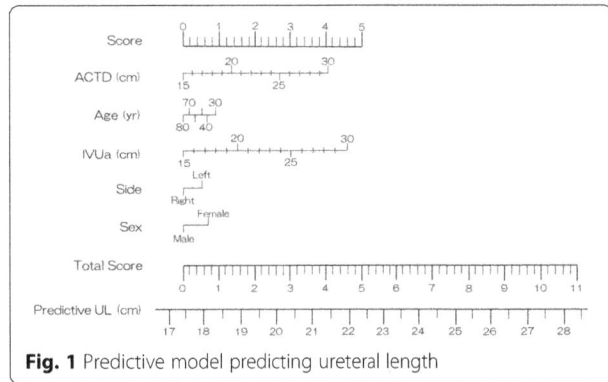

Fig. 1 Predictive model predicting ureteral length

with a ureteral catheter is thought to be the optimal method for selecting the appropriate length of ureteral stent, but the patient and operator are exposed to additional radiation and an extra procedure is required. Thus, while the direct measurement of the ureteral length is ideal, this predictive model may represent a new, more accurate method for estimating the ureteral length.

It is easy to apply the BH in predicting the ureteral length. Various studies have shown the association between BH and the ureteral length or the ureteral stent position [3, 16, 19, 20]. However, Shah et al. demonstrated that they were not significantly associated [21]. Gregory et al. reported the association of some variables, including body habitus, with ureteral lengths based on Vitruvius' and da Vinci's theories of proportion [22]. The AUL was significantly correlated with the BH, followed by the distances from the xyphoid process to the umbilicus (X-P) and from the shoulder to wrist (S-W), but they concluded that it was difficult to predict the ureteral length.

We previously investigated to define the best modality for estimating ureteral length in patients undergoing ureteral stent placement [17]. ACTD showed the strongest correlation ($R^2 = 0.381$) with AUL, compared with IVUa ($R^2 = 0.274$), IVUb ($R^2 = 0.230$), IVUc ($R^2 = 0.206$), BH ($R^2 = 0.098$), and body surface area ($R^2 = 0.095$). However, when inserting loop-type ureteral stent, more accurate methods for predicting ureteral length are needed because of easy to migrate to the ureter, because the differences of 1 cm might change the risk of migration and increase the ureteral stent related symptoms.

In the current study, we developed a predictive model using the preoperative factors identified by multiple regression analysis: age, side, sex, length measured by IVU, and ACTD. Interestingly, IVUc which is a trace of the whole ureteral length (according to the curve of ureter) did not show a stronger correlation with the AUL. We hypothesize that when we measured the AUL, the ureteral catheter straightened the ureter, causing the AUL to shorten. We chose IVUa because it was most highly correlated with the AUL and because it was strongly

Table 2 Multiplelinear regression for ureteral length (cm)

Variables	Coefficients	Standard error	P value
Intercept	10.130	1.580	<0.0001
Age	-0.016	0.009	0.010
Sex	0.716	0.259	0.007
Side	0.504	0.247	0.043
IVUa	0.302	0.054	<0.0001
ACTD	0.027	0.005	<0.0001

correlated with each of the IVU methods. To our knowledge, this is the first report of a predictive model that predicts ureteral length. This predictive model showed the coefficient of determination ($R^2 = 0.566$).

There are limitations in the present study. The endpoint of this predictive model was ureteral length, but not stent position or ureteral stent-related symptoms. We are now conducting a study to assess the stent position, using this predictive model. Furthermore, when a validated ureteral stent symptom questionnaire (USSQ) becomes available in Japan, we plan to conduct another study. The second limitation is that this predictive model is for patients who received both CT and IVU, not CT or IVU only. We previously showed the formula for estimating the actual ureteral length; however, this predictive model was found to have greater accuracy [17]. The third limitation is that we did not assess the background characteristics of the patients, including whether they were pregnant or had a history of radiation treatment, which might have influenced the length of the ureter. In this study, we only obtained data from patients who were treated for stone disease. We therefore speculate that these patients did not have a significant effect on the predictive model. On the other hand, this predictive model is not suitable for use with pregnant patients or patients undergoing radiation therapy. The forth one is that the same data was used for both variable selection and parameter estimation there is a risk that overfitting has occurred. Until an external validation is conducted model fit estimates are like to be inflated.

Conclusion

We have developed a predictive model, for the first time, which can precisely predict ureteral length, using the five preoperative clinical and radiographical factors. This predictive model may thus be a useful tool to help determine the optimal length of a ureteral stent.

Abbreviation

ACTD: Actual CT distance; AUL: Actual ureteral length; IVU: Intravenous urography; UPJ: Uretero pelvic junction; UVJ: Uretero vesicle junction

Acknowledgements

TK received a research grant from the Japanese Foundation for Research and Promotion of Endoscopy (2014).

Funding

The present study received funding in the form of grants from KAKENHI and grants (16 K20152) from the Ministry of Education, Culture, Sports, Science and Technology (MEXT) of Japan.

Authors' contributions

TK, HI, SK, HT, and JM performed the operation. TK conceived the study, participated in its design and wrote the manuscript. KM, HU, HM, and MY analyzed the data and corrected the draft. KS created and validated the predictive model. All of the authors read and approved the final manuscript.

Competing interests

The authors declare that they have no competing interests.

Author details

[1]Department of Urology, Yokohama City University, Graduate School of Medicine, 3-9 Fukuura, Kanazawa-ku, Yokohama, Kanagawa 2360004, Japan. [2]Departments of Biostatistics, Yokohama City University Graduate School of Medicine, Yokohama, Japan. [3]Department of Urology, Ohguchi Higashi General Hospital, Yokohama, Japan. [4]Departments of Pathology and Urology, Johns Hopkins University School of Medicine, Baltimore, USA.

References

1. Zimskind PD, Fetter TR, Wilkerson JL. Clinical use of long-term indwelling silicone rubber ureteral splints inserted cystoscopically. J Urol. 1967;97(5):840–4.
2. Borboroglu PG, Kane CJ. Current management of severely encrusted ureteral stents with a large associated stone burden. J Urol. 2000;164(3 Pt 1):648–50.
3. Ho CH, Huang KH, Chen SC, Pu YS, Liu SP, Yu HJ. Choosing the ideal length of a double-pigtail ureteral stent according to body height: study based on a Chinese population. Urol Int. 2009;83(1):70–4. doi:10.1159/000224872.
4. Joshi HB, Stainthorpe A, MacDonagh RP, Keeley Jr FX, Timoney AG, Barry MJ. Indwelling ureteral stents: evaluation of symptoms, quality of life and utility. J Urol. 2003;169(3):1065–9. doi:10.1097/01.ju.0000048980.33855.90. discussion 1069.
5. Pollard SG, Macfarlane R. Symptoms arising from Double-J ureteral stents. J Urol. 1988;139(1):37–8.
6. Kawahara T, Ito H, Terao H, Yoshida M, Matsuzaki J. Ureteral Stent Encrustation, Incrustation, and Coloring: Morbidity Related to Indwelling Times. J Endourol. 2011. doi:10.1089/end.2011.0385.
7. Kawahara T, Ishida H, Kubota Y, Matsuzaki J. Ureteroscopic removal of forgotten ureteral stent. BMJ case reports. 2012. doi:10.1136/bcr.02.2012.5736.
8. Kawahara T, Ito H, Terao H, Yamagishi T, Ogawa T, Uemura H, Kubota Y, Matsuzaki J. Ureteral stent retrieval using the crochet hook technique in females. PLoS One. 2012;7(1), e29292. doi:10.1371/journal.pone.0029292.
9. Kawahara T, Ito H, Terao H, Yamashita Y, Tanaka K, Ogawa T, Uemura H, Kubota Y, Matsuzaki J. Ureteral stent exchange under fluoroscopic guidance using the crochet hook technique in women. Urol Int. 2012;88(3):322–5. doi:10.1159/000336870.
10. Slaton JW, Kropp KA. Proximal ureteral stent migration: an avoidable complication? J Urol. 1996;155(1):58–61.
11. Breau RH, Norman RW. Optimal prevention and management of proximal ureteral stent migration and remigration. J Urol. 2001;166(3):890–3.
12. Wills MI, Gilbert HW, Chadwick DJ, Harrison SC. Which ureteric stent length? Br J Urol. 1991;68(4):440.
13. Pocock RD, Stower MJ, Ferro MA, Smith PJ, Gingell JC. Double J stents. A review of 100 patients. Br J Urol. 1986;58(6):629–33.
14. Chin JL, Denstedt JD. Retrieval of proximally migrated ureteral stents. J Urol. 1992;148(4):1205–6.
15. Kawahara T, Ito H, Terao H, Yoshida M, Ogawa T, Uemura H, Kubota Y, Matsuzaki J. Choosing an appropriate length of loop type ureteral stent using direct ureteral length measurement. Urol Int. 2012;88(1):48–53. doi:10.1159/000332431.
16. Pilcher JM, Patel U. Choosing the correct length of ureteric stent: a formula based on the patient's height compared with direct ureteric measurement. Clin Radiol. 2002;57(1):59–62. doi:10.1053/crad.2001.0737.
17. Kawahara T, Ito H, Terao H, Yoshida M, Ogawa T, Uemura H, Kubota Y, Matsuzaki J. Which is the best method to estimate the actual ureteral length in patients undergoing ureteral stent placement? Int J Urol. 2012;19(7):634–8. doi:10.1111/j.1442-2042.2012.02998.x.
18. Kawahara T, Ito H, Terao H, Ogawa T, Uemura H, Kubota Y, Matsuzaki J. Changing to a loop-type ureteral stent decreases patients' stent-related symptoms. Urol Res. 2012;40(6):763 7. doi:10.1007/s00240-012-0500-4.

19. Paick SH, Park HK, Byun SS, Oh SJ, Kim HH. Direct ureteric length measurement from intravenous pyelography: does height represent ureteric length? Urol Res. 2005;33(3):199–202. doi:10.1007/s00240-004-0461-3.

20. Lee BK, Paick SH, Park HK, Kim HG, Lho YS. Is a 22 cm Ureteric Stent Appropriate for Korean Patients Smaller than 175 cm in Height? Korean J Urol. 2010;51(9):642–6. doi:10.4111/kju.2010.51.9.642.

21. Shah J, Kulkarni RP. Height does not predict ureteric length. Clin Radiol. 2005;60(7):812–4. doi:10.1016/j.crad.2004.08.018.

22. Hruby GW, Ames CD, Yan Y, Monga M, Landman J. Correlation of ureteric length with anthropometric variables of surface body habitus. BJU Int. 2007; 99(5):1119–22. doi:10.1111/j.1464-410X.2007.06757.x.

Sacral neuromodulation for the treatment of neurogenic lower urinary tract dysfunction caused by multiple sclerosis

Daniel S. Engeler[1*], Daniel Meyer[1], Dominik Abt[1], Stefanie Müller[2] and Hans-Peter Schmid[1]

Abstract

Background: Sacral neuromodulation is well established in the treatment of refractory, non-neurogenic lower urinary tract dysfunction, but its efficacy and safety in patients with lower urinary tract dysfunction of neurological origin is unclear. Only few case series have been reported for multiple sclerosis. We prospectively evaluated the efficacy and safety of sacral neuromodulation in patients with multiple sclerosis.

Methods: Seventeen patients (13 women, 4 men) treated with sacral neuromodulation for refractory neurogenic lower urinary tract dysfunction caused by multiple sclerosis were prospectively enrolled (2007–2011). Patients had to have stable disease and confirmed neurogenic lower urinary tract dysfunction. Voiding variables, adverse events, and subjective satisfaction were assessed.

Results: Sixteen (94 %) patients had a positive test phase with a >70 % improvement. After implantation of the pulse generator (InterStim II), the improvement in voiding variables persisted. At 3 years, the median voided volume had improved significantly from 125 (range 0 to 350) to 265 ml (range 200 to 350) ($p < 0.001$), the post void residual from 170 (range 0 to 730) to 25 ml (range 0 to 300) ($p = 0.01$), micturition frequency from 12 (range 6 to 20) to 7 (range 4 to 12) ($p = 0.003$), and number of incontinence episodes from 3 (range 0 to 10) to 0 (range 0 to 1) ($p = 0.006$). The median subjective degree of satisfaction was 80 %. Only two patients developed lack of benefit. No major complications occurred.

Conclusions: Chronic sacral neuromodulation promises to be an effective and safe treatment of refractory neurogenic lower urinary tract dysfunction in selected patients with multiple sclerosis.

Keywords: Sacral neuromodulation, Sacral nerve stimulation, Neurologic disease, Lower urinary tract dysfunction, Multiple sclerosis

Background

Between 50 and 90 % of patients with multiple sclerosis (MS) develop lower urinary tract symptoms (LUTS) in the course of the disease [1, 2]. These symptoms are distressing and have a major impact on quality of life. Treatment of associated lower urinary tract dysfunction (LUTD) is often difficult and may fail. Underlying urodynamic abnormalities include neurogenic detrusor overactivity, detrusor sphincter dyssynergia and detrusor underactivity. These often lead to chronic urinary retention, urge urinary incontinence, and recurrent urinary tract infection. Oral antimuscarinics and, more recently, repeat intradetrusor botulinum toxin type A injections are the most frequent treatment for detrusor overactivity. Many patients need to perform intermittent self-catheterization because of urinary retention, and may eventually need an indwelling catheter or suprapubic cystostomy due to sensorimotor or visual deficits.

Sacral neuromodulation (SNM) has become a well-established approach over the past few years for patients with refractory idiopathic urinary urge incontinence,

* Correspondence: daniel.engeler@kssg.ch
[1]Department of Urology, Cantonal Hospital St. Gallen, St. Gallen, Switzerland
Full list of author information is available at the end of the article

urgency-frequency syndrome and non-obstructive chronic urinary retention [1–4]. Originally, SNM was not considered an option for neurogenic LUTD, but studies suggest that it is also effective in this these patients [5, 6]. Although LUTS are highly prevalent in patients with MS, only limited case series from 1 to 15 patients treated with SNM have been reported in the literature [7–17]. This low number may be explained partly by the fear of treatment failure due to disease progression.

SNM is minimally invasive and reversible, and may be a valuable treatment option for neurogenic LUTD in MS before resorting to more invasive procedures. The aim of our prospective study was the evaluation of efficacy and safety of sacral neuromodulation in patients with multiple sclerosis based on our experience.

Methods
Patient selection
Patients were enrolled prospectively on inclusion in an online registry run by the Swiss Society for Sacral Neuromodulation (SSSNM) founded as a requirement of the Swiss National Department of Health for quality control reasons. All patients had to have MS diagnosed using McDonald criteria [18] and a diagnosis of neurogenic LUTD due to MS confirmed by urodynamic examination. The symptoms could comprise either storage symptoms caused by detrusor overactivity with or without incontinence, or voiding symptoms caused by detrusor underactivity or detrusor sphincter dyssynergia, or both. Exclusion criteria were cognitive impairment precluding the ability to give informed consent for the intervention, progression of MS during the last twelve months, and an expanded disability status scale (EDSS) ≥ 8 preventing independent toilet transfer to enable voiding.

Assessments at baseline and follow-up
A complete neurourological evaluation was performed at baseline, including a history with clinical examination, assessment of the EDSS, bladder diary, urinalysis, cystoscopy and multichannel urodynamics with electromyogram of the pelvic floor using superficial electrodes (Duet® Encompass™ System, Mediwatch, Rugby, UK). Micturition frequency, voided volume, post void residual and the number of incontinence episodes were recorded as objective variables at baseline and during follow-up, based on a 72-h micturition diary. Incomplete voiding was defined as a repeat post void residual of more than 50 ml. The values of the individual micturition parameters were calculated as means from the diary. Patients rated their grade of satisfaction with the treatment in percent. Clinical data were collected preoperatively after a test phase, and in patients receiving implants, after 6 weeks, and then yearly.

Test phase
Before permanent implantation, all patients underwent a staged procedure with temporary percutaneous stimulation to assess their response to treatment. This test phase was performed using the definitive tined lead electrode model 3889 (Medtronic Inc., Minneapolis, MN, USA). The procedure was done under local or general anaesthesia with the patient in the prone position. A single intravenous infusion of 2 g cefamandole and 500 mg metronidazole was given as perioperative antibiotic prophylaxis. The test needle and the electrode were positioned under fluoroscopy using the bony landmarks to identify the level of the S3 foramen. After puncture of the S3 foramen on both sides with the test needle, the motor response to electrical stimulation was demonstrated by visible pulling in of the anus to ensure optimal placement of the needle. Monolateral implantation of the quadripolar tined lead electrode was performed on the side with the lower amplitude level for adequate motor response. The lead wire then was tunnelled to the right side in right-handers and to the left side in left-handers. A subcutaneous pocket was created in the posterior gluteal area, and the temporary external wire was connected and tunnelled to the contralateral lumbar side. If the response at both S3 foramina was inadequate, the same procedure was performed on the S4 foramen. Postoperatively, the subacute test phase was conducted with continuous neuromodulation at a sensory amplitude sufficient to induce a light vibratory sensation in the perineum, vagina, bladder or penis. Patients with >70 % improvement in voiding and storage symptoms were regarded as suitable for placement of the permanent pulse generator. If the result was unclear or negative, a second test using an additional contralateral electrode was recommended.

Implantation of the InterStim II pulse generator
After the test phase, the temporary external wire was cut at the skin level and the InterStim II pulse generator was placed under local or general anaesthesia. A single infusion of 2 g cefamandole was given as perioperative antibiotic prophylaxis. After locating the connecting cluster, the temporary external wire was removed and the InterStim II pulse generator connected, before placing it in the subcutaneous pocket and closing the wound.

Statistical analysis
GraphPad Prism Version 5.0d (GraphPad Software, Inc., California) was used for the statistical analysis. Outcome data were reported as medians and ranges. The Mann–Whitney and Spearman rank tests were used as appropriate. A p value <0.05 was considered statistically significant.

Ethical approval

Although ethical approval was not sought in advance, the cantonal ethical committee of St. Gallen has evaluated the study (EKSG 15/024) and has confirmed that there is no legal opportunity to approve a study retrospectively. However, upon evaluation of the project, the independent ethical committee has stated that the ethical requirements of this study would have been fulfilled.

Results

Patient characteristics at baseline

All 17 patients included prospectively from July 2007 to November 2011 fulfilled the study inclusion and exclusion criteria. The subtype of MS at baseline was relapsing-remitting in 9 (53 %) patients, secondary progressive in 7 (41 %) patients, and primary progressive in 1 (6 %) patient. Most were women (13/17, 76 %). The median age at inclusion was 46.3 years (range 16.9 to 74.6), the median duration of MS was 8 years (range 3 to 46), and the median EDSS at baseline was 5 (range 3 to 7.5).

Incomplete voiding measured by ultrasound or intermittent self-catheterization was present in 16 (94 %) patients. One woman needed an indwelling catheter because of incomplete voiding (>700 ml post void residual) and inability to self-catheterize. The median number of voids per day in the other patients was 12 (range 6 to 20) with a median voided volume of 130 ml (range 70 to 350). The previous urinary tract infection rate was two or more per year in 5 (29 %) patients. The median number of incontinence episodes was 3.5 (range 0 to 10). Five of the patients performed self-catheterization with a median number of 4 per day (range 3 to 6). All patients had failed or not tolerated previous antimuscarinic treatment. One patient had had intradetrusor injection of 200 U onabotulinum toxin A 20 months before developing urinary retention and undergoing temporary cystostomy placement. Three patients also had associated neurogenic faecal incontinence.

Neurogenic LUTD caused by MS was confirmed by urodynamic testing (Table 1). Detrusor overactivity was shown in 15 (88 %) patients, which was phasic in 9, and only terminal in 6 patients. Detrusor overactivity incontinence was present in 9 (53 %) patients. In addition, detrusor sphincter dyssynergia was demonstrated in 7 (41 %) patients.

Test phase outcome

Implantation of the tined lead for the test phase was done under local ($N = 7$) or general ($N = 10$) anaesthesia according to patient preference, as described in the methods section. The first test phase was successful in 14 (82 %) patients with an objective improvement of >70 %. One patient had a clearly negative first test phase.

Table 1 Urodynamic variables at baseline

Characteristic	Median value (range)
First urge to void (ml)	107 (38-276)
Strong urge to void (ml)	187 (47-777)
Reflex volume (ml)	80 (8-319)
Maximum cystometric capacity	254 (48-778)
Compliance (ml/cmH$_2$O)	10.3 (0.5-80)
Maximum urinary flow (ml/s)	10.3 (0-33.7)
Maximum detrusor pressure during voiding (cmH$_2$O)	38 (8-85)
Detrusor pressure at maximum urinary flow (cmH$_2$O)	20 (4-200)
Voided volume (ml)	101 (0-414)
Post void residual (ml)	83 (0-778)

This patient refused further testing. Two patients with an equivocal result were tested twice, including the contralateral side. This decision was made after an improvement of less than 70 % during the first test phase. These two patients had better results with bilateral testing. Overall, the test phase was successful in 16 (94 %) patients. The median test duration was 22.3 days (range 3 to 70) and the median period from test start to implantation was 28.5 days (range 3 to 87). No complications occurred during the test phase.

Implantation

All 16 patients with a positive test phase underwent implantation of the InterStim II pulse generator under local ($N = 11$) or general ($N = 5$) anaesthesia according to patient preference. Two were implanted bilaterally using two InterStim II pulse generators in opposite gluteal positions. Low stimulation amplitudes (<1 V) were achieved in all patients (Table 2). This low level was the result of our attempting to minimize amplitudes and also using subsensory thresholds for stimulation to reduce battery consumption. No perioperative complications occurred.

Table 2 Implantation characteristics

Characteristic	Value
Unilateral implantation – N/total N (%)	14/16 (88)
Sacral foramen S3 - N/total N (%)	13/16 (81)[a]
Sacral foramen S4 - N/total N (%)	3/16 (19)[a]
Amplitude – Volt, median (range)	0.58 (0.2-0.9)
Impulse width – μs, median (range)	210 (210-210)
Stimulation frequency – Hertz, median (range)	14 (9-21)
Subsensory stimulation - N/total N (%)	13/16 (81)

[a]one bilaterally

Follow-up

Fourteen (88 %) patients reached the 3-year follow-up time point. Two had had their device for only 2 years at last follow-up. The maximum follow-up was 6 years. The configuration of electrodes was changed at least once in all 16 patients during follow-up. Several also underwent multiple reprogramming to optimize the treatment effect and reach low amplitudes. The median amplitude used with the InterStim II pulse generator was 0.70 V (range 0.2 to 1.3) after 6 weeks, 0.85 (range 0.35 to 1.5) after 1 year, 0.9 (range 0.6 to 1.2) after 2 years, and 0.85 (range 0.6 to 1.55) after 3 years.

Micturition parameters had improved statistically significantly at all measuring times (Fig. 1). At 3 years after implantation, the voided volume had improved significantly from a median of 125 ml (range 0 to 350) before treatment to 265 ml (range 200 to 350) ($p < 0.001$), the median post void residual was reduced from 170 (range 0 to 730) to 25 ml (range 0 to 300) ($p = 0.01$), the median micturition frequency from 12 (range 6 to 20) to 7 (range 4 to 12) ($p = 0.003$), and the median number of incontinence episodes from 3 (range 0 to 10) to 0 (range 0 to 1) ($p = 0.006$).

Subjective assessment of success showed a persistently high degree of satisfaction with a median of 80 % (range 0 to 100) after up to three years. As mentioned above, the effect of the SNM subsided as the disease progressed. Patients with baseline EDSS scores <6 (i.e. able to walk 100 m or more unaided) showed a statistically significantly greater degree of satisfaction after three

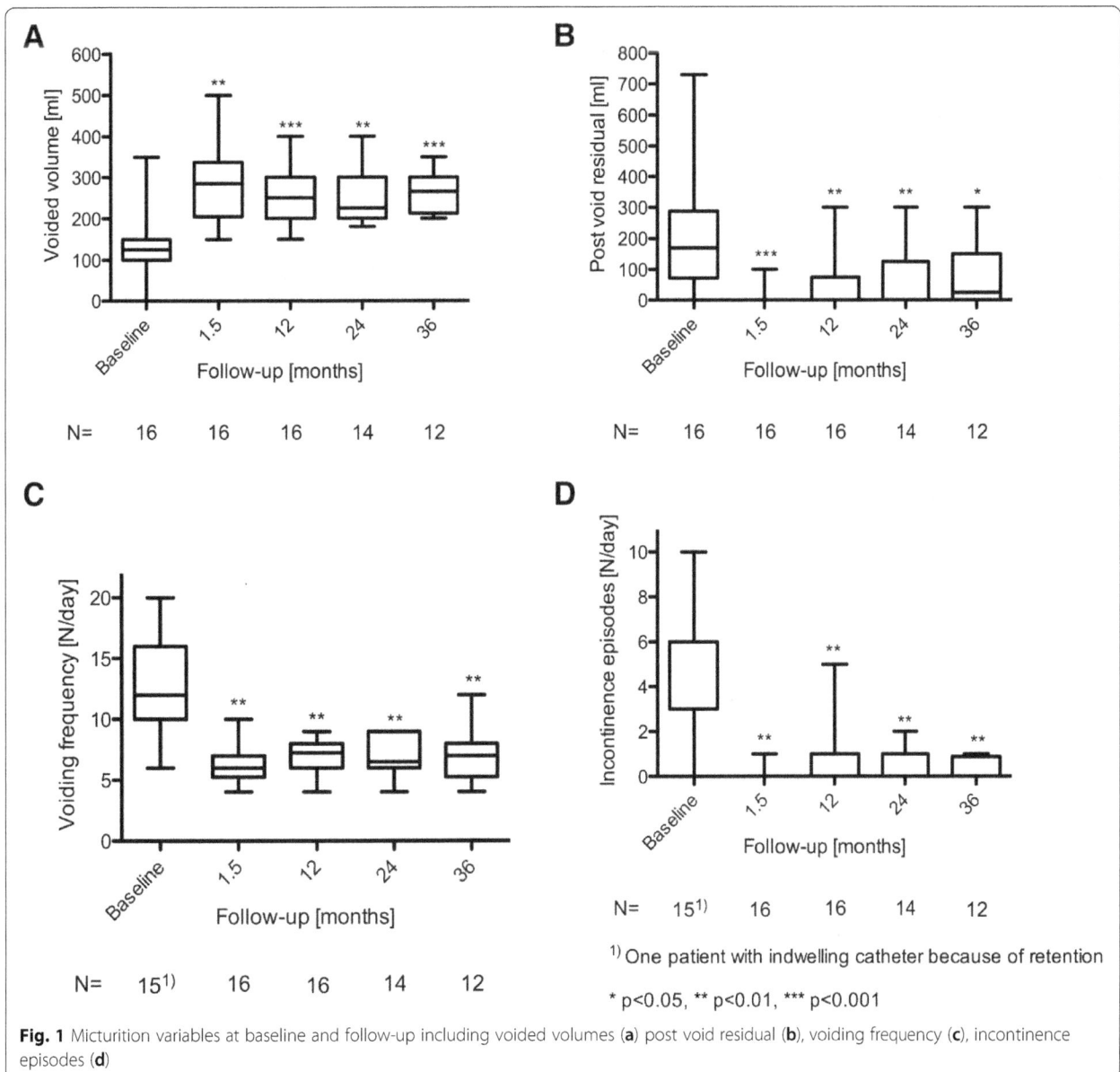

Fig. 1 Micturition variables at baseline and follow-up including voided volumes (**a**) post void residual (**b**), voiding frequency (**c**), incontinence episodes (**d**)

year's follow-up than those with EDSS scores ≥ 6 ($N = 8$ vs. 5, respectively; $p = 0.025$).

Adverse events

Overall, 5 (31 %) patients underwent revision during follow-up because of problems at the electrode site. There were 2 cases (at 7 and 24 months) of electrode dysfunction with high electrode impedance (>4000 Ohm) for all electrode combinations, loss of sensory response, and clinical impairment of micturition. One patient had a bilateral fracture of the electrodes at 24 months because of a traumatic transverse fracture of the sacrum. Two additional patients had dislocation of their electrode at 18 and 31 months. Revision with exchange of electrodes was successful in all of these cases. One additional patient developed loss of effect during the third year of treatment and decided against reoperation. Another was treated by cystostomy placement because of increasing motor disabilities, and implantation was assessed as a failure because the patient was no longer benefiting. None of the devices were explanted during follow-up. No other complications were observed.

Discussion

Neurogenic LUTD has a major impact on quality of life in MS patients. The incidence of urinary symptoms increases with disease duration and involvement of the motor system [19]. The anatomic lesions responsible are most often located in the spinal cord [20], although some urinary tract symptoms may also be due to cortical involvement [21].

Treatment options for neurogenic LUTD in MS depend on concomitant motor dysfunction and goal of treatment. Although frequently used and recommended by a UK consensus on the management of the bladder in MS [22] and by the EAU Guidelines on neuro-urology [23] for neurogenic detrusor overactivity, evidence for the use of antimuscarinics is very limited. In MS, disease-specific factors may accentuate LUTS and the side effects of medications, and render symptom management increasingly difficult, including reduced patient compliance. A Cochrane review concluded that anticholinergics (i.e. antimuscarinics) could not be recommended in MS [24]. Other options recommended by the consensus include pelvic floor exercises in patients with mild disability, intermittent self-catheterization if the post void residual is more than 100 ml, and intradetrusor botulinum toxin A injections.

A more recent option is percutaneous tibial nerve stimulation. Clinical improvement in about 80 % of cases has been reported from two prospective non-comparative studies using daily or weekly stimulation schedules [25, 26]. However, treatment effects were assessed over only 3 months.

A minimally invasive approach like SNM that restores the ability to reach the toilet in time and enables complete emptying of the bladder would be a major factor in improving quality of life.

In our patient series treated with SNM, we found a high success rate after failure of conservative treatment options, in agreement with small, previously published series [7–17]. Our test phase was successful (objective improvement >70 %) in a high percentage of patients (94 %). In 6 patients, the test phase was longer than 4 weeks, reflecting our caution in determining the result as positive. However, more prolonged testing did not lead to infectious complications. After implantation, transient deteriorations in effect were generally managed by adaptation of the stimulation parameters and electrode configuration.

A major advantage of SNM over other treatment options is that it not only improves the volume voided, urgency and urge urinary incontinence, but also reduces the post void residual. These effects were achieved early in treatment and remained stable throughout follow-up of up to 3 years.

It is important to note that the degree of subjective satisfaction during follow-up was negatively correlated to the degree of disability at the time of implantation. Not surprisingly, worse motor function at the time of implantation limits the benefits to physical micturition that can be regained. This must be considered when selecting MS patients for SNM.

Our results demonstrate that SNM can be effective even in patients with progressive MS. Even patients with long-standing disease (up to 46 years in our series) can benefit from SNM. Complications we observed were associated with dysfunction or dislocation of electrodes in 5 (31 %) patients, all of which were managed simply by changing the electrodes. Only one patient had complete loss of effect during follow-up, and one other was no longer benefiting from treatment because of motor disabilities.

We included patients prospectively, and follow-up was complete without dropouts over time. A positive treatment effect was evident, despite previous conservative treatment having failed. Nevertheless, the conclusions that can be drawn from this small sample size are limited.

As an implication for research, our findings and those made by others warrant a randomized controlled study to investigate the beneficial effect of SNM in this indication. A Swiss multicentre trial with SNM in patients with neurogenic LUTD is at present under way and we are contributing patients [27].

Thanks to its low associated morbidity, SNM can be considered an option for carefully selected patients with neurogenic LUTD caused by MS. Patients should have failed previous conservative treatment and have stable disease without major motor dysfunction. At best, candidates should be able to walk unaided and should be likely to be able to regain physiological control over micturition. The advent of a number of new disease-modifying medical treatments for relapsing-remitting MS may contribute to prolonging benefit from treatment of their LUTD by SNM.

Conclusions

Our own mid-term experience and work from others suggests that SNM for refractory neurogenic LUTD due to MS is a good option in carefully selected patients with a high probability of objective and subjective success, including improvement of quality of life. Confirmation in a randomized, controlled trial is needed.

Abbreviations
EDSS: Expanded disability status scale; LUTD: Lower urinary tract dysfunction; LUTS: Lower urinary tract symptoms; MS: Multiple sclerosis; SNM: Sacral neuromodulation.

Competing interests
DSE has received speaker honoraria from Medtronic Inc. and has participated in a trial by this company. All other authors declare that they have no competing interests.

Authors' contributions
DSE and HPS designed the study. DSE, DM and DA acquired the data. DSE did the statistical analysis of the data. DSE, DM, DA and SM interpreted the data. DSE, DM and DA drafted the manuscript. SM and HPS provided a critical revision of the manuscript. All authors read and approved the final manuscript.

Acknowledgments
The authors thank Alistair Reeves for editing the manuscript.

Funding
There was no external funding.

Author details
[1]Department of Urology, Cantonal Hospital St. Gallen, St. Gallen, Switzerland. [2]Department of Neurology, Cantonal Hospital St. Gallen, St. Gallen, Switzerland.

References
1. Hennessey A, Robert NP, Swingler R, Compston DA. Urinary, faecal and sexual dysfunction in patients with multiple sclerosis. J Neurol. 1999;246:1027–32.
2. Koldewijn EL, Hommes OR, Lemmens WA, Debruyne FM, van Kerrebroeck PE. Relationship between lower urinary tract abnormalities and disease-related parameters in multiple sclerosis. J Urol. 1995;154:169–73.
3. Brazzelli M, Murray A, Fraser C. Efficacy and safety of sacral nerve stimulation for urinary urge incontinence: a systematic review. J Urol. 2006;175:835–41.
4. Herbison GP, Arnold EP. Sacral neuromodulation with implanted devices for urinary storage and voiding dysfunction in adults. Cochrane Database Syst Rev 2009;(2):CD004202. doi:10.1002/14651858.CD004202.pub2.
5. Kessler TM, Buchser E, Meyer S, Engeler DS, Al-Khodairy AW, Bersch U, et al. Sacral neuromodulation for neurogenic lower urinary tract dysfunction: systematic review and meta-analysis. Eur Urol. 2010;58:865–74.
6. van Kerrebroeck PE, van Voskuilen AC, Heesakkers JP, Nijholt AA L a, Siegel S, Jonas U, et al. Results of sacral neuromodulation therapy for urinary voiding dysfunction: outcomes of a prospective, worldwide clinical study. J Urol. 2007;178:2029–34.
7. Wallace PA, Lane FL, Noblett KL. Sacral nerve neuromodulation in patients with underlying neurologic disease. Am J Obstet Gynecol. 2007;197:96;e1-96.e5.
8. Hohenfellner M, Schultz-Lampel D, Dahms S, Matzel K, Thuroff JW. Bilateral chronic sacral neuromodulation for treatment of lower urinary tract dysfunction. J Urol. 1998;160:821–4.
9. Chartier-Kastler EJ, Ruud Bosch JL, Perrigot M, Chancellor MB, Richard F, Denys P. Long-term results of sacral nerve stimulation (S3) for the treatment of neurogenic refractory urge incontinence related to detrusor hyperreflexia. J Urol. 2000;164:1476–80.
10. Spinelli M, Bertapelle P, Cappellano F, Zanollo A, Carone R, Catanzaro F, et al. Chronic sacral neuromodulation in patients with lower urinary tract symptoms: results from a national register. J Urol. 2001;166:541–5.
11. Spinelli M, Giardiello G, Gerber M, Arduini A, van den Hombergh U, Malaguti S. New sacral neuromodulation lead for percutaneous implantation using local anaesthesia: description and first experience. J Urol. 2003;170:1905–7.
12. Lavano A, Volpentesta G, Aloisi M, Veltri C, Piragine G, Signorelli CD. Use of chronic sacral nerve stimulation in neurological voiding disorders. J Neurosurg Sci. 2004;48:157–9.
13. Minardi D, Muzzonigro G. Lower urinary tract and bowel disorders and multiple sclerosis: role of sacral neuromodulation: a preliminary report. Neuromodulation. 2005;8:176–81.
14. Sutherland SE, Lavers A, Carlson A, Holtz C, Kesha J, Siegel SW. Sacral nerve stimulation for voiding dysfunction: One institution's 11-year experience. Neurourol Urodyn. 2007;26:1–28.
15. Lombardi G, Mondaini N, Macchiarella A, Cilotti A, Del Popolo G. Clinical female sexual outcome after sacral neuromodulation implant for lower urinary tract symptoms (LUTS). J Sex Med. 2008;5:1411–7.
16. Marinkovic SP, Gillen LM. Sacral neuromodulation for multiple sclerosis patients with urinary retention and clean intermittent catheterization. Int Urogynecol J. 2010;21:223–8.
17. Minardi D, Muzzonigro G. Sacral neuromodulation in patients with multiple sclerosis. World J Urol. 2012;30:123–8.
18. Polman CH, Reingold SC, Edan G, Filippi M, Hartung HP, Kappos L, et al. Diagnostic criteria for multiple sclerosis: 2005 revisions to the "McDonald Criteria". Ann Neurol. 2005;58:840–6.
19. Giannanoni A, Scivoletto G, Di Stasi SM, Grasso MG, Vespasiani G, Castellano V. Urological dysfunctions and upper urinary tract involvement in multiple sclerosis patients. Neurourol Urodyn. 1998;17:89–98.
20. Littwiller SE, Frohman EM, Zimmern PE. Multiple sclerosis and the urologist. J Urol. 1999;161:743–57.
21. Giannantoni A, Scivoletto G, Di Stasi SM, Grasso MG, Finazzi Agrò E, Collura G, et al. Lower urinary tract dysfunction and disability status in patients with multiple sclerosis. Arch Phys Med Rehabil. 1999;80:437–41.
22. Fowler CJ, Panicker JN, Drake M, Harris C, Harrison SC, Kirby M, et al. A UK consensus on the management of the bladder in multiple sclerosis. J Neurourol Neurosurg Psychiatry. 2009;80:470–7.
23. Blok B, Pannek J, Castro Diaz D, del Popolo G, Groen J, Hamid R, et al. Guidelines on Neuro-Urology. EAU Guidelines 2015 edition. http://uroweb.org/guideline/neuro-urology/. Accessed 15 May 2015.
24. Nicholas RS, Friede T, Hollis S, Young CA. Anticholinergics for urinary symptoms in multiple sclerosis. Cochrane Database Syst Rev. 2009;(2):CD004202. doi:10.1002/14651858.CD004202.pub2.
25. De Seze M, Rabaut P, Gallien P, Even-Schneider A, Denys P, Bonniaud V, et al. Transcutaneous posterior tibial nerve stimulation for treatment of the overactive bladder syndrome in multiple sclerosis: Results of a multicentre prospective study. Neurourol Urodyn. 2011;30:306–11.
26. Gobbi C, Digesu GA, Khullar V, Elneil S, Caccia Z, Zecca C. Percutaneous posterior tibial nerve stimulation as an effective treatment of refractory lower urinary tract symptoms in patients with multiple sclerosis: preliminary data from a multicentre, prospective, open label trial. Mult Scler. 2011;17:1514–9.
27. Knüpfer SC, Liechti MD, Mordasini L, Abt D, Engeler DS, Wöllner J, et al. Protocol for a randomized, placebo-controlled, double-blind clinical trial investigating sacral neuromodulation for neurogenic lower urinary tract dysfunction. BMC Urol. 2014;14:65.

Design of a single-arm clinical trial of regenerative therapy by periurethral injection of adipose-derived regenerative cells for male stress urinary incontinence in Japan: the ADRESU study protocol

Shinobu Shimizu[1*], Tokunori Yamamoto[2], Shinobu Nakayama[1,8], Akihiro Hirakawa[1,9], Yachiyo Kuwatsuka[1], Yasuhito Funahashi[2], Yoshihisa Matsukawa[2], Keisuke Takanari[3], Kazuhiro Toriyama[3,4], Yuzuru Kamei[3], Kazutaka Narimoto[5], Tomonori Yamanishi[6], Osamu Ishizuka[7], Masaaki Mizuno[1] and Momokazu Gotoh[2*]

Abstract

Background: Male stress urinary incontinence is a prevalent condition after radical prostatectomy. While the standard recommendation for the management of urine leakage is pelvic floor muscle training, its efficacy is still unsatisfactory. Therefore, we have focused on regenerative therapy, which consists of administering a periurethral injection of autologous regenerative cells from adipose tissue, separated using the Celution® system. Based on an interim data analysis of our exploratory study, we confirmed the efficacy and acceptable safety profile of this treatment. Accordingly, we began discussions with Japanese regulatory authorities regarding the development of this therapy in Japan. The Ministry of Health, Labour and Welfare suggested that we implement a clinical trial of a new medical device based on the Pharmaceutical Affaires Act in Japan. Next, we discussed the design of this investigator-initiated clinical trial (the ADRESU study) aimed at evaluating the efficacy and safety of this therapy, in a consultation meeting with the Pharmaceuticals and Medical Device Agency.

Methods: The ADRESU study is an open-label, multi-center, single-arm study involving a total of 45 male stress urinary incontinence patients with mild-to-moderate urine leakage persisting more than 1 year after prostatectomy, in spite of behavioral and pharmacological therapies. The primary endpoint is the rate of patients at 52 weeks with improvement of urine leakage volume defined as a reduction from baseline greater than 50% by 24-h pad test. Our specific hypothesis is that the primary endpoint result will be higher than a pre-specified threshold of 10%.

Discussion: The ADRESU study is the first clinical trial of regenerative treatment for stress urinary incontinence by adipose-derived regenerative cells using the Celution® system based on the Japanese Pharmaceutical Affaires Act.
(Continued on next page)

* Correspondence: s-shimizu@med.nagoya-u.ac.jp; gotoh@med.nagoya-u.ac.jp
[1]Center for Advanced Medicine and Clinical Research, Nagoya University Hospital, 65 Tsurumai-cho, Showa-ku, Nagoya, Aichi 466-8560, Japan
[2]Department of Urology, Nagoya University Graduate School of Medicine, 65 Tsurumai-cho, Showa-ku, Nagoya, Aichi 466-8550, Japan
Full list of author information is available at the end of the article

(Continued from previous page)

We will evaluate the efficacy and safety in this trial to provide an adequate basis for marketing approval with the final objective of making this novel therapy widely available for Japanese patients.

Keywords: Stress urinary incontinence, Lower urinary tract symptoms, Regenerative medicine, Cell therapy, Prostatectomy, Adipose-derived regenerative cells

Background

Male stress urinary incontinence (SUI) is a secondary intrinsic sphincter deficiency and a prevalent condition after radical prostatectomy [1–5]. Individuals with SUI may limit activities of daily living to reduce the chance of urine leakage; hence, SUI can have a major impact on the quality of life (QOL) of patients. The standard therapy of male SUI is pelvic floor muscle training, and clenbuterol hydrochloride, which is solely approved for SUI indication in Japan; however, the efficacy of these treatments is still unsatisfactory. Another potential therapy is periurethral injection of collagen, but its efficacy has only been shown in short-term trials [6, 7], and this treatment is not currently approved for SUI in Japan. Another potential alternative involves the implantation of an artificial urinary sphincter, which is recommended for patients with severe incontinence [8–10]. Unfortunately, according to a Japanese report from the Office of Pharmaceutical Industry Research (OPIR News No.45), new pharmaceutical agents for SUI have not been developed in Japan as of 2015.

Meanwhile, we have focused on regenerative cell therapy of urethral sphincter deficiency based on several experimental studies [11–16]. We previously confirmed that periurethral injection of cultured adipose-derived stem cells improved leak point pressure in an SUI animal model [17]. Therefore, we planned a preliminary clinical study with the objective of developing a novel treatment using autologous adipose-derived regenerative cells (ADRCs) without cell culture. In other words, the ADRCs are isolated in a few hours by the Celution® system (Cytori Therapeutics, Inc., San Diego, CA, USA). That study was approved by the Ethics Committee of the Nagoya University Graduate School of Medicine, and also by the committee of the Japanese Ministry of Health, Labour and Welfare (MHLW) according to the Guidelines on Clinical Research using Human Stem Cells [18], and registered at the University Hospital Medical information Network Clinical Trial Registry (UMIN-CTR Unique ID: UMIN000006116). Based on an interim data analysis of that exploratory clinical study, we obtained preliminary evidence confirming that the periurethral injection of isolated ADRCs is effective and safe for use in the male SUI patients [19, 20]. However, the Celution® system is not currently available for

treatment purposes in Japan. This system is only currently approved for use in clinical research under the Japanese 'Act on the Safety of Regenerative Medicine'. Therefore, as our objective is to disseminate this novel therapy throughout Japan as soon as possible, we prepared a confirmatory study protocol and began discussions with the Japanese regulatory authorities to build a bridge from 'benchside to bedside to community' in cooperation with Cytori Therapeutics, Inc.

In this article, we provide the detailed design of this investigator-initiated clinical trial in male SUI patients as a pivotal study for the licensure of this therapy in Japan (the ADRESU study). Incidentally, the main design of this trial is undergoing the process of approval by the Pharmaceuticals and Medical Device Agency (PMDA), which is responsible for reviewing new pharmaceuticals, medical devices, and regenerative medicines; however, whether the final approval by PMDA is granted or not will depend on the data obtained in this study.

Methods/Design
Overall design and objective

The primary objective of this trial is to evaluate the efficacy and safety of periurethral injection of autologous ADRCs separated with the Celution® system in male SUI patients. The ADRESU study is an open-label, multicenter, single-arm study involving a total of 45 male patients with stress urinary incontinence, with mild-to-moderate urine leakage persisting more than 1 year after prostatectomy that achieved insufficient symptom improvement by behavioral and pharmacologic therapies. The primary endpoint of this study is the rate of patients with improvement in urine leakage volume. Our specific hypothesis is that the rate of patients with improvement in urine leakage volume, defined as a reduction greater than 50% from baseline by 24-h pad test, is higher than a pre-specified threshold of 10%. Additionally, we will consider whether or not patients with symptom improvement will also show improvement in QOL scores.

Selection of subjects

First, we decided to select male patients with SUI as our patient population, not only because urinary incontinence mechanisms differ by sex, but also because few female data were available in our former study. Next, we considered prior incontinence history, in other words, duration and severity of incontinence after surgery. Regarding the duration of incontinence, there is enough evidence to show that patients who develop post-prostatectomy incontinence persisting for a period longer than 1 year are unlikely to recover function thereafter [1–5]. With respect to incontinence severity, we restricted our population to patients with mild-to-moderate urinary incontinence based on subgroup analysis of our available data in comparison with more severe patients. The mean reduction rate of leakage volume at 12 months of patients with mild-to-moderate and severe urinary incontinence was 62.6% and 18.0%, respectively (Table 1).

The detailed inclusion criteria are as follows:

1) Males with stress urinary incontinence persisting more than 1 year after either of the following surgical procedures, with insufficient improvement of symptoms by behavioral and pharmacological therapies:
   i. Patients with symptoms after radical prostatectomy for localized prostate cancer and currently without relapse/metastasis, and prostate specific antigen (PSA) level less than 0.1 ng/mL for over 1 year
   ii. Patients with symptoms after transurethral prostatectomy or laser prostatectomy for prostatic hyperplasia and PSA level less than 4.0 ng/mL over 1 year
2) Age of 20 years or above
3) Mild-to-moderate urinary incontinence by the 24-h pad test
4) Patients who can keep a bladder diary in a satisfactory manner
5) Patients that can provide a signed informed consent

The main exclusion criteria are as follows:

1) Concurrent with any other types of urinary incontinence
2) History of urinary or reproductive surgery within 6 months
3) History of behavioral therapy or pharmacotherapy initiation within 3 months
4) Concurrent with diabetes insipidus

5) History of radiotherapy in the lower urinary tract
6) History of ADRCs treatment for stress urinary incontinence
7) History of any type of cell therapy within 6 months
8) Participation in any other clinical trial within 3 months
9) Concurrent with lower urinary tract obstruction
10) Concurrent with urolithiasis, urinary tract infection or interstitial cystitis
11) History of recurrent urinary tract infection
12) History or suspicion of malignant neoplasm within the last 5 years
13) Any other patients whom the trial investigator deems ineligible for this study

Selection of patients for the control group

In general, a concurrent control group is needed for a clinical trial as the most common clinical trial designs for a confirmatory trial is a randomized, controlled, parallel-group design [21, 22]. Potential candidates for the control group include those receiving approved treatment (pharmaceuticals, behavioral therapy, or surgical procedure), placebo, sham treatment, or no treatment.

Regarding approved treatments, as shown in 'Selection of subjects', there is no conventional therapy in Japan for patients eligible for this study. To select placebo or sham treatment as a control group is not acceptable for clinical and ethical reasons given the invasive nature of the periurethral injection and liposuction. While a no-treatment group may be effective as a potential comparator, such a comparison is not always necessary because patients with post-prostatectomy incontinence persisting for 1 year are unlikely to improve from 1 year onward [1–5]. Therefore, we decided to implement a confirmatory single-arm study.

Registration and informed consent

Patients are registered temporarily as candidates for this study after providing written informed consent and the investigators have confirmed that they meet most of the eligibility criteria. Thereafter, an investigator reviews the patient's urination diary, the method of data collection, that is that the patient measures the weight of the urination pad, the number of incontinence episodes, and the number of pads used, and then records it at home for 7

Table 1 Reduction rate of urine leakage volume from baseline by 24-h pad test in exploratory study

	Daily urine leakage volume at baseline	Reduction rate of daily urine leakage volume			
		1 month	3 months	6 months	12 months
Severe SUI ($n = 5$)	531.1 ± 229.2 g	−40.0 ± 62.6%	−6.2 ± 56.2%	2.9 ± 58.3%	18.0 ± 46.9%
Mild-to-moderate SUI ($n = 9$)	85.2 ± 55.0 g	17.0 ± 66.1%	32.2 ± 54.7%	27.6 ± 50.5%	62.6 ± 19.0%

Each data point represents the mean ± SD

consecutive days. Then, these data are assessed to determine eligibility by the inclusion criteria no. 3. After all eligibility criteria are confirmed, the patients are enrolled via electronic data capture system (Viedoc™, PCG Solutions Ab. Uppsala, Sweden), with the subsequent initialization of the treatment process.

Preparation and injection of ADRCs

About 250 to 300 mL and an additional 20 to 30 mL of adipose tissue are manually suctioned from subcutaneous layer in abdominal wall or hip under general or spinal anesthesia. About 250 to 300 mL of extracted adipose tissue are applied into the Celution® system. This system is an apparatus designed to isolate ADRCs from human suctioned fat semi-automatically in 1 to 2 h. Collected ADRCs by the Celution® system are composed of a heterogeneous cell population, including adipose-derived stem cells, endothelial (progenitor) cells and vascular smooth muscle cells [23]. Finally, we will obtain a 5-mL ADRCs solution including about 1×10^7 nucleated cells.

For periurethral injection, we will prepare two materials: one consists of 1 mL of ADRCs solution for direct injection into the sphincter, and the other is a 20 mL mixture comprising 4 mL of ADRCs solution with 16 mL of fat for injection into the submucosal spaces. A 'NUU Device'™ (Hakko Co. Ltd. Bunkyo-ku, Tokyo, Japan), which is a puncture needle of 38 cm in length, is inserted through the endoscope into the urethra under direct endoscopic vision. Initially, 1 mL of ADRC solution are injected using the 22 G puncture needle to a 5- to 10-mm depth into the rhabdosphincter at 5 and 7 o'clock positions. Subsequently, a 20-mL mixture of ADRCs and fat is administered with an 18 G puncture needle to about a 10-mm depth into the submucosal spaces at the 4 and 8 o'clock positions (if needed 6 o'clock position) at the external urethral sphincter area. Detailed procedures for the preparation and injection of ADRC solutions are provided in previous reports [19, 20].

Response variables (outcomes)

Patients will be followed-up for 52 weeks after injection of ADRCs. The ADRESU study schedule is shown in Table 2.

As a general rule, the primary endpoint should reflect clinically relevant and meaningful effects [24]. The USA Food and Drug Administration (FDA), which is the regulatory authority of the USA, recommends commonly used effectiveness endpoints for SUI listed as follows: amount of urine leakage (1-h pad weight test, 24-h pad test), number of incontinence episodes, number of pads used, QOL, and urodynamic measurements [25]. However, the FDA insists that dryness is the ultimate goal of treatment for SUI. The FDA also recognizes that

many patients are satisfied even if they only experience a reduction in urine leakage. Accordingly, the FDA recommends defining the clinically meaningful level as improvement in pad weight or improvement in the number of incontinence episodes defined as a reduction from baseline greater than 50%. Based on interim data of improvement in pad weight in the exploratory study, we selected the rate of patients with improvement in urine leakage volume (defined as reduction from baseline greater than 50% by 24-h pad test) at 52 weeks (last observation carried forward) as the primary endpoint of the ADRESU study.

The secondary endpoints are as follows:

1) Rate of patients at each evaluation time point with reduction in urine leakage volume greater than 50% from baseline by 24-h pad test
2) Urine leakage volume at each evaluation time point by 24-h pad test
3) Rate of patients at each evaluation time point with a reduction greater than 50% from baseline in the number of incontinence episodes per day
4) Number of incontinence episodes per day at each evaluation time point
5) Number of pads used per day at each evaluation time point
6) QOL score (International Consultation on Incontinence Questionnaire-Short Form [ICIQ-SF] and King's Health Questionnaire [KHQ]) at each evaluation time point
7) Overall patient satisfaction at each evaluation time point
8) Urodynamic parameters (maximum urethral closing pressure, functional profile length, and abdominal leak point pressure) at each evaluation time point
9) Blood flow at the injection site measured by transrectal enhanced ultrasonography at each evaluation time point
10) Injection site evaluated by pelvic magnetic resonance imaging (MRI) scan at each evaluation time point

We also plan confirm the improvement tendency on QOL scores in SUI patients who satisfy the primary endpoint (defined as 'Responders'), that is, that a point estimation of reduction rate on ICIQ-SF score is greater than 0%.

Number of subjects

Our specific hypothesis is that the rate of 'Responders' as a primary endpoint, is higher than a pre-specified threshold of 10% given the poor likelihood of natural recovery of incontinence in these subjects [1–5].

Table 2 The ADRESU study data collection schedule

	Screening period		Operation	Observation period							
	Provisional registration	Registration	Day 0	Day 1	At end of hospitalization	Week 2	Week 4	Week 12	Week 26	Week 38	Week 52
Eligibility criteria	X	X									
Vital signs[a]			X	X	X	X					
Oxygen saturation			X	X	X	X					
Laboratory tests											
Infections[b]		X									
Hematology[c], Biochemistry[d], CRP, Coagulation[e], Urinalysis[f]		X		X	X	X	X	X	X		X
PSA		X						X	X		X
12 Lead electrocardiography		X		X	X	X					
Chest X-rays		X									
Urination diary[g]		X				X	X	X	X	X	X
QOL scores[h]		X							X		X
Patient overall satisfaction		X							X		X
Urodynamic parameters[i]		X				X	X	X	X		X
Transrectal ultrasonography		X						X	X		X
MRI		X				X			X		X
Liposuction			X								
Periurethral injection of ADRCs, and mixture of ADRCs and fat			X								
Concomitant therapies	X	X	X	X	X	X	X	X	X	X	X
Adverse events	X	X	X	X	X	X	X	X	X	X	X

[a] Blood pressure, pulse rate, body temperature
[b] HBs antigen, HCV antibody, HIV antibody, serologic test of syphilis
[c] Red blood, hemoglobin, hematocrit, white blood cell count, fraction of leucocytes (basophil, eosinophil, neutrophil, lymphocyte, monocyte), platelet count
[d] Total protein, albumin, total cholesterol, blood urea nitrogen, creatinine, uric acid, sodium, chloride, potassium, calcium, phosphate, lactate dehydrogenase, aspartate aminotransferase, alanine aminotransferase, alkaline phosphatase, gamma-glutamyl transferase, total bilirubin, creatinine kinase
[e] Prothrombin time, activated partial thromboplastin time, fibrinogen
[f] pH, protein, glucose, urobilinogen, occult blood
[g] Urine leakage volume, number of incontinence episodes, number of pads used
[h] International Consultation on Incontinence Questionnaire-Short Form, King's Health Questionnaire
[i] Maximum urethral closing pressure, functional profile length, abdominal leak point pressure
Abbreviations: CRP C-reactive protein, *PSA* Prostate-Specific Antigen, *QOL* quality of life, *MRI* magnetic resonance imaging, *ADRCs* adipose-derived regenerative cells

Conservatively, the expected effectiveness rate is 30% because the rate of 'Responders' on interim analysis is 33.3% at 6 months and 66.7% at 12 months. Using two-side testing at a 5% significant level, we estimated that a sample of 41 patients was needed to achieve a 90% power of detection based on statistical calculations. Accordingly, a sample size of 45 patients was set in the ADRESU study anticipating a 10% loss to follow-up.

Statistical analysis

Analysis of this trial is based on an intention to treat principle. The primary analysis is performed in the Full Analysis Set that consists of all the enrolled subjects who injected ADRCs. The rate of 'Responders' for the primary endpoint and the secondary endpoints of 1) and

3) were estimated and their 95% confidence intervals are calculated using the Clopper-Pearson method. The descriptive statistics (e.g., mean, standard deviation, minimum, median, and maximum) of the secondary endpoints of 2) and 4)-10) are provided at each evaluation time point.

Discussion

Radical prostatectomy for male prostate cancer or prostatic hyperplasia causes a urethral sphincter dysfunction that can lead to persistent urinary incontinence. The underlying causes are thought to be the reduction of skeletal and smooth muscle, decreased blood flow, and denervation at the sphincter. We focused on adipose-derived stem cells for the functional recovery of the urethral sphincter because adipose tissue has more abundant multipotent stem cells than the bone marrow. Our basic research revealed that cultured adipose-derived stem cells improved leak point pressure and the amount of smooth muscle cells in an SUI rat model [17]. These promising basic research results drove us to implement a clinical exploratory study. However, when using cultured adipose stem cells, quality management of cell products is the hurdle in cell therapy for clinicians. The Celution System has a CE Mark approval in Europe, and it is a useful research tool for physicians. The Celution system is of particular interest to us for the application of this regenerative therapy. To the best of our knowledge, no previous studies have focused on the treatment of SUI with selected ADRCs prepared using the Celution systems. The interim result of this proof of concept clinical study for SUI patients showed the potential efficacy of ADRCs isolated by the Celution® system. As a new therapy for male SUI has not been developed in Japan as far as 2015, we aim to make our novel therapy widely available in Japan. As the following step, we discussed a development strategy of this novel therapy and the key design of the next pivotal study with the MHLW and PMDA. The MHLW suggested that we implement a clinical trial of the injection of ADRCs separated by the Celution® system as a new medical device based on the Pharmaceutical Affaires Act in Japan. Thus, we discussed the design of the investigator-initiated clinical trial (the ADRESU study) in a consultation meeting with PMDA. We constructed the rationale of the main design as a single-arm clinical trial for SUI in men based on several guidelines and previous research. As a result of a series of discussions in the consultation meeting, PMDA accepted our proposal.

Ethics approval and current status on this trial

This study protocol is in accordance with the Declaration of Helsinki [26] and the Pharmaceutical Affaires Act in Japan. The protocol of this trial was approved by the following Institutional Review Boards: Nagoya University Hospital (No. 272001), Kanazawa University Hospital (No. 9009), Shinshu University Hospital (No. 1483), and Dokkyo Medical University Hospital (No. S-288). In June 2015, a clinical trial notification as a new medical device, much like a U.S. Investigational Device Exemption application, was accepted by the MHLW. The first patient completed the provisional registration in August 20, 2015 and received transplantation of ADRCs in September 1, 2015. The ADRESU study has currently enrolled 33 patients and is still recruiting patients from the four institutes (Nagoya University Hospital, Kanazawa University Hospital, Dokkyo Medical University Hospital, and Shinshu University Hospital). We are planning to enroll 45 patients as the full analysis set. The limit of enrollment will be December 2017, and the planned study end is March 2019.

Conclusion

Herein, we present the overall design of this open-label, multi-center, single-arm study to evaluate the efficacy and safety of the periurethral injection of autologous ADRCs separated by the Celution® system in male SUI patients. In this article, we provide the key considerations regarding the overall study design, selection of subjects, selection of a control group, registration, response variables (endpoints), number of subjects and statistical analysis.

The ADRESU study is the first investigator-initiated clinical trial of a regenerative treatment for SUI patients using ADRCs separated by the Celution® system based on the Japanese Pharmaceutical Affaires Act. We will evaluate efficacy and safety in this trial to provide an adequate basis for marketing approval with the objective of disseminating this novel therapy to Japanese SUI patients. We believe that this translational medicine approach, often referred to as 'from benchside to bedside to community', has given rise to a novel treatment alternative for SUI in Japan.

Abbreviations

ADRCs: Adipose-derived regenerative cells; FDA: Food and Drug Administration; ICIQ-SF: International Consultation on Incontinence Questionnaire-Short Form; KHQ: King's Health Questionnaire; MHLW: Ministry of Health, Labour and Welfare; MRI: Magnetic resonance imaging; PMDA: Pharmaceuticals and Medical Devices Agency; PSA: Prostate specific antigen; QOL: Quality of life; SUI: Stress urinary incontinence

Acknowledgments

We would like to acknowledge the support of the staff in the participating institutes (Nagoya University Hospital, Nagoya, Aichi, Japan; Kanazawa University Hospital, Kanazawa, Ishikawa, Japan; Shinshu University Hospital, Matsumoto, Nagano, Japan; Dokkyo Medical University, Mibu, Tochigi, Japan) particularly for their assistance in this study. We would also like to thank the Cytori Therapeutics, Inc. for provide the Celution® system plus all required accessories free of charge, as well as the safety information of previous studies using the Celution® system for the execution of the ongoing ADRESU trial.

Funding

This research is supported and funded by the Project for Early-phase/ Exploratory or International-standard Clinical Research, and the Research Project for Practical Applications of Regenerative Medicine from the Japan Agency for Medical Research and Development (AMED).

Authors' contributions

MG is the principle investigator of this trial and performed the submission to the regulatory authorities. SS, SN, AH, TY, and MG designed the trial. YK is responsible for the data management, and AH supervised the statistical analysis. SS, SN, and MM supported preparation and management of this trial. KN, TY, OI, and MG are investigators in each institutions, and they participated in the submissions to the Institutional Review Board. YF YM TY, KN, TY, OI, and MG contribute to recruitment of patients and evaluation. KT, KT, and YK advise regarding the manipulation of liposuction at all institutes. SS wrote the final manuscript. All authors have read and approved the final manuscript.

Competing interests

The authors declare no conflicts of interest regarding this manuscript or the work described herein.

Author details

[1]Center for Advanced Medicine and Clinical Research, Nagoya University Hospital, 65 Tsurumai-cho, Showa-ku, Nagoya, Aichi 466-8560, Japan. [2]Department of Urology, Nagoya University Graduate School of Medicine, 65 Tsurumai-cho, Showa-ku, Nagoya, Aichi 466-8550, Japan. [3]Department of Plastic and Reconstructive Surgery, Nagoya University Graduate School of Medicine, 65 Tsurumai-cho, Showa-ku, Nagoya, Aichi 466-8550, Japan. [4]Department of Plastic and Reconstructive Surgery, Nagoya City University Hospital, 1-Kawasumi, Mizuho-cho, Mizuho-ku, Nagoya, Aichi 467-8602, Japan. [5]Department of Integrative Cancer Therapy and Urology, Kanazawa University Graduate School of Medical Sciences, 13-1 Takara-machi, Kanazawa, Ishikawa 920-8640, Japan. [6]Department of Urology, Continence Center, Dokkyo Medical University, 880 Kita-Kobayashi, Mibu-machi, Shimotsuga-gun, Tochigi 321-0293, Japan. [7]Department of Urology, Shinshu University School of Medicine, 3-1-1 Asahi, Matsumoto 390-8621, Japan. [8]Department of Clinical Research Management, Clinical Research Center, National Hospital Organization Nagoya Medical Center, 4-1-1, Sannomaru, Naka-ku, Nagoya Aichi 460-0001, Japan. [9]Department of Biostatistics and Bioinformatics, Graduate School of Medicine, The University of Tokyo, 7-3-1 Hongo, Bunkyo-ku, Tokyo 113-0033, Japan.

References

1. Prabhu V, Sivarajan G, Taksler GB, Laze J, Lepor H. Long-term continence outcomes in men undergoing radical prostatectomy for clinically localized prostate cancer. Eur Urol. 2014;65:52–7.
2. Namiki S, Kaiho Y, Mitsuzuka K, Saito H, Yamada S, Nakagawa H, Ito A, Arai Y. Long-term quality of life after radical prostatectomy: 8-year longitudinal study in Japan. Int J Urol. 2014;21:1220–6.
3. Parker WR, Wang R, He C, Wood DP Jr. Five year expanded prostate cancer index composite-based quality of life outcomes after prostatectomy for localized prostate cancer. BJU Int. 2011;107:585–90.
4. Namiki S, Kwan L, Kagawa-Singer M, Terai A, Arai Y, Litwin MS. Urinary quality of life after prostatectomy or radiation for localized prostate cancer: a prospective longitudinal cross-cultural study between Japanese and U.S. men. Urology 2008;71:1103–1108.
5. Saranchuk JW, Kattan MW, Elkin E, Touijer AK, Scardino PT, Eastham JA. Achieving optimal outcomes after radical prostatectomy. J Clin Oncol. 2005;23:4146–51.
6. Reek C, Noldus J, Huland H. Experiences with local collagen injection in male stress incontinence. Urologe A. 1997;36:40–3.
7. Faerber GJ, Richardson TD. Long-term results of transurethral collagen injection in men with intrinsic sphincter deficiency. J Endourol. 1997;11:273–7.
8. Lucas MG, Bedretdinova D, Berghmans LC, Bosch JLHR, Burkhard FC, Druz F, Nambiar AK, Nilsson CG, Tubaro A, Pickard RS. Guidelines on Urinary Incontinence; European Association of Urology 2015. http://uroweb.org/wp-content/uploads/20-Urinary-Incontinence_LR1.pdf. Accessed 22 Sept 2017.
9. Bettez M, Tu le M, Carlson K, Corcos J, Gajewski J, Jolivet M, Bailly G. 2012 update: guidelines for adult urinary incontinence collaborative consensus document for the canadian urological association. Can Urol Assoc J. 2012;6:354–63.
10. Bauer RM, Bastian PJ, Gozzi C, Stief CG. Postprostatectomy incontinence: all about diagnosis and management. Eur Urol. 2009;55:322–33.
11. Wu G, Song Y, Zheng X, Jiang Z. Adipose-derived stromal cell transplantation for treatment of stress urinary incontinence. Tissue Cell. 2011;43:246–53.
12. Kim SO, Na HS, Kwon D, Joo SY, Kim HS, Ahn Y. Bone-marrow-derived mesenchymal stem cell transplantation enhances closing pressure and leak point pressure in a female urinary incontinence rat model. Urol Int. 2011;86:110–6.
13. Roche R, Festy F, Fritel X. Stem cells for stress urinary incontinence: the adipose promise. J Cell Mol Med. 2010;14:135–42.
14. Smaldone MC, Chancellor MB. Muscle derived stem cell therapy for stress urinary incontinence. World J Urol. 2008;26:327–32.
15. Praud C, Sebe P, Biérinx AS, Sebille A. Improvement of urethral sphincter deficiency in female rats following autologous skeletal muscle myoblasts grafting. Cell Transplant. 2007;16:741–9.
16. Kwon D, Kim Y, Pruchnic R, Jankowski R, Usiene I, de Miguel F, Huard J, Chancellor MB. Periurethral cellular injection: comparison of muscle-derived progenitor cells and fibroblasts with regard to efficacy and tissue contractility in an animal model of stress urinary incontinence. Urology. 2006;68:449–54.
17. Watanabe T, Maruyama S, Yamamoto T, Kamo I, Yasuda K, Saka Y, Ozaki T, Yuzawa Y, Matsuo S, Gotoh M. Increased urethral resistance by periurethral injection of low serum cultured adipose-derived mesenchymal stromal cells in rats. Int J Urol. 2011;18:659–66.
18. Ministry of Health, Labour and Welfare. Guidelines on Clinical Research using Human Stem Cells. July 3, 2016. http://www.mhlw.go.jp/english/policy/health-medical/medical-care/dl/guidelines.pdf. Accessed 22 Sept 2017.
19. Gotoh M, Yamamoto T, Kato M, Majima T, Toriyama K, Kamei Y, Matsukawa Y, Hirakawa A, Funahashi Y. Regenerative treatment of male stress urinary incontinence by periurethral injection of autologous adipose-derived regenerative cells: 1-year outcomes in 11 patients. Int J Urol. 2014;21:294–300.
20. Yamamoto T, Gotoh M, Kato M, Majima T, Toriyama K, Kamei Y, Iwaguro H, Matsukawa Y, Funahashi Y. Periurethral injection of autologous adipose-derived regenerative cells for the treatment of male stress urinary incontinence: Report of three initial cases. Int J Urol. 2012;19:652–9.
21. International Conference on Harmonisation. Statistical Principles for Clinical Trials E9. http://www.ich.org/fileadmin/Public_Web_Site/ICH_Products/Guidelines/Efficacy/E9/Step4/E9_Guideline.pdf. Accessed 22 Sept 2017.
22. International Conference on Harmonisation. Choice of Control Group and Related Issues in Clinical Trials E10. http://www.ich.org/fileadmin/Public_Web_Site/ICH_Products/Guidelines/Efficacy/E10/Step4/E10_Guideline.pdf. Accessed 22 Sept 2017.
23. Lin K, Matsubara Y, Masuda Y, Togashi K, Ohno T, Tamura T, Toyoshima Y, Sugimachi K, Toyoda M, Marc H, Douglas A. Characterization of adipose tissue-derived cells isolated with the Celution system. Cytotherapy. 2008;10:417–26.
24. International Conference on Harmonisation. General Considerations for Clinical Trials E8. http://www.ich.org/fileadmin/Public_Web_Site/ICH_Products/Guidelines/Efficacy/E8/Step4/E8_Guideline.pdf. Accessed 22 Sept 2017.
25. U.S. Department of Health and Human Services Food and Drug Administration Center for Devices and Radiological Health. Guidance for Industry and Food and Drug Administration Staff. Clinical Investigation of Devices Indicated for the Treatment of Urinary Incontinence. March 8, 2011. http://www.fda.gov/downloads/MedicalDevices/DeviceRegulationandGuidance/GuidanceDocuments/ucm070854.pdf. Accessed 22 Sept 2017.
26. World Medical Association. Declaration of Helsinki Ethical Principles for Medical Research Involving Human Subjects. October 2013. http://dl.med.or.jp/dl-med/wma/helsinki2013e.pdf. Accessed 22 Sept 2017.

Protocol for a prospective, randomized study on neurophysiological assessment of lower urinary tract function in a healthy cohort

Stéphanie van der Lely[1], Martina Stefanovic[1], Melanie R. Schmidhalter[1], Marta Pittavino[2], Reinhard Furrer[2], Martina D. Liechti[1], Martin Schubert[3], Thomas M. Kessler[1] and Ulrich Mehnert[1*]

Abstract

Background: Lower urinary tract symptoms are highly prevalent and a large proportion of these symptoms are known to be associated with a dysfunction of the afferent pathways. Diagnostic tools for an objective and reproducible assessment of afferent nerve function of the lower urinary tract are missing. Previous studies showed first feasibility results of sensory evoked potential recordings following electrical stimulation of the lower urinary tract in healthy subjects and patients. Nevertheless, a refinement of the methodology is necessary.

Methods: This study is a prospective, randomized trial conducted at Balgrist University Hospital, Zürich, Switzerland. Ninety healthy subjects (forty females and fifty males) without lower urinary tract symptoms are planned to be included in the study. All subjects will undergo a screening visit (including standardized questionnaires, 3-day bladder diary, urinalysis, medical history taking, vital signs, physical examination, neuro-urological examination) followed by two measurement visits separated by an interval of 3 to 4 weeks. Electrical stimulations (0.5Hz-5Hz, bipolar, square wave, pulse width 1 ms) will be applied using a custom-made transurethral catheter at different locations of the lower urinary tract including bladder dome, trigone, proximal urethra, membranous urethra and distal urethra. Every subject will be randomly stimulated at one specific site of the lower urinary tract. Sensory evoked potentials (SEP) will be recorded using a 64-channel EEG cap. For an SEP segmental work-up we will place additional electrodes on the scalp (Cpz) and above the spine (C2 and L1). Visit two and three will be conducted identically for reliability assessment.

Discussion: The measurement of lower urinary tract SEPs elicited by electrical stimulation at different locations of the lower urinary tract has the potential to serve as a neurophysiological biomarker for lower urinary tract afferent nerve function in patients with lower urinary tract symptoms or disorders. For implementation of such a diagnostic tool into clinical practice, an optimized setup with efficient and reliable measurements and data acquisition is crucial. In addition, normative data from a larger cohort of healthy subjects would provide information on variability, potential confounding factors and cut-off values for investigations in patients with lower urinary tract dysfunction/symptoms.

Keywords: Sensory evoked potential, Electroencephalography, Lower urinary tract, Urinary bladder, Urethra, Randomized, Lower urinary tract dysfunction, Current perception threshold, A-delta afferent fibers, Electrical stimulation

* Correspondence: ulrich.mehnert@balgrist.ch
[1]Neuro-Urology, Spinal Cord Injury Center & Research, University of Zürich, Balgrist University Hospital, Forchstrasse 340, 8008 Zürich, Switzerland
Full list of author information is available at the end of the article

Background

Lower urinary tract symptoms (LUTS) such as urinary urgency, frequency and incontinence, imply a massive impairment of quality of life [1, 2].

LUTS are highly prevalent and a large proportion of LUTS are found to be associated with afferent nerve dysfunction [1, 3–5]. Assessment of afferent pathways in patients with LUTS is however a challenge. Specific diagnostic tools for an objective and reproducible measurement of bladder and urethral afferent nerve function are missing. Yet, filling cystometry (FC) is the standard method used in clinical practice for the assessment of bladder sensations [6–10]. Nevertheless, FC largely depends on the subjective perceptions and collaboration of the patient and is hence not an objective measurement of bladder sensations. In addition, the reliability of the FC is questionable and its variability and outcome resolution is too large to detect differences smaller than 100 mL [11, 12]. Moreover, FC only covers sensory information from the bladder but not from the urethra.

Current perception threshold (CPT) testing is another method of assessing sensations from the lower urinary tract (LUT). CPT testing is performed by asking the subject to indicate the onset of sensation when an increasing electrical stimulus is applied [13]. It was shown that this method is safe and well tolerated by healthy subjects and patients, but still, it provides only semi-quantitative information on sensations of the LUT [14–16]. In addition, local factors such as distance of electrodes to the mucosa and the mucosal condition itself can significantly affect CPTs [14, 17, 18].

A more objective and qualitative assessment of afferent nerve function are sensory evoked potentials (SEP) that are routinely used in neurophysiology to detect afferent nerve conduction qualities and integrity from different parts of the human body. By analysing the latencies and amplitudes of the SEPs (Fig. 1), information on nerve fiber integrity, conduction velocity and fiber type can be obtained [19, 20]. SEPs from the LUT would be useful not only for an assessment of LUT sensory function, to amend findings from previous investigations (i.e. history, neurologic examination, urodynamic examination), but also as a surrogate marker and outcome measure for treatments targeting afferent LUT pathways [21]. However, SEP measurements stimulating the LUT are more challenging than SEP measurements for cutaneous sites due to less direct control of electrode placement and potential changes of bladder volume with time, which can influence the SEP measurement. Furthermore, bladder SEPs may be less synchronized as they are likely mediated by poorly or non-myelinated fibres leading to less distinct summation of sensory potentials. Nevertheless, previous studies reported first feasibility results of SEP recordings from the LUT following

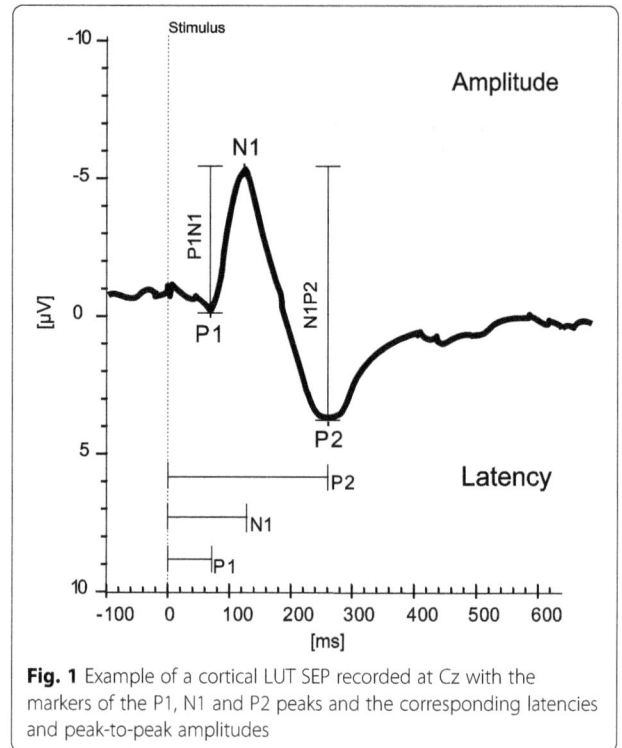

Fig. 1 Example of a cortical LUT SEP recorded at Cz with the markers of the P1, N1 and P2 peaks and the corresponding latencies and peak-to-peak amplitudes

electrical stimulation in healthy subjects [22–26] and patients [20, 27–29]. However, due to heterogeneous measurement settings and study populations, a clear conclusion cannot be drawn from these data. Currently, there is no standard for SEP measurements for the LUT. Hence, optimal stimulation and recording procedures as well as parameters still need to be determined.

In this study we would like to advance the evaluation of viscero-sensory afferent pathways of the LUT and to refine the methodology of LUT SEPs in healthy subjects. We aim to get more knowledge on the impact of different stimulation parameters (e.g. stimulation frequency) on the reliability, shape, latency, amplitude and topographical distribution of SEPs recorded during electrical stimulation of the LUT. In a first step it is our goal to find a frequency that allows a faster acquisition of reliable SEPs than the previously used 0.5 Hz [25, 26] and to obtain normative LUT SEP data for the different localizations in the LUT from different gender groups. In a second step we aim to implement the optimized methodology into clinical practice to use it as an objective marker of pathological LUT conditions and to show distinction of healthy LUT neurophysiology and function.

Methods and design
Study design

This study is a prospective, randomized trial conducted as a single center study at the Spinal Cord Injury Center & Research Lab, Balgrist University Hospital, University of Zürich, Zürich, Switzerland. The study comprises three visits of which the first will be a screening visit followed by two measurement visits separated by an interval of 3–4 weeks (Fig. 2). The site of stimulation will be indicated by random group assignment (in females and males: dome, trigone, proximal urethra, distal urethra; in males additionally: membranous urethra). Consequently, ten females and ten males will be allocated to one localization. In addition, the frequencies used for the stimulation of the LUT and thereafter the SSEP measurements will be randomly applied.

Study population and recruitment

The volunteers will be recruited via announcements at the University of Zürich, internet platforms (i.e. www.marktplatz.uzh.ch, www.tutti.ch, www.ronorp.net) and personal contacts. According to the inclusion- and exclusion criteria (Table 1), healthy female and male subjects without any LUTS will be included. Health is defined as the absence of any health troubles, as assessed by a complete medical history, standardized questionnaires, physical, neurological and neuro-urological examinations (Table 2). The absence of LUTS will be determined by uroflowmetry, a 3-day bladder diary and standardized urological questionnaires (FLUTS [30] /MLUTS [31]; Qualiveen [32]; IPSS [33]; Swiss German OAB [34]) (Table 2).

Investigations and procedures
Screening (visit one)
The content and purpose of the study will be explained in written and oral form to all recruited subjects. Those subjects providing written informed consent will be screened for in- and exclusion criteria by using the tests, questionnaires, and examinations listed in Table 2. Subjects who are eligible for study participation according to the in- and exclusion criteria (Table 1) will be invited for visit two and three (Fig. 2).

Measurement visits (visit two and three)
Prior to each measurement, the urine of the volunteers is analyzed to exclude signs suggestive for asymptomatic bacteriuria, microhaematuria, and (in women only) pregnancy. Both measurements consist of a resting electroencephalogram (EEG) measurement followed by recordings of SEPs elicited by transurethral electrical stimulation at a specific LUT site indicated by the group assignment. Each measurement includes recordings of the electrooculogram (left and right eye), electrocardiogram, and electroencephalogram using a 64 Ag/AgCl surface electrodes system comprising a cap-based extended international 10–20 montage (Easy cap, Easy cap GmbH, Herrsching, Germany). Electrode impedances are constantly kept below 20kΩ. Six additional electrodes are placed at Cpz (reference: Fz), C2 (reference: Fz) and L1 (reference: iliac crest), respectively, for segmental assessment. LUT electrical stimulation will be applied transurethrally with a custom-made 14 Ch catheter (Unisensor AG, Attikon, Switzerland), using frequencies between 0.5Hz and 5Hz (bipolar, square wave, pulse width 1 ms). Stimulation intensities are adapted to the 3 to 4× CPT, which is determined using the method of limits prior to each SEP measurement [13]. The catheter includes platinum electrodes and a radiopaque marker, which allows precise catheter positioning under fluoroscopic guidance. After each stimulation, the bladder will be emptied and filled with 60 mL of contrast medium (Ultravist® 150™, Bayer AG, Switzerland). Consequent to LUT SEPs, SEPs elicited by transcutaneous stimulation of the tibial and pudendal nerves will be recorded in random order. These standard neurophysiological measurements will serve as comparators to the

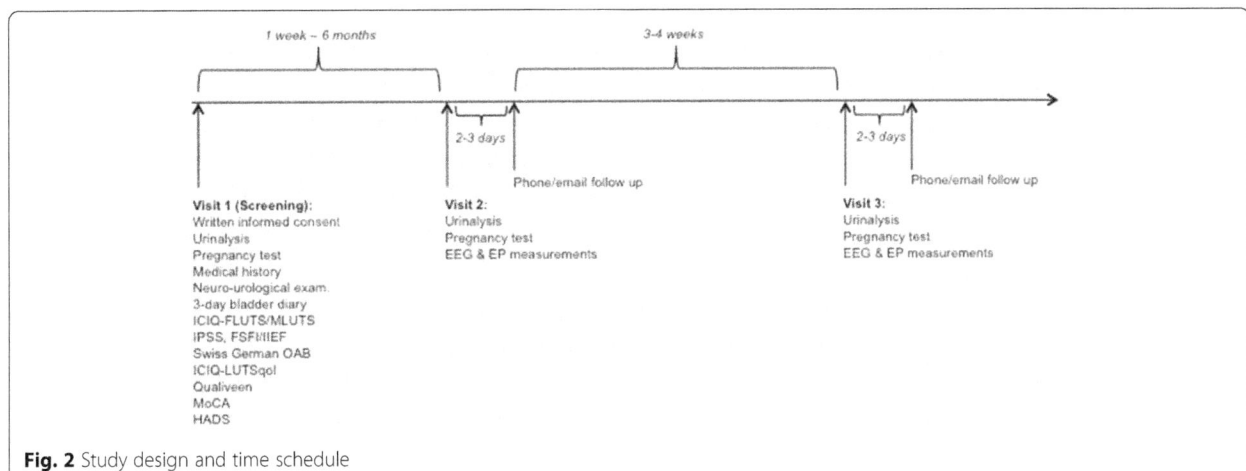

Fig. 2 Study design and time schedule

Table 1 Inclusion and exclusion criteria for healthy female and male volunteers

Inclusion criteria	Exclusion criteria
Written informed consent	Any lower urinary tract symptoms[d, f, c]
Good mental[a] and physical health[c]	Any neurological or urological pathology [e, f, c]
Age > 18 years[c]	Current pregnancy[bc], lactation[c]
No regular intake of medication[c]	UTI[b, c, f]
Bladder capacity <150 mL or SDV already at 60mL[d, e, g]	Hematuria[b]
Number of voids per day <8, number of voids per night <2[d, f, c]	Any anatomical anomaly/malignancy of the LUT or genitalia [e, c]
	Any previous pelvic, spine or craniocerebral surgery[c]

LUT lower urinary tract, *SDV* strong desire to void, *UTI* urinary tract infection
[a]assessed by MoCA and HADS; [b]excluded by urine dipstick test; [c]assessed by history taking; [d]assessed by 3-day bladder diary; [e]assessed by neuro-urological examination [f]assessed by standardized urological questionnaires (FLUTS, MLUTS, IPSS, Qualiveen, Swiss-German OAB questionnaire); [g]assessed by uroflowmetry

LUT SEPs. Visits two and three will be performed identically with an interval of 3 to 4 weeks (Fig. 3).

Follow-up

Two to three days after each measurement visit, a follow-up interview is performed to evaluate the general well-being of the volunteers. In case of any side effects, such as dysuria, the subjects are appointed to an extra medical visit for further evaluation, investigation and, if necessary, medical treatment.

Safety

During the first visit, all subjects are carefully screened to exclude subjects with neurological and/or urological pathology or any regular medication intake. At the beginning of every visit an urinalysis and pregnancy test (in females only) is performed to exclude signs suggestive for asymptomatic bacteriuria, microhaematuria and pregnancy, respectively. Pregnancy leads to study exclusion and referral to a gynecologist for further evaluation. In case of a positive urine

Table 2 Overview of the screening procedure

Tests	Questionnaires / Bladder diary
Urine dipstick	FLUTS [28] / MLUTS [29]
Pregnancy	Qualiveen [30]
	ICIQ-LUTSqol [35]
	IPSS [31] (only for males)
Examinations	Swiss German OAB questionnaire (short form) [32]
Bulbocavernosus reflex	FSFI [34] / IIEF [33]
Anal reflex	HADS [36]
Pin-prick of S2-S5 dermatomes	MoCA [37]
Uroflowmetry	3-day bladder diary
Assessment of medical history	
Physical examination	

dipstick test suspicious for asymptomatic bacteriuria or urinary tract infection (UTI), the measurement will be postponed until the dipstick test result becomes negative or UTI has been treated. In case of a dipstick test indicating microhaematuria, subjects can choose to repeat the test at a later time-point or to directly have the result verified by clean catheterization. If clean catheterization still indicates microhaematuria, subjects will be excluded from study participation and referred to their general practitioner or urologist for further evaluation.

Two or three days after the measurement visits, a follow-up interview will be conducted to assess general well-being and document possible adverse events or symptoms. In case of an adverse event, additional tests or medical interventions will be initiated as necessary and subjects might be referred to a general physician or medical specialist for further investigations and/or treatment. All responsible authorities will be informed about any adverse events (AE) or severe adverse events (SAE). These events will be observed and followed until complete cure. To decrease the radiation dose during visits two and three, we will not perform full radiographs but fluoroscopy with a reduced field of view focusing on the LUT only. For a protection of the male gonads, men will wear a gonad shielding.

Endpoints of the study

Primary endpoint: N1 responder rate / latency of N1 – as the most prominent peak of LUT SEPs.

Secondary endpoints: A) Latencies (P1, P2), amplitudes (P1, N1, P2, P1N1, N1P2), topographies and source localizations of LUT SEPs; B) CPTs; C) latencies, amplitudes, topographies and source localization of tibial, pudendal SSEPs; D) 3-day bladder diary, scores of questionnaires (i.e. ICIQ-FLUTS [30]/ICIQ-MLUTS [31], IPSS [33], IIEF [35] /FSFI [36], Swiss German OAB [34], ICIQ-LUTSqol [37], Qualiveen [32], HADS [38], MoCA [39]).

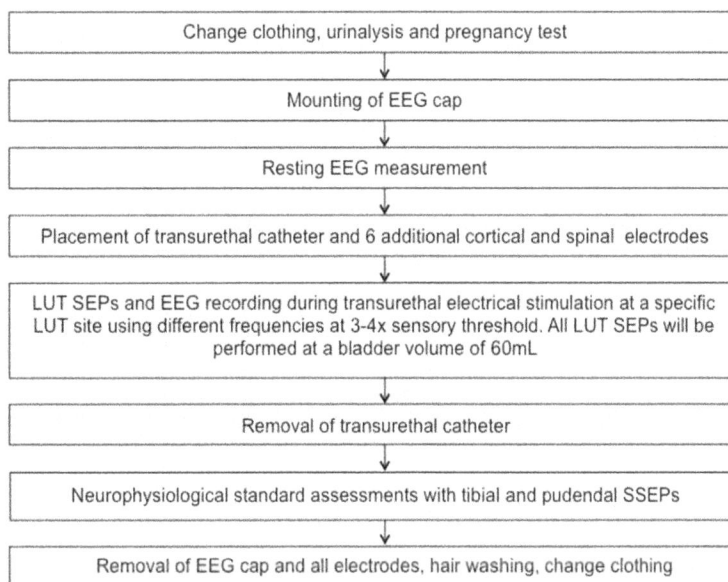

Fig. 3 Flowchart of the measurement visits (visits two and three)

Determination of sample size

Based on data from a previous study [25], the sample size was determined using a non-parametric approach [40]. Non-parametric smoothing estimates (kernel smooth) were iteratively compared for subsets of individuals in order to establish the smallest subset (sample size) in which a significant outcome was observed. Determined using cross-validation [41], the smoothing parameter was set to 20. From the smoothed curves, the empirical second derivatives (as an expression of the 'information', i.e. latency, amplitude and dispersion, contained therein) were used, the estimates of which were computed and standardized by the absolute value of their mean. The difference between the two frequencies (0.5Hz and 3Hz) was taken into account, to allow for a standardized vector summary of the curve. Normality was tested using the Kolmogorov-Smirnov method and no evidence against was revealed. A t-test based on this standardized vector was subsequently conducted. Power analysis was performed using a bootstrapping technique [42, 43]. For each different sample size combination, the difference between the two frequencies, contained in the standardized vector, was analyzed. The bootstrap simulations were executed at the individual level. All elements of the standardized vector summary were first subsampled before results were presented based on the mean p-values for all possible combinations. To ensure robustness of the results, four different criteria – standard deviation, variance, total variance (sum of the absolute values) and *wigglyness* (sum of the absolute values of the second derivatives) – were applied to the standardized vector. The aforementioned procedure was repeated for the different study visits and simulation sites. This resulted in a required sample size of 50 male and 40 female subjects, taking into account potential dropouts.

Data management and analysis

All EEG data will be filtered and segmented using Brain Vision Analyzer 2 (Version 2.1.0.327, Brain Products, Gilching, Germany). The segments will be averaged and the P1, N1, P2 latencies as well as the P1N1 and N1P2 amplitudes will be determined.

Study data will be collected and managed using the Research Electronic Data Capture Tool (REDCap, Version 6.12.1, Vanderbilt University) electronic data capture tools hosted at Balgrist University Hospital [44]. REDCap is a secure, web-based application designed to support data capture for research studies, providing 1) an intuitive interface for validated data entry; 2) audit trails for tracking data manipulation and export procedures; 3) automated export procedures for seamless data downloads to common statistical packages; and 4) procedures for importing data from external sources.

Primarily, all data will be examined using exploratory data analysis (EDA) methods and described providing mean and standard deviation (or median and range where appropriate). ANOVAs or independent sample t-tests (or Kruskal-Wallis test or Mann-Whitney tests where appropriate) will be performed to compare participant characteristics between groups or to detect gender differences. Linear mixed effects models will be used to compare the two measurement visits. The level of significance will be 5% (alpha = 0.05). Regression techniques will be taken into account, if needed. All the statistical analyses will be performed with the software RStudio (Version 0.98.1083) [45].

Discussion

This clinical trial will investigate the effect of several stimulation frequencies at different locations of the LUT. Since it was already shown that SEPs could be reproducibly recorded from the LUT [25], we now aim to optimize the settings to achieve a faster acquisition of reliable SEPs, which is important for implementation into clinical diagnostics and to minimize measurement bias through changes that occur over time such as bladder volume.

The assessment of normative values of LUT SEPs in healthy male and female subjects will give us more knowledge on the variability of LUT SEPs, as well as potential factors that may influence the shape and the reliability of the SEPs. Cut-offs for amplitude and latency values can be defined for future investigations in patients with LUT dysfunction. The advancement of neurophysiological assessment methods for the LUT will significantly influence the evaluation of afferent nerve function in the LUT and has the potential to serve as a clinical diagnostic tool complementary to standard urodynamic investigations. After having refined our methodology, we would like to apply LUT SEPs with the optimized stimulation frequency in different patient groups suffering from LUTS, including patients with spinal cord injury and multiple sclerosis. Established cut-off amplitudes and latency values from this study should then be used to relate LUT symptoms and dysfunction in patients with LUT SEP data, thus amending FC findings with an objective evaluation of afferent LUT nerve function in these disorders.

Trial status

At the time of manuscript submission, first subjects have been recruited, included and investigated.

Abbreviations

AE: Adverse event; CPT: Current perception threshold; EDA: Exploratory data analysis; EEG: Electroencephalography / electroencephalogram; FC: Filling cystometry; GCP: Good clinical practice; LUTS: Lower urinary tract symptoms; OAB: Overactive bladder; SAE: Severe adverse event; SDV: Strong desire to void; SEP: Sensory evoked potential; UTI: Urinary tract infection

Funding

The study is made possible through funding from the Swiss National Science Foundation (grant number: 32003B_149628) and the Swiss Continence Foundation.

Authors' contributions

SvdL, UM participated in designing protocol of the study. SvdL, MRS, MP, UM drafted the manuscript. MSt, RF, MDL, MS, TMK critically revised the manuscript. MS, TMK, UM obtained the funding of this study. SvdL, MSt, MRS collect the data of the study. All the authors read and approved the final manuscript.

Competing interests

The authors declare that they have no competing interests.

Ethics approval and consent to participate

The study was approved by the local ethics committee (Kantonale Ethikkommission Zürich, KEK-ZH-Nr. 2013-0518) and is performed according to the (World Medical Association) Declaration of Helsinki [46], the guidelines for Good Clinical Practice (GCP) [47], and the guidelines of the Swiss Academy of Medical Sciences [48]. Written informed consent is required for study participation. All personal data are handled according to the federal law of data protection in Switzerland [49].

Author details

[1]Neuro-Urology, Spinal Cord Injury Center & Research, University of Zürich, Balgrist University Hospital, Forchstrasse 340, 8008 Zürich, Switzerland. [2]Institute of Mathematics, University of Zürich, Winterthurerstrasse 190, 8057 Zürich, Switzerland. [3]Neurophysiology, Spinal Cord Injury Center & Research, University of Zürich, Balgrist University Hospital, Forchstrasse 340, 8008 Zürich, Switzerland.

References

1. Coyne KS, Wein AJ, Tubaro A, Sexton CC, Thompson CL, Kopp ZS, Aiyer LP. The burden of lower urinary tract symptoms: evaluating the effect of LUTS on health-related quality of life, anxiety and depression: EpiLUTS. BJU Int. 2009;103 Suppl 3:4–11.
2. Irwin DE, Milsom I, Kopp Z, Abrams P, Cardozo L. Impact of overactive bladder symptoms on employment, social interactions and emotional well-being in six European countries. BJU Int. 2006;97(1):96–100.
3. Irwin DE, Kopp ZS, Agatep B, Milsom I, Abrams P. Worldwide prevalence estimates of lower urinary tract symptoms, overactive bladder, urinary incontinence and bladder outlet obstruction. BJU Int. 2011;108(7):1132–8.
4. Yoshimura N. Lower urinary tract symptoms (LUTS) and bladder afferent activity. Neurourol Urodyn. 2007;26(6 Suppl):908–13.
5. Fowler CJ. Bladder afferents and their role in the overactive bladder. Urology. 2002;59(5 Suppl 1):37–42.
6   Schafer W, Abrams P, Liao L, Mattiasson A, Pesce F, Spangberg A, Sterling AM, Zinner NR, van Kerrebroeck P, International Continence S. Good urodynamic practices: uroflowmetry, filling cystometry, and pressure-flow studies. Neurourol Urodyn. 2002;21(3):261–74.
7   Heeringa R, van Koeveringe GA, Winkens B, van Kerrebroeck PE, de Wachter SG. Degree of urge, perception of bladder fullness and bladder volume– how are they related? J Urol. 2011;186(4):1352–7.
8   Erdem E, Akbay E, Doruk E, Cayan S, Acar D, Ulusoy E. How reliable are bladder perceptions during cystometry? Neurourol Urodyn. 2004;23(4):306–9.
9   De Wachter S, Van Meel TD, Wnydaele JJ. Can a faked cystometry deceive patients in their perception of filling sensations? A study on the reliability of spontaneously reported cystometric filling sensations in patients with non-neurogenic lower urinary tract dysfunction. Neurourol Urodyn. 2008;27(5): 395–8.
10 Groen J, Pannek J, Castro Diaz D, Del Popolo G, Gross T, Hamid R, Karsenty G, Kessler TM, Schneider M, t Hoen L, et al. Summary of European Association of Urology (EAU) guidelines on Neuro-Urology. Eur Urol. 2016; 69(2):324–33.
11 Virseda M, Salinas J, Esteban M, Mendez S. Reliability of ambulatory urodynamics in patients with spinal cord injuries. Neurourol Urodyn. 2013;32(4):387–92.
12 Bellucci CH, Wollner J, Gregorini F, Birnbock D, Kozomara M, Mehnert U, Kessler TM. Neurogenic lower urinary tract dysfunction–do we need same session repeat urodynamic investigations? J Urol. 2012;187(4):1318–23.
13 Yarnitsky D. Quantitative sensory testing. Muscle Nerve. 1997;20(2):198–204.
14 De Wachter S, Wyndaele JJ. Quest for standardisation of electrical sensory testing in the lower urinary tract: the influence of technique related factors on bladder electrical thresholds. Neurourol Urodyn. 2003;22(2):118–22.
15 De Laet K, De Wachter S, Wyndaele JJ. Current perception thresholds in the lower urinary tract: Sine- and square-wave currents studied in young healthy volunteers. Neurourol Urodyn. 2005;24(3):261–6.
16 Ulrich Mehnert, André Reitz, Maya Ziegler, Peter A. Knapp, Brigitte Schurch. Does Tolterodine Extended Release Affect the Bladder Electrical Perception

Threshold? A Placebo Controlled, Double-Blind Study With 4 and 8 mg in Healthy Volunteers. The Journal of Urology. 2007;178(6):2495-2500.

17 Ukimura O, Ushijima S, Honjo H, Iwata T, Suzuki K, Hirahara N, Okihara K, Mizutani Y, Kawauchi A, Miki T. Neuroselective current perception threshold evaluation of bladder mucosal sensory function. Eur Urol. 2004;45(1):70–6.

18 Knupfer SC, Liechti MD, Gregorini F, De Wachter S, Kessler TM, Mehnert U. Sensory function assessment of the human male lower urinary tract using current perception thresholds. Neurourol Urodyn. 2016 [Epub ahead of print].

19 Cruccu G, Aminoff MJ, Curio G, Guerit JM, Kakigi R, Mauguiere F, Rossini PM, Treede RD, Garcia-Larrea L. Recommendations for the clinical use of somatosensory-evoked potentials. Clin Neurophysiol. 2008;119(8):1705–19.

20 Deltenre PF, Thiry AJ. Urinary bladder cortical evoked potentials in man: suitable stimulation techniques. Br J Urol. 1989;64(4):381–4.

21 Chiappa KH, Ropper AH. Evoked potentials in clinical medicine (first of two parts). N Engl J Med. 1982;306(19):1140–50.

22 Ganzer H, Madersbacher H, Rumpl E. Cortical evoked potentials by stimulation of the vesicourethral junction: clinical value and neurophysiological considerations. J Urol. 1991;146(1):118–23.

23 Hansen MV, Ertekin C, Larsson LE. Cerebral evoked potentials after stimulation of the posterior urethra in man. Electroencephalogr Clin Neurophysiol. 1990;77(1):52–8.

24 Sarica Y, Karacan I, Thornby JI, Hirshkowitz M. Cerebral responses evoked by stimulation of vesico-urethral junction in man: methodological evaluation of monopolar stimulation. Electroencephalogr Clin Neurophysiol. 1986;65(2):130–5.

25 Gregorini F, Wollner J, Schubert M, Curt A, Kessler TM, Mehnert U. Sensory evoked potentials of the human lower urinary tract. J Urol. 2013;189(6):2179–85.

26 Flavia Gregorini, Stephanie C. Knüpfer, Martina D. Liechti, Martin Schubert, Armin Curt, Thomas M. Kessler, Ulrich Mehnert. Sensory evoked potentials of the bladder and urethra in middle-aged women: the effect of age. BJU International. 2015;115:18-25.

27 Sarica Y, Karatas M, Bozdemir H, Karacan I. Cerebral responses elicited by stimulation of the vesico-urethral junction (VUJ) in diabetics. Electroencephalogr Clin Neurophysiol. 1996;100(1):55–61.

28 Badr G, Carlsson CA, Fall M, Friberg S, Lindstrom L, Ohlsson B. Cortical evoked potentials following stimulation of the urinary bladder in man. Electroencephalogr Clin Neurophysiol. 1982;54(5):494–8.

29 Hansen MV, Ertekin C, Larsson LE, Pedersen K. A neurophysiological study of patients undergoing radical prostatectomy. Scand J Urol Nephrol. 1989;23(4):267–73.

30 Brookes ST, Donovan JL, Wright M, Jackson S, Abrams P. A scored form of the Bristol female lower urinary tract symptoms questionnaire: data from a randomized controlled trial of surgery for women with stress incontinence. Am J Obstet Gynecol. 2004;191(1):73–82.

31 Donovan JL, Peters TJ, Abrams P, Brookes ST, de aa Rosette JJ, Schafer W. Scoring the short form ICSmaleSF questionnaire. International Continence Society. J Urol. 2000;164(6):1948–55.

32 Costa P, Perrouin-Verbe B, Colvez A, Didier J, Marquis P, Marrel A, Amarenco G, Espirac B, Leriche A. Quality of life in spinal cord injury patients with urinary difficulties. Development and validation of qualiveen. Eur Urol. 2001;39(1):107–13.

33 Barry MJ, Fowler Jr FJ, O'Leary MP, Bruskewitz RC, Holtgrewe HL, Mebust WK, Cockett AT. The American Urological Association symptom index for benign prostatic hyperplasia. The measurement committee of the American Urological Association. J Urol. 1992;148(5):1549–57. discussion 1564.

34 Coyne KS, Thompson CL, Lai JS, Sexton CC. An overactive bladder symptom and health-related quality of life short-form: validation of the OAB-q SF. Neurourol Urodyn. 2015;34(3):255–63.

35 Rosen RC, Riley A, Wagner G, Osterloh IH, Kirkpatrick J, Mishra A. The international index of erectile function (IIEF): a multidimensional scale for assessment of erectile dysfunction. Urology. 1997;49(6):822–30.

36 Rosen R, Brown C, Heiman J, Leiblum S, Meston C, Shabsigh R, Ferguson D, D'Agostino Jr R. The Female Sexual Function Index (FSFI): a multidimensional self-report instrument for the assessment of female sexual function. J Sex Marital Ther. 2000;26(2):191–208.

37 Kelleher CJ, Cardozo LD, Khullar V, Salvatore S. A new questionnaire to assess the quality of life of urinary incontinent women. Br J Obstet Gynaecol. 1997;104(12):1374–9.

38 Zigmond AS, Snaith RP. The hospital anxiety and depression scale. Acta Psychiatr Scand. 1983;67(6):361–70.

39 Nasreddine ZS, Phillips N, Chertkow H. Normative data for the Montreal Cognitive Assessment (MoCA) in a population-based sample. Neurology. 2012;78(10):765–6. author reply 766.

40 Silverman BW. Some aspects of the spline smoothing approach to non-parametric regression curve fitting. J R Stat Soc B Methodol. 1985;47(1):1–52.

41 Abraham B, Ledolter J. Introduction To Regression Modeling. 2006.

42 Davidson AC, Hinkley DV. Bootstrap Methods and Their Application. Cambridge University Press. 1997;48.

43 Efron B. Bootstrap methods: another look at the jackknife. Annals of Statistics. 1979;7(1):1–26.

44 Harris PA, Taylor R, Thielke R, Payne J, Gonzalez N, Conde JG. Research electronic data capture (REDCap)–a metadata-driven methodology and workflow process for providing translational research informatics support. J Biomed Inform. 2009;42(2):377–81.

45 R Development Core Team. R. A Language and Environment for Statistical Computing. Vienna: R Foundation for Statistical Computing;2015.

46 World Medical Association. World Medical Association Declaration of Helsinki: ethical principles for medical research involving human subjects. JAMA. 2013;310(20):2191–4.

47 International conference on harmonisation. Good clinical practice guideline. http://www.ich.org/products/guidelines/efficacy/article/efficacy-guidelines.html.

48 Swiss Academy of Medical Sciences. Guideline-concerning scientific research involving human beings. 2009:http://www.samw.ch/de/ Publikationen/Leitfaden-fuer-die-Praxis.html. Accessed 22 Nov 2016.

49 The Federal Authorities of the Swiss Confederation. Bundesgesetz über den Datenschutz (DSG) vom 19. Juni 1992, Stand. 01.01.2014. 1992: https://www. admin.ch/opc/de/classified-compliation/19920153/index.html#app1. Accessed 22 Nov 2016.

25

Sociodemographic correlates of urine culture test utilization in Calgary, Alberta

Thomas P. Griener[1,3], Christopher Naugler[1,2], Wilson W. Chan[1,3] and Deirdre L. Church[1,3,4,5]*

Abstract

Background: Many clinical practice guidelines encourage diagnosis and empiric treatment of lower urinary tract infection without laboratory investigation; however, urine culture testing remains one of the largest volume tests in the clinical microbiology laboratory. In this study, we sought to determine if there were specific patient groups to which increased testing was directed. To do so, we combined laboratory data on testing rates with Census Canada sociodemographic data.

Methods: Urine culture testing data was obtained from the Calgary Laboratory Services information system for 2011. We examined all census dissemination areas within the city of Calgary and, for each area, testing rates were determined for age and gender cohorts. We then compared these testing rates to sociodemographic factors obtained from Census Canada and used Poisson regression and generalized estimating equations to test associations between testing rates and sociodemographic variables.

Results: Per capita urine culture testing is increasing in Calgary. For 2011, 100,901 individuals (9.2% of all people) received urine cultures and were included in this analysis. The majority of cultures were received from the community (67.9%). Substantial differences in rate of testing were observed across the city. Most notably, urine culture testing was drastically lower in areas of high ($\geq$ \$100000) household income (RR = 0.07, $p < 0.0001$) and higher employment rate (RR = 0.36, $p < 0.0001$). Aboriginal – First Nations status (RR = 0.29, $p = 0.0008$) and Chinese visible minority (RR = 0.67, $p = 0.0005$) were also associated with decreased testing. Recent immigration and visible minority status of South Asian, Filipino or Black were not significant predictors of urine culture testing. Females were more likely to be tested than males (RR = 2.58, $p < 0.0001$) and individuals aged 15–39 were the most likely to be tested (RR = 1.69, $p < 0.0001$).

Conclusions: Considerable differences exist in urine culture testing across Calgary and these are associated with a number of sociodemographic factors. In particular, areas of lower socioeconomic standing had significantly increased rates of testing. These observations highlight specific groups that should be targeted to improve healthcare delivery and, in turn, enhance laboratory utilization.

Background

Lower urinary tract infection (LUTI, cystitis) can be reliably diagnosed without laboratory investigation based on a focused history of urinary symptoms (frequency, urgency and dysuria) in the absence of urethral discharge or vaginal irritation. Adult women with symptomatic, uncomplicated LUTI should receive short-course empiric antibiotic therapy and do not require urinalysis or urine culture for diagnostic confirmation of bacteriuria or pyuria. Numerous clinical practice guidelines support this and encourage the use of urine culture testing in the adult population primarily for bacterial identification and antibiotic sensitivity testing in patients not responding to therapy or with recurrent disease [1–4]. However, urine culture testing is necessary in all cases of upper urinary tract infection (pyelonephritis) and screening cultures for asymptomatic bacteriuria is also indicated in pregnancy and for those undergoing urologic procedure where bleeding is anticipated [5].

These recommendations are largely based on the following important considerations. Bacteriuria is not itself a disease state and is typically not an indication for

---

* Correspondence: Deirdre.church@albertahealthservices.ca
[1]Department of Pathology and Laboratory Medicine, University of Calgary, Calgary, AB, Canada
[3]Division of Microbiology, Department of Pathology and Laboratory Medicine, University of Calgary, Calgary, AB, Canada
Full list of author information is available at the end of the article

antibiotic therapy [5]. Asymptomatic bacteriuria is particularly common in the elderly population, with prevalence estimates of 3.6–19% in those aged 70 or over and living in the community [5, 6]. In nursing home residents, prevalence is estimated at up to 50%. It is not associated with increased morbidity or mortality [7]. Guidelines from the Infectious Disease Society of America (IDSA) and Choosing Wisely initiatives emphasize that even in the presence of pyuria, asymptomatic bacteriuria does not normally require treatment [5, 8]. The clinical significance of bacteriuria is therefore defined by patient signs and symptoms. Furthermore, the majority of urine specimens submitted for culture are the midstream portion of voided urine and culture results from these minimally-invasive collections have poor specificity, with a false positive rate of over 40% when compared to suprapubic needle aspiration or catheterization as gold standard [3, 9]. A positive urine culture therefore does not prove true bacteriuria, and certainly does not prove the presence of a urinary tract infection. Several strategies have been adopted by clinical microbiology laboratories to minimize reporting of contaminated specimens. The most common method is reporting of quantitative culture, for which there are established thresholds of bacterial quantity which define clinical significance [3, 5, 10]. However, in symptomatic patients, colony count thresholds likely underestimate the clinical significance of certain potential urinary pathogens while overestimating others [11]. For example, *Escherichia coli* can be associated with symptomatic disease even when isolated at quantities that are orders of magnitude below these thresholds. These combined factors minimize the value of urine culture results in both asymptomatic and symptomatic individuals.

Despite these problems, urine culture remains an important test that directs antibiotic therapy and further investigations in certain clinical settings. However, there is substantial practice variation in the use of diagnostic tests in LUTI and urine culture remains one of the highest volume tests in clinical microbiology laboratories [12]. Inappropriate testing is not without consequence as positive urine culture results likely drive unnecessary antibiotic treatment and contribute to rising rates of antibiotic resistance and other adverse events associated with antibiotic usage including *Clostridium difficile* infection [13–18]. We undertook the current ecological study to determine what variation in urine cultures testing existed across Calgary, Alberta and to determine what sociodemographic factors were associated with increased urine culture testing. Such information will allow targeted investigation into causes of potential over-utilization and more focused intervention strategies.

Methods

The study protocol was approved by the University of Calgary Conjoint Health Review Ethics Board and a waiver of consent was granted (ID#REB15–0629).

This observational study combined laboratory data with variables obtained from the 2011 Census Canada Canadian Household Survey, the most recent such survey at the time this study was completed. The study population consisted of all individuals within Calgary, Alberta who underwent urine culture testing between January 1, 2011 and December 31, 2011. All urine culture testing at Calgary Laboratory Services (CLS) is performed as part of routine patient care and samples are analyzed in a single laboratory. CLS is the only testing laboratory in Calgary, Alberta and data from the CLS laboratory information system (LIS) therefore represents a comprehensive view of urine culture testing in the entire city (2011 population 1.1 million). In addition to data for the 2011 year, the number of monthly urine cultures collected from the LIS for each month from January 2010 to December 2013 in order to measure trends in urine culture ordering.

Each patient was included only once in the analysis to avoid pseudo-replication. For each test record, the following information was extracted from the laboratory information system: urine culture result, age, sex and health care number. Health care number was used as a linking variable to determine subject postal codes from an Alberta Health database, which were then converted to their corresponding geographic coordinates and census dissemination areas (CDA). CDAs are the smallest geographic groupings used for Canadian census data and contain 300–700 individuals. The data was then permanently de-identified. We included only individuals living within the City of Calgary.

For each CDA, the following sociodemographic variables were linked from the Canadian Household Survey: median household income ≥ $CDN 100,000 (overall median household income in Calgary for 2011 was $93,410), level of education (percent with university education), percent of individuals of Aboriginal - First Nations descent (North American Indian, as defined by Statistics Canada [19]), percent of individuals immigrating to Canada within the past 5 years and percent of individuals of Chinese, South Asian (primarily Indian, Pakistani and Sri Lankan), Filipino or Black visible minority status (the four most common statuses in Calgary, as defined by Statistics Canada [20]). We then examined these data-sets for associations between these sociodemographic variables and urine culture testing rate.

For per capita testing rate (Fig. 1), the total number of urine culture tests for each year was divided by the total Calgary population as reported by the annual City of Calgary Civic census (http://www.calgary.ca). To calculate the

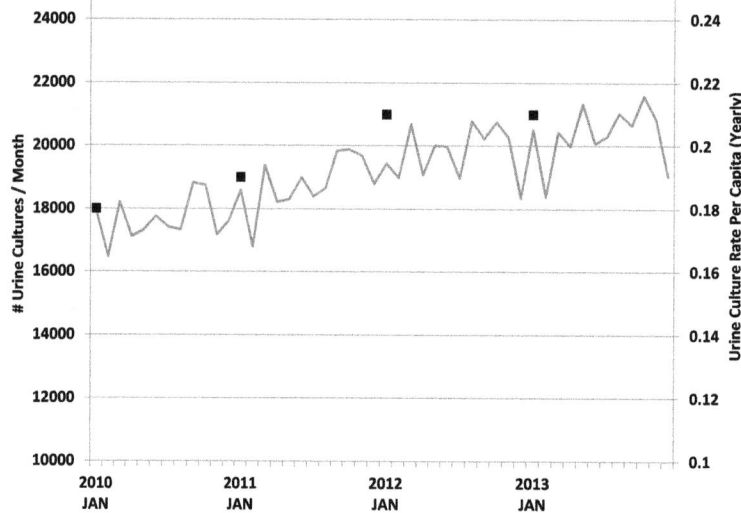

Fig. 1 Urine culture testing at CLS from January 1, 2010 to December 31, 2013 presented as the number of urine culture tests per month (grey line) and the yearly per capita urine culture test rate (black squares)

percent of testing within each age and gender group (Table 1), the total number of individuals within each group who received at least one urine culture was divided by the total population within that group in Calgary according to the 2011 Canadian census. To calculate the testing frequency for the age and gender group in each CDA, the number of individuals that received testing from that group was divided by the total number of that age group in the dissemination area. For visual representation of the data, the values were then plotted onto a

dissemination area map for Calgary using the ArcGIS v9.3 geo-mapping software (Environmental System Research Institute, Redlands, California). This software tool uses Getis-Ord Gi* statistic to produce z-scores and identify statistically significant hot (increased testing) and cold (decreased testing) spots depending on how many standard deviations the data is removed from the mean [21]. Statistical inference regarding sociodemographic variables associated with testing rate was performed using the generalized estimating equations version of Poisson regression in SAS v9.4. The reported relative risks refer to the independent contribution of each variable with the other categorical variables (age, gender, group) held constant at an arbitrary reference value. The differences in testing rates are reported as relative risk (RR) for the independent contribution of that variable to the analysis and results were considered statistically significant at a p-value of 0.05.

Results

Increased testing volumes and per capita testing rates have been reported in most laboratory divisions [22]. Urine culture testing, which is the highest volume microbiology test at CLS, has seen a similar rise that exceeds Calgary's population growth (Fig. 1). Linear regression analysis of this data shows statistically significant increases in test volumes ($R^2 = 0.68$, $P < 0.001$) and year over year per capita test rates ($R^2 = 0.96$, $P = 0.002$).

Data on 225,473 urine culture results were available in our LIS for 2011, which represented 133,464 individuals who underwent urine culture testing. After excluding individuals where no postal code was available and those with postal codes outside the city of Calgary, 100,901

Table 1 Frequency of Urine culture testing in Calgary, Alberta for 2011

	Number of Tests	Individuals Tested	Total Population	Percent Tested
Total	219,015	100,901	1,096,830	9.2%
Male	40,294	23,009	547,475	4.2%
<15	4999	3752	100,450	3.7%
15-39	6046	4410	208,840	2.1%
40-49	4083	2653	86,935	3.1%
50-59	6130	3407	77,460	4.4%
60-69	5870	3129	41,920	7.4%
≥70	13,166	5658	31,875	17.8%
Female	132,388	77,892	549,360	14.2%
<15	10,292	7105	95,970	7.4%
15-39	53,888	34,282	205,995	16.6%
40-49	14,449	9393	84,950	11.1%
50-59	14,110	8716	75,415	11.6%
60-69	11,755	6437	43,075	15.0%
≥70	27,894	11,959	43,940	27.2%

individuals remained and were included in our study. The majority of specimens were received from patients in the community (67.9%) and the emergency department (19.3%), with the remainder from nursing homes (2.3%), inpatients (5.3%) and various outpatient settings including pre-admission clinics and subspecialty clinics (collectively 5.2%). Overall, 9.2% of individuals in the city of Calgary were tested during the study period, including 4.2% of males and 14.2% of females (Table 1). For males and females, the highest testing rate was in individuals ≥70 years (17.8% and 27.2%, respectively), however the greatest number of specimens were received from females aged 15–39. In part, this increased testing rate is likely accounted for by screening for asymptomatic bacteriuria in pregnancy but such clinical information was not available in our study.

The ArcGIS hot spot analysis mapping illustrates significant differences in screening rates across the city (Fig. 2). Significantly increased testing is observed in the inner city and northeast quadrants of the city. The median urine culture testing rates among neighbourhoods was 9.1% with 7.5% and 10.9% as the lower and upper quartiles, respectively.

The association between sociodemographic variables and urine culture test rates are shown in Table 2 and many inequities are present. The regression model showed that females were significantly more likely to be tested than males (RR = 2.58, $p < 0.0001$). As seen in Table 2, individuals aged 15–39 were the most likely to be tested (RR = 1.69, $p < 0.0001$), followed by those ≥70 years of age (analysis control, RR = 1.0). Decreased urine culture testing was associated with higher (≥ $100000) household income (RR = 0.07, $p < 0.0001$) and higher employment rate (RR = 0.36, $p < 0.0001$). No association between university education and testing was detected. Aboriginal – First Nations individuals (RR = 0.29, $p = 0.0008$) and individuals of Chinese descent (RR = 0.672, $p = 0.0005$) were also less likely to be tested. Interestingly, recent immigration (≤ 5 years), South Asian descent, Filipino descent or Black visible minority status were not significant predictors of urine culture testing.

Discussion

Our data reveal a drastically lower rate of urine culture testing with higher household income (≥ $100000) and higher employment rate. In previous studies, we demonstrated that these factors were associated with increased 25-hydroxyvitamin D and prostate specific antigen (PSA) testing and we hypothesized that this was possibly due to greater access to health care and patient-requested testing [23, 24]. The differences in urine culture testing identified in the present study appears contrary to that hypothesis. Why such drastic differences in urine testing rates exist between higher and lower

socioeconomic status groups is unclear. One possibility is that the testing differences are warranted and reflect increased rates of LUTI, complicated urinary tract infection or antibiotic resistance in lower income earners. Previous studies have demonstrated a modest association between lower household income and community-acquired urinary tract infections and asymptomatic bacteriuria [25–27]. Increased incidence of other genitourinary tract infections causing similar symptoms, such as *Neisseria gonorrhoeae* or *Chlamydia trachomatis* urethritis/vulvovaginitis, could result in greater urine culture testing as well. In support of this, an earlier study showed a similar association between lower socioeconomic indicators and prevalence of these infections in Calgary [28].

It is also possible that discrepancies in urine culture ordering are unrelated to genitourinary tract infection, but instead result from differences in the prevalence of diseases with overlapping clinical presentation. Irritative lower urinary tract symptoms (urinary urgency, incontinence and frequency) consistent with overactive bladder syndrome (OAB) and/or benign prostatic hyperplasia (BPH) increase with age and may elicit urine culture testing [29]. Previous studies have demonstrated a relationship between higher income, higher levels of education and employment status and fewer of these symptoms in both women and men [30, 31]. The authors of these studies speculated that the reduced symptoms were the result of regular health check-ups, earlier recognition of symptoms and prior treatment. This could also explain our findings as patients of lower socioeconomic status may have more persistent urinary symptoms and have more urine cultures performed while not receiving appropriate therapy for these non-infectious conditions as a result of less consistent healthcare contact. Further studies are needed to determine whether this is indeed the case, as appropriate intervention would substantially improve patient care while also reducing microbiologic testing.

Concern regarding antibiotic resistant organisms could also drive increased urine culture utilization and clinical guidelines support the use of urine cultures in these instances. Resistant rates vary throughout the world; however, the Study for Monitoring Antimicrobial Resistance Trends (SMART) has established that the highest levels of antimicrobial resistance exist in the Asia-Pacific region where as many as 28.2% of LUTI pathogens possess extended spectrum β-lactamases [32]. South Asian, Chinese and Filipino people are strongly represented in Calgary's visible minority population, and increased urine culture test rates would be expected if there were concerns about antimicrobial resistance. In fact, our data reveal the opposite trend with Chinese ethnicity associated with a statistically significant decrease in testing,

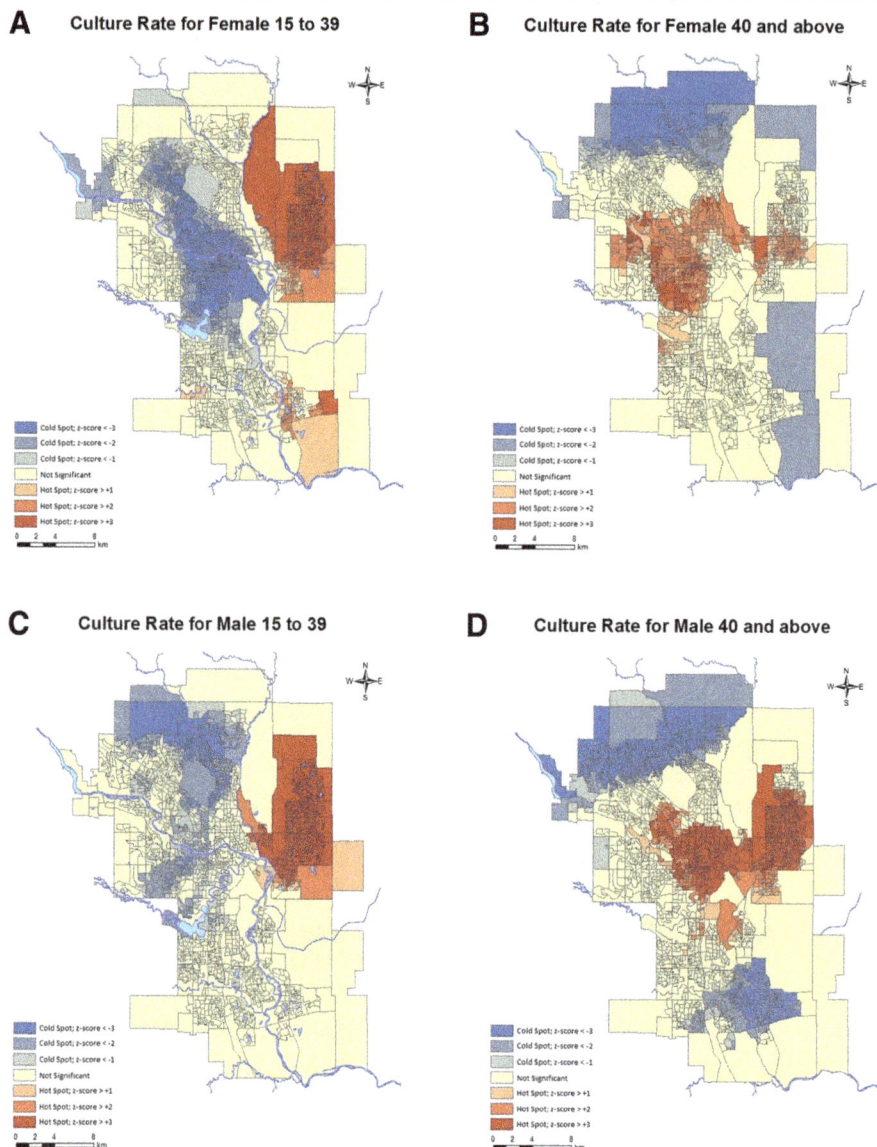

Fig. 2 Hotspot maps representing the frequency of urine culture test ordering in four age/gender groups. The testing rate (individuals tested / total individuals in dissemination area) is represented by the number of standard deviations (z-score) it is removed from the mean (yellow/beige) in the positive (red, increased testing) and negative (blue, decreased testing) direction. Culture rates are shown for Females aged 15–39 (**a**), Females aged ≥40 (**b**), Males aged 15–39 (**c**), Males aged ≥40 (**d**). Maps generated using ArcGIS v9.3 geo-mapping software

and no relationship between test rate and recent immigration, South Asian or Filipino ethnicity. The cause of this decreased testing is unclear, but could represent barriers preventing health care access. Given the risk of resistance, this is a potential cause for concern.

The main strength of this study is the large sample of patients and, because our laboratory performs testing for all of Calgary, the data presented herein represents a complete view of urine culture testing on the adult (>15) population of the city. However, the limitations of this study must be recognized when interpreting these results. Because this study was retrospective and

involved a very large number of patients, we were unable to collect clinical information or assess other concurrent laboratory testing (such as urinalysis or testing for sexually transmitted infection). As a result, we cannot ascertain the clinical appropriateness of urine culture testing. However, the variability in test ordering across the city without clear explanation is highly suggestive of inappropriate utilization. Patients with underlying disease may necessitate increased urine culture testing and such patients were certainly included in this study. We attempted to minimize the impact of such patients by counting a single urine culture per individual. As well,

Table 2 Sociodemographic variables and Urine culture testing rates in Calgary, Alberta for 2011

Socio-demographic Variable	Relative Risk (RR)	RR 95% Confidence Interval		Parameter Estimate	P-value
Female	2.583	2.539	2.629	0.9491	<0.0001
Male[a]	1.000	Reference		Reference	Reference
Age < 15	0.586	0.548	0.627	−0.534	<0.0001
Age 15–39	1.689	1.587	1.797	0.524	<0.0001
Age 40–49	0.624	0.587	0.663	−0.472	<0.0001
Age 50–59	0.660	0.623	0.700	−0.415	<0.0001
Age 60–69	0.550	0.520	0.581	−0.599	<0.0001
Age ≥ 70[b]	1.000	Reference		Reference	Reference
Median Household Income ≥$100,000	0.074	0.038	0.147	−2.600	<0.0001
Employment Rate	0.367	0.251	0.537	−1.002	<0.0001
University Education	1.091	0.864	1.377	0.087	0.464
Recent Immigrant (≤ 5 years)	0.678	0.440	1.044	−0.389	0.077
Aboriginal – First Nations	0.289	0.140	0.596	−1.240	0.0008
Chinese	0.672	0.536	0.842	−0.398	0.0005
South Asian	0.924	0.779	1.097	−0.079	0.3656
Filipino	0.791	0.563	1.111	−0.235	0.1761
Visible Minority - Black	0.878	0.392	1.965	−0.130	0.7515

[a]Males were used as reference for females
[b]Age group ≥70 was used as a reference for the other age groups

as this is an ecological study, inferences are made based on group level variables that may not accurately represent individual level variables. Some of the differences identified may be the result of confounding variables that are not captured in this study. It is also unknown what degree of urine testing is driven by patient or physician characteristics (generalist versus specialist practice, experience, location of training, etc.) and physician variables were not controlled for in the current study. Despite these deficits, we have identified several sociodemographic groups with significantly increased rates of testing and have demonstrated substantial variation in urine culture utilization across Calgary.

Further work will be to expand these studies to investigate for mismatch between urine culture ordering practices and clinical utility. Assessment of urine culture positivity rates and antibiotic resistance rates and how they align with the test utilization rates presented in the current study will provide useful information to direct intervention strategies to improve appropriate urine culture usage.

Conclusions

Despite clinical practice guidelines recommending limited use of urine culture in diagnosing LUTI, we have shown that test rates continue to increase in Calgary and that substantial heterogeneity exists in test utilization across the city. We have also identified several patient groups with greatly increased or decreased test rates that may be indicative of inappropriate test utilization. Future investigations will now be focused on these patient groups to ascertain specific explanations for the potential over-utilization observed herein.

Abbreviations
CDA: Census dissemination area; CLS: Calgary Laboratory Services; IDSA: Infectious Disease Society of America; LIS: Laboratory Information System; LUTI: Lower urinary tract infection; RR: Relative Risk

Acknowledgments
We would like to acknowledge the crucial contributions of Jeannine Viczko, who acquired the data from the Calgary Laboratory Services laboratory information system, and Maggie Guo, who assisted with the statistical analysis and geo-mapping of the data.

Funding
This work was supported by a Canadian Institutes of Health Research foundation scheme grant to CN [RN254781–333204]. The funding agency had no input on the study.

Authors' contributions

TPG, DLC and CN conceived of the study, participated in its design. TPG analysed the data. TPC, DLC, CN and WWC all participated in interpretation of data, as well as drafting the manuscript and revising it critically. All authors have read and approve of the final manuscript.

Competing interests

The authors declare that they have no competing interests.

Author details

[1]Department of Pathology and Laboratory Medicine, University of Calgary, Calgary, AB, Canada. [2]Department of Family Medicine, University of Calgary, Calgary, AB, Canada. [3]Division of Microbiology, Department of Pathology and Laboratory Medicine, University of Calgary, Calgary, AB, Canada. [4]Department of Medicine, University of Calgary, Calgary, AB, Canada. [5]1W-410, Diagnostic and Scientific Centre, 9-3535 Research Road NW, Calgary, AB T2L 2K8, Canada.

References

1. Bonkat MG, Pickard R, Bartoletti R, Bruyère F, Geerlings SE, Wagenlehner F, Wullt W. members of the EAU Urological Infections Guidelines Panel. EAU Urological Infections Guidelines. Retrieved from: https://uroweb.org/guideline/urological-infections//. Accessed 5 Jan 2018.
2. Colgan R, Williams M. Diagnosis and treatment of acute uncomplicated cystitis. Am Fam Physician. 2011;84:771–6.
3. Scottish Intercollegiate Guidelines Network. Management of suspected bacterial urinary tract infection in adults. 2012;SIGN no 88.
4. American College of Obstetricians and Gynecologists. Treatment of Urinary Tract Infections in Nonpregnant Women, ACOG Pract. Bull. No 91, vol. 111; 2008. p. 785–94.
5. Nicolle LE, Bradley S, Colgan R, Rice JC, Schaeffer A, Hooton TM. Infectious Diseases Society of America guidelines for the diagnosis and treatment of asymptomatic bacteriuria in adults. Clin Infect Dis. 2005;40:643–54.
6. Nicolle LE. Asymptomatic bacteriuria in the Eldery. Infect Dis Clin N Am. 1997;11:647–62.
7. Nicolle LE, Bjornson J, Harding GK, MacDonell JA. Bacteriuria in elderly institutionalized men. N Engl J Med. 1983;309:1420-5.
8. Infectious Diseases Society of America. Five things physicians and patients should question. 2015. http://www.choosingwisely.org/societies/infectious-diseases-society-of-america/. Accessed 5 Jan 2018.
9. Campbell-Brown M, McFadyen IR. Bacteriuria in pregnancy treated with a single dose of cephalexin. Br J Obstet Gynaecol. 1983;90:1054–9.
10. Hooton TM, Bradley SF, Cardenas DD, Colgan R, Geerlings SE, Rice JC, et al. Diagnosis, prevention, and treatment of catheter-associated urinary tract infection in adults: 2009 international clinical practice guidelines from the Infectious Diseases Society of America. Clin Infect Dis. 2010;50:625–63.
11. Hooton TM, Roberts PL, Cox ME, Stapleton AE. Voided midstream urine culture and acute cystitis in premenopausal women. N Engl J Med. 2013;369:1883–91.
12. Llor C, Rabanaque G, López A, Cots JM. The adherence of GPs to guidelines for the diagnosis and treatment of lower urinary tract infections in women is poor. Fam Pract. 2011;28:294–9.
13. McIsaac WJ, Hunchak CL. Overestimation error and unnecessary antibiotic prescriptions for acute cystitis in adult women. Med Decis Mak. 2011;31:405–11.
14. Trautner BW. Asymptomatic bacteriuria: when the treatment is worse than the disease. Nat Rev Urol. 2011;9:85–93.
15. Phillips CD, Adepoju O, Stone N, Moudouni DKM, Nwaiwu O, Zhao H, et al. Asymptomatic bacteriuria, antibiotic use, and suspected urinary tract infections in four nursing homes. BMC Geriatr. 2012;12:73.
16. Werner NL, Hecker MT, Sethi AK, Donskey CJ. Unnecessary use of fluoroquinolone antibiotics in hospitalized patients. BMC Infect Dis. 2011;11:187.
17. Cai T, Mazzoli S, Mondaini N, Meacci F, Nesi G, D'Elia C, et al. The role of asymptomatic bacteriuria in young women with recurrent urinary tract infections: to treat or not to treat? Clin Infect Dis. 2012;55:771–7.
18. Cai T, Nesi G, Mazzoli S, Meacci F, Lanzafame P, Caciagli P, et al. Asymptomatic bacteriuria treatment is associated with a higher prevalence of antibiotic resistant strains in women with urinary tract infections. Clin Infect Dis. 2015;61:1655–61.
19. Aboriginal Group Definition. 2016; Available from: http://www12.statcan.gc.ca/nhs-enm/2011/ref/dict/pop144-eng.cfm
20. Visible Minority Definition. 2016. Available from: http://www12.statcan.gc.ca/nhs-enm/2011/ref/dict/pop127-eng.cfm
21. Mitchell A. The ESRI Guide to GIS Analysis, Volume 2: Spatial Measurements and Statistics. Redlands: 1st ed. ESRI Press; 2005.
22. Rockey M, Naugler C, Sidhu D. Laboratory utilization trends : past and future. Can Pathol. 2013;5:65–72.
23. de Koning L, Henne D, Woods P, Hemmelgarn BR, Naugler C. Sociodemographic correlates of 25-hydroxyvitamin D test utilization in Calgary, Alberta. BMC Health Serv Res. 2014;14:339.
24. Gorday W, Sadrzadeh H, de Koning L, Naugler C. Association of sociodemographic factors and prostate-specific antigen (PSA) testing. Clin Biochem. 2014;47:164–9.
25. Turck M, Goffe BS, Petersdorf RG. Bacteriuria of pregnancy. N Engl J Med. 1962;266:857–60.
26. Emiru T, Beyene G, Tsegaye W, Melaku S. Associated risk factors of urinary tract infection among pregnant women at Felege Hiwot referral hospital, Bahir Dar, north West Ethiopia. BMC Res Notes. 2013;6:292.
27. Jeon CY, Muennig P, Furuya EY, Cohen B, Nash D, Larson EL. Burden of present-on-admission infections and health care-associated infections, by race and ethnicity. Am J Infect Control. 2014;42:1296–302.
28. Bush KR, Henderson EA, Dunn J, Read RR, Singh A. Mapping the core: chlamydia and gonorrhea infections in Calgary, Alberta. Sex Transm Dis. 2008;35:291–7.
29. Wang Y, Xu K, Hu H, Zhang X, Wang X, Na Y, et al. Prevalence, risk factors, and impact on health related quality of life of overactive bladder in China. Neurourol Urodyn. 2011;30:1448–55.
30. Kim JH, Ham BK, Shim SR, Lee WJ, Kim HJ, Kwon S-S, et al. The association between the self-perception period of overactive bladder symptoms and overactive bladder symptom scores in a non-treated population and related sociodemographic and lifestyle factors. Int J Clin Pract. 2013;67:795–800.
31. Joseph MA, Harlow SD, Wei JT, Sarma AV, Dunn RL, Taylor JMG, et al. Risk factors for lower urinary tract symptoms in a population-based sample of African-American men. Am J Epidemiol. 2003;157:906–14.
32. Lu PL, Liu YC, Toh HS, Lee YL, Liu YM, Ho CM, et al. Epidemiology and antimicrobial susceptibility profiles of Gram-negative bacteria causing urinary tract infections in the Asia-Pacific region: 2009–2010 results from the Study for Monitoring Antimicrobial Resistance Trends (SMART). Int J Antimicrob Agents. 2012;40:S37–43.

26

An observational study of the use of beclomethasone dipropionate suppositories in the treatment of lower urinary tract inflammation in men

Giorgio Bozzini[1*], Marco Provenzano[2], Nicolò Buffi[3], Mauro Seveso[1], Giovanni Lughezzani[3], Giorgio Guazzoni[2,3], Alberto Mandressi[1] and Gianluigi Taverna[1]

Abstract

Background: Nonbacterial prostatitis, together with chronic pelvic pain syndrome, accounts for 90–95 % of prostatitis cases. Anti-inflammatory medications are commonly used to reduce storage/inflammatory symptoms that can deteriorate quality of life. The purpose of this study was to observe the efficacy and safety of beclomethasone dipropionate rectal suppositories (Topster®) in inflammations of the lower urinary tract in men.

Methods: Patients underwent diagnostic and therapeutic protocols according to current evidence-based practice. Efficacy assessments: voiding parameters, perineal pain, International Prostate Symptom Score (IPSS), digital rectal examination (DRE). Adverse events and patient compliance were recorded throughout the study.

Results: One hundred eighty patients were enrolled, mean age 52 ± 14.97. Most frequent diagnosis: nonbacterial prostatitis (85 %). All patients completed visits 1 and 2. All patients were treated with beclomethasone dipropionate (BDP) suppositories, 136/180 also with *Serenoa repens* (SR) extract. Antibiotics were rarely required. 162/180 patients presented clinically significant improvements and terminated treatment.
Mean change vs. baseline in voiding frequency: -3.55 ± 2.70 n/day in patients taking only BDP and -3.68 ± 2.81 n/day in those taking both BDP and SR ($P<.0001$ in both groups). Uroflowmetry improved significantly; change from baseline 3.26 ± 5.35 ml/s in BDP only group and 5.61 ± 7.32 ml/s in BDP + SR group ($P = 0.0002$ for BDP, $P<.0001$ for BDP + SR). Urine stream normal in 35 % of patients at visit 1 and 57.22 % of patients at visit 2. Mean change in perineal pain, on 0–10 VAS, -0.66 ± 2.24 for BDP only group ($P = 0.0699$) and -1.37 ± 2.40 for BDP + SR group ($P<.0001$). IPSS increased at visit 2. No adverse events were reported.
For all parameters, none of the comparisons between groups was found to be statistically significant.

Conclusion: This study confirmed the drug's good safety profile. We also observed an improvement in the main storage symptoms and clinical findings associated with lower urinary tract inflammation in patients treated with beclomethasone dipropionate suppositories.

Keywords: Nonbacterial prostatitis, Beclomethasone dipropionate, Lower urinary tract inflammation

* Correspondence: gioboz@yahoo.it
[1]Departmentt of Urology, Humanitas Mater Domini, Via Gerenzano 2, I -
21053 Castellanza, Varese, Italy
Full list of author information is available at the end of the article

Background

Inflammation of the lower urinary tract, especially of the prostate, commonly affects men of a wide age range, with detrimental repercussions on quality of life [1–3]. Symptoms include pelvic pain and a variable degree of voiding and sexual dysfunction [4, 5].

Although prostatitis is historically considered mainly a bacterial disease, its most common form is chronic prostatitis/chronic pelvic pain syndrome, accounting for 90–95 % of prostatitis cases [1, 2, 6].

Traditional medical therapy for prostatitis is centered on treating infection with antimicrobials, although less than 10 % of prostatitis cases are bacterial, and on alleviating symptoms with NSAIDS, alpha-blockers, 5-Alpha-Reductase Inhibitors, and phytotherapy [2, 6, 7].

Currently, corticosteroids are not considered "standard of care" for treating prostatitis. However, in a double-blinded, randomized, parallel study, 160 patients presenting with chronic nonbacterial prostatitis received prednisone and levofloxacin or levofloxacin and placebo; significant differences between the two groups as well as between pre- and post-treatment ($P < 0.01$) were found for total NIH-CPSI score, pain index, voiding index and quality of life [5]. Currently beclomethasone dipropionate suppositories is a part of the standard practice in the hospital.

Furthermore, new formulations of corticosteroids have been developed to limit systemic activity and reduce corticosteroid adverse events [8–12]. Second-generation oral or rectal corticosteroids such as beclomethasone dipropionate have high topical anti-inflammatory efficacy in the gut and minimal systemic bioavailability due to low absorption and highly efficient first-pass hepatic inactivation [10, 11]. A systematic review of rectal therapies for distal forms of ulcerative colitis found that a greater percentage of patients receiving 5-aminosalicylic acid or corticosteroid rectal formulations obtained therapeutic benefit after treatment compared with placebo [13]. The overall safety profile of rectal therapies was favorable and treatment with beclomethasone dipropionate did not increase the incidence of steroid-related adverse events [9, 10, 12, 13].

The objectives of this study were to collect safety data and observe the effects of beclomethasone dipropionate (Topster®, SOFAR S.p.A., Milan, Italy) rectal suppositories on symptoms associated with lower urinary tract inflammation.

Methods

This was a prospective, observational, single-center study performed on outpatients referred to a high-volume academic teaching hospital in Italy. The study was approved by the local Ethics Committee and written informed consent was obtained from all patients.

Male patients presenting with storage/inflammatory symptoms of the lower urinary tract (pelvic pain, voiding and sexual dysfunction) were observed as they underwent diagnostic and therapeutic protocols according to clinical practice. Subjects affected by coagulation impairments, cardiovascular or pulmonary comorbidities were excluded from the observation, along with those who had undergone a prostatic biopsy within the previous 14 days.

Semen and urine cultures were performed at baseline to determine if the inflammation was triggered by an infection, and whether an antibiotic was therefore indicated.

The following parameters were assessed at each visit: voiding frequency, uroflowmetry, urine stream, perineal pain, prostate-specific antigen (PSA), International Prostate Symptom Score (IPSS) [14] and digital rectal examination (DRE) (evaluation of prostate size, temperature and consistency).

At visit 1, baseline clinical assessments were performed and therapy was prescribed according to current evidence-based practice [1, 2, 15, 16]. Patients were then re-evaluated at visit 2, after the end of the treatment course.

A patient was considered "responder" to therapy following a clinically significant improvement of the evaluated parameters (i.e. voiding frequency, uroflowmetry, urine stream, perineal pain) and the patient's impression of a good clinical outcome.

Drugs prescribed and rationale

Beclomethasone dipropionate (BDP) rectal suppositories (3 mg, 1 supp. once a day) were prescribed for the relief of inflammation-related storage symptoms. The duration of treatment varied depending on the patient's conditions: 10-day courses were prescribed to patients with mild symptoms (e.g. perineal pain on a 0–10 VAS between 4 and 6, voiding frequency less than 10 times a day) or to those expected not to comply with longer treatment; 20-day courses in other cases (severe symptoms, high compliance expected).

Serenoa repens (SR) 320 mg (1 tab. a day for 60 days) was suggested as adjuvant treatment for voiding and storage symptoms due to prostatic hypertrophy and inflammation. We used the only formulation registered as a drug (and not as a dietary supplement) in Italy (Permixon 320 mg®), as requested by the Ethics committee due to the current Literature evidence. It was not prescribed in patients who had already undergone this treatment with unsatisfactory outcomes.

An antibiotic course was prescribed in case of bacterial infection (positive seminal fluid and/or urine cultures). The specific antibiotic was recommended according to antibiogram results, patient preference regarding route of administration and current guidelines for the outpatient treatment of lower urinary tract infections [15, 16].

A diet (no alcohol, beer or spicy food) and/or hygiene rules (e.g. avoid cycling/riding, prolonged/interrupted sexual intercourse, constipation/diarrhea) were also recommended.

Safety monitoring consisted in gathering all adverse reactions occurring during the study.

All statistical tables, figures, listings and analyses were produced using SAS® for Windows release 9.4 (64-bit) or later (SAS Institute Inc., Cary, NC, USA). Box plots for IPSS score, uroflowmetry, urination frequency, PSA and perineal pain were produced by visit and by type of therapy (BDP suppositories only for patients in group A, or BDP suppositories plus SR for patients in group B). Differences between visit 2 and baseline were analyzed by means of a paired t-test in case of normal data distribution, or a non-parametric Wilcoxon signed rank sum test otherwise. A two independent samples t-test was performed in order to compare the two treatment groups if the changes vs. baseline were normally distributed. Otherwise, the analogous non-parametric test (Wilcoxon-Mann–Whitney test) was used.

Results

One hundred eighty patients were enrolled in this study between January and December 2013 and all of them completed both visit 1 and visit 2. One hundred thirty-six patients were treated with both BDP and SR (Group B), whereas 44 were treated with BDP only (Group A).

Patients averaged 52 years of age (SD 14.9, range 22–87) and nonbacterial prostatitis was by far the most frequent diagnosis, affecting 89.7 % of patients treated with BDP + SR (Group B) and 70.4 % of those treated with BDP (Group A) (Table 1). The mean duration of symptoms was 2.7 ± 1.8 months (range 1–12 months) and the number of previous episodes 1.2 ± 1.2 (range 0–6).

Approximately 26 % of patients had undergone previous treatment with antibiotics, of which ciprofloxacin, cefixime and levofloxacin were the most commonly prescribed. Urine and semen cultures at visit 1 were positive in 13 (7.2 %) and 12 (6.6 %) patients respectively.

All 180 patients underwent at least one course of therapy with BDP suppositories. Serenoa repens 320 mg (saw palmetto extract) was prescribed to 136 patients. Antibiotics were prescribed to only one patient (Table 2). The other patients with positive urine or semen cultures were already taking the proper antibiotic prescribed by their general practicner.

At visit 2, all patients reported being compliant with the prescribed therapies and suggestions concerning diet and lifestyle.

Mean time elapsed between visits was 99.6 ± 38.3 days (range 27–179 days).

Efficacy results
One hundred sixty-two of the 180 patients treated with BDP presented clinically significant improvements and terminated treatment. Further therapeutic interventions were required for only 18 patients.

The study evidenced noteworthy improvements in voiding parameters. Considering voiding frequency, the changes from baseline were found to be statistically significant ($P<.0001$) in both groups (-3.5 ± 2.7 n/day in patients taking only BDP suppositories and -3.6 ± 2.8 n/day in those taking both BDP and SR), whereas the difference in mean change between the two groups was not (p-value = 0.8560) (Fig. 1).

Uroflowmetry values also improved considerably, with mean values increasing of 3.26 ± 5.35 mL/s in the Group A and 5.6 ± 7.3 mL/s in the Group B. The difference between the two groups was again not statistically significant ($P = 0.0638$) (Fig. 2).

Uroflowmetry data reported in Table n°3 are also matched with voided volume and post voided residual

Table 1 Diagnosis

		Total (N = 181)		Treatment			
				Group A (N = 45)		Group B (N = 136)	
		N	%	N	%	N	%
Diagnosis at Baseline	Chlamydial Urethritis	2	1.10	1	2.27	1	0.74
	Chronic Nonbacterial Prostatitis	3	1.66	0	0.00	3	2.21
	Nonbacterial Prostatitis	154	85.08	31	70.45	122	89.71
	Nonbacterial Prostatitis (First episode)	3	1.66	1	2.27	2	1.47
	Post Endoscopic Resection Urethritis	11	6.08	7	15.91	4	2.94
	Results of pyelonephritis	1	0.55	0	0.00	1	0.74
	Urethritis	7	3.87	4	9.09	3	2.21

Table 2 Prescribed medications

			Total (N = 181)		Treatment Group A (N = 45)		Group B (N = 136)	
			N	%	N	%	N	%
Visit	Drug	Dosage	181	-	45	-	136	-
Visit 1	Patients visited -	-						
	Doxycycline 400	1 tab for 7 days	1	0.55	1	2.27	0	0.00
	Serenoa repens 320 mg	1 tab for 40 days	30	16.67	0	0.00	30	22.06
		1 tab for 60 days	106	58.89	0	0.00	106	77.94
	Beclomethasone dipropionate suppositories	1 supp. for 10 days	28	15.56	1	2.27	27	19.85
		1 supp. for 20 days	152	84.44	43	97.73	109	80.15

(PVR) to assess the improvements from baseline. The percentage of patients reporting normal urine stream increased significantly, from 43.1 % at baseline to 54.5 % at visit 2 in Group A patients, and from 32.3 to 58.1 % in Group B patients.

At visit 2, patients reported feeling less perineal pain, assessed by means of a Visual Analogue Scale of 0–10. The t-test for the difference between groups was not statistically significant although the p-value (0.0787) suggested a slightly stronger decrease among patients administered both BDP and SR (Fig. 3).

DREs were performed to evaluate prostate volume, temperature and consistency. A clear trend was not apparent for size; an enlarged prostate was detected in

50.5 % of the patients at visit 1, and 60.5 % at visit 2. On the contrary, the number of patients with a warm prostate decreased from 42.7 % of the patients at visit 1 to 5.5 % of the patients at visit 2. Clinical evidence of an inflamed prostate at DRE was reported in 83.8 % of the patients at visit 1, whereas 87.7 % of the patients presented a normal prostate at visit 2.

The mean change from baseline in IPSS was 2.1 ± 7.9 ($P = 0.0767$) in Group A patients and 4.7 ± 7.9 ($P < .0001$) in Group B patients, which could suggest a worsening of IPSS score over time, although a temporary rise in score prior to final improvement is quite common in this pathology. The difference in the mean changes from baseline between the two groups was not statistically

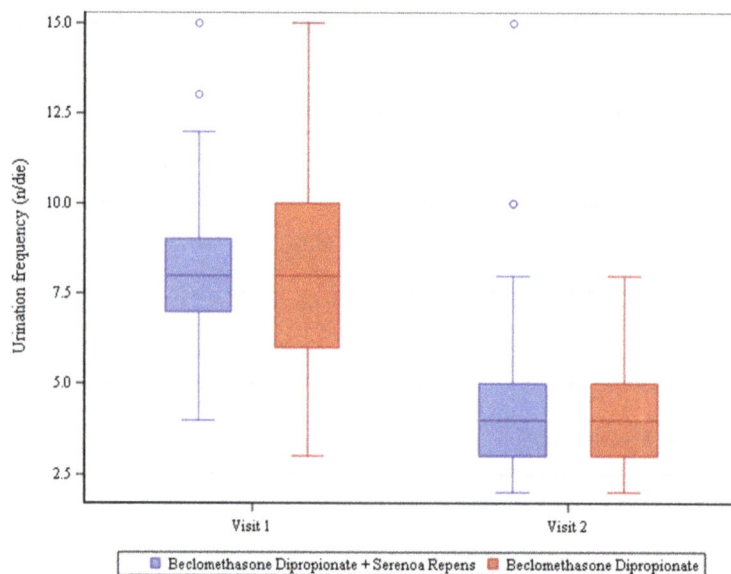

Fig. 1 Voiding frequency. The bottom of each box is the 25th percentile (Q1), the top is the 75th percentile (Q3), and the internal line is the median. The whiskers indicate variability outside the upper and lower quartiles, i.e. scores outside the middle 50 %. A circle outside of this range is an outlier, an observation that is distant from others

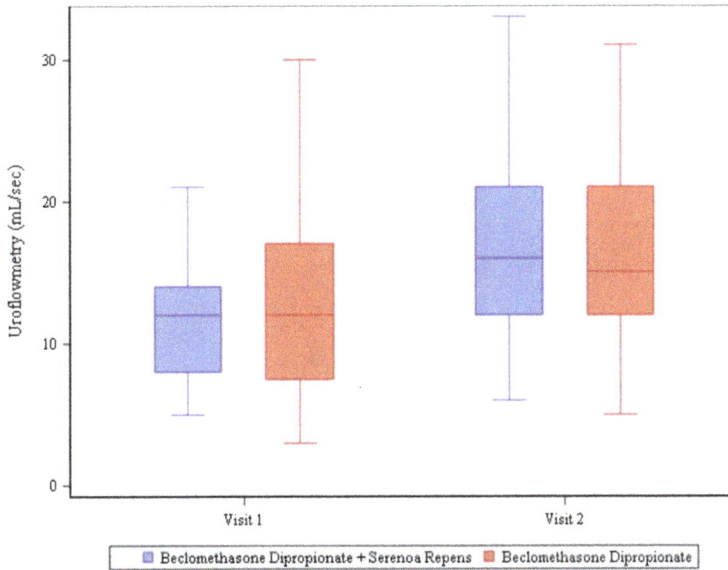

Fig. 2 Uroflowmetry. The bottom of each box is the 25th percentile (Q1), the top is the 75th percentile (Q3), and the internal line is the median. The whiskers indicate variability outside the upper and lower quartiles, i.e. scores outside the middle 50 %. A circle outside of this range is an outlier, an observation that is distant from others

significant although a more marked increase of IPSS was present among those patients who took both treatments (Fig. 4).

PSA levels remained stable and below 4.0 ng/mL, dropping slightly from 3.4 ± 3.2 ng/mL (range 0.07– 21 ng/mL) at visit 1 to 3.07 ± 2.35 at visit 2 (range 1.10– 21.00 ng/mL).

Table 3 contains a summary of all the main efficacy results of the study, comparing the two groups of patients.

No adverse reactions or adverse events were reported.

Discussion

Chronic inflammation plays an important role in the initiation and progression of a wide spectrum of diseases with

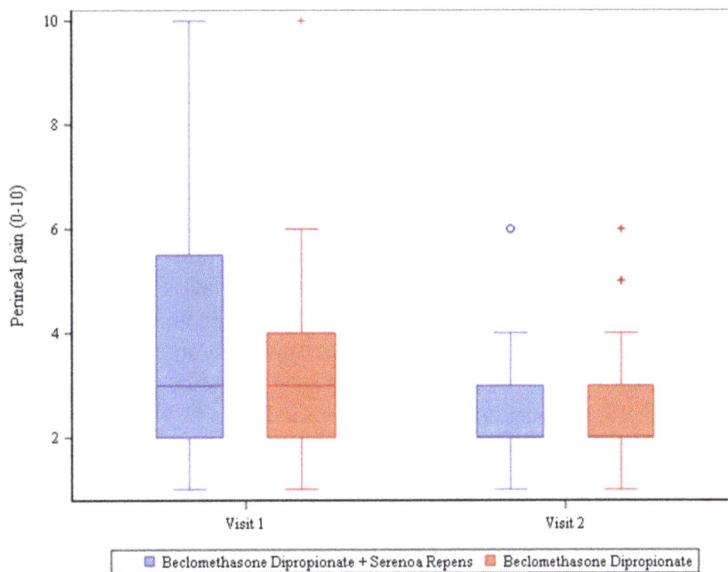

Fig. 3 Perineal pain. The bottom of each box is the 25th percentile (Q1), the top is the 75th percentile (Q3), and the internal line is the median. The whiskers indicate variability outside the upper and lower quartiles, i.e. scores outside the middle 50 %. A circle outside of this range is an outlier, an observation that is distant from others

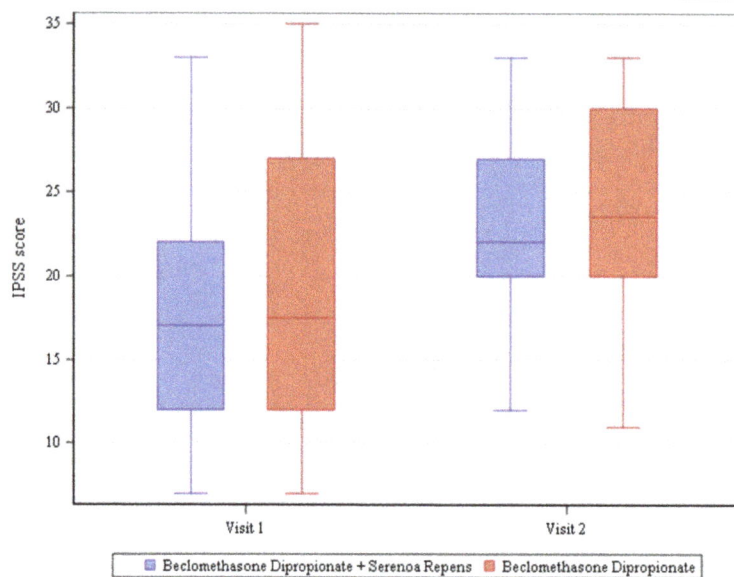

Fig. 4 IPSS score. The bottom of each box is the 25th percentile (Q1), the top is the 75th percentile (Q3), and the internal line is the median. The whiskers indicate variability outside the upper and lower quartiles, i.e. scores outside the middle 50 %. A circle outside of this range is an outlier, an observation that is distant from others

prostate involvement [17]. Therefore, anti-inflammatory medications are commonly used in clinical practice for the treatment of several prostatic diseases, including nonbacterial prostatitis. These therapies aim principally at reducing symptoms caused by inflammation (e.g. pelvic pain, voiding dysfunction) that can significantly impair a patient's quality of life [1, 5, 6].

The vast majority of our patients presenting with lower urinary tract inflammation were affected with nonbacterial prostatitis (85 %). This was an expected result given the high prevalence of this pathological condition [2, 6, 7]. In fact, nearly 50 % of all men experience prostatitis-like symptoms at least once during their lifetime and 90 % of those have abacterial prostatitis [2, 6, 7].

The majority of patients (152/180) underwent a 20-day course of therapy with BDP suppositories because of the severity of symptoms and the high compliance expected.

Treatment with Serenoa repens is very common and is driven by evidence-based practice to treat voiding and mainly storage symptoms of the lower urinary tract [18–20]. Its widespread use in clinical practice for the treatment of voiding symptoms is also described in several studies [21, 22]. Its beneficial effects are linked mainly to its pro-apoptotic and anti-proliferative properties, which are mediated by various mechanisms including inhibition of 5α-reductase, competition with dihydrotestosterone for binding to its receptor and inhibition of fibroblast-growth factor.

BDP suppositories were already found to be a safe and well-tolerated medication in previous studies [10, 11]. One-hundred percent treatment compliance and the absence of adverse reactions in our study substantiate its good safety profile also in inflammations of the lower urinary tract.

The vast majority of patients showed a clinically significant improvement of symptoms at visit 2. In fact, voiding parameters (frequency, uroflowmetry and urine stream) and perineal pain significantly improved during the study, likely with a positive effect on patients' quality of life and perception of good clinical outcome.

We were not able to define a clear trend of improvement of the parameters evaluated by DRE because of the non-standardizable nature of the assessment. However, we did observe a tendency toward normalization in temperature and consistency of the prostate. As expected, PSA levels remained stable since it is not a specific parameter for lower urinary tract inflammation.

In our patients, IPSS increased at visit 2. This was however expected as it is a consequence of the way IPSS is intended to be used in common clinical practice [14]. The mean change from baseline was 2.1 ± 7.9 ($P = 0.0767$) in patients taking only BDP and 4.7 ± 7.9 ($P<.0001$) in patients also taking SR. This may indicate a worsening of IPSS, especially in patients taking both treatments, although a temporary increase in score prior to final improvement is quite common in inflammations of the lower urinary tract [23]. In fact, IPSS is more accurate for the evaluation of voiding symptoms, whereas BDP is an

Table 3 Summary table

Variable	Treatment	
	Group A (N = 45)	Group B (N = 136)
Age	53.3 ± 15.1	51.8 ± 14.9
IPSS		
Baseline value	21.6 ± 7.2	18.3 ± 6.4
Value at visit 2	23.7 ± 6.1	23.1 ± 5.7
Change from baseline	2.1 ± 7.9	4.7 ± 7.9
Test of change from baseline	$P = 0.0767$	$P < .0001$
Change vs baseline – test between two groups Two-Sample T-Test	$P = 0.0593$	
Voiding frequency (n/day)		
Baseline value	7.7 ± 2.5	7.8 ± 2.1
Value at visit 2	4.2 ± 1.4	4.1 ± 1.9
Change from baseline	−3.5 ± 2.7	−3.6 ± 2.8
Test of change from baseline	$P < .0001$	$P < .0001$
Change vs baseline – test between two groups Two-Sample T-Test	$P = 0.8560$	
Uroflowmetry (ml/s)		
Baseline value	13.1 ± 6.5	11.6 ± 3.8
Value at visit 2	16.4 ± 6.7	17.2 ± 6.5
Change from baseline	3.2 ± 5.3	5.6 ± 7.3
Test of change from baseline	$P = 0.0002$	$P < .0001$
Change vs baseline – test between two groups Two-Sample T-Test	$P = 0.0638$	
Voided volume and post voided residual PVR (ml)		
Baseline value	98.7 ± 20.5 45 ± 9.7	112.7 ± 19.3 51 ± 9.3
Value at visit 2	137.3 ± 33.9 32.4 ± 9.9	139.2 ± 25.3 30.1 ± 12.0
Change from baseline	38.6 ± 26.3 12.6 ± 9.1	26.5 ± 23.7 20.9 ± 11.4
Test of change from baseline	$P = 0.0002$	$P < .0001$
Change vs baseline – test between two groups Two-Sample T-Test	$P = 0.0478$	
Perineal pain		
Baseline value	3.2 ± 1.8	3.8 ± 2.0
Value at visit 2	2.5 ± 1.2	2.4 ± 1.1
Change from baseline	−0.6 ± 2.2	−1.3 ± 2.4
Test of change from baseline	$P = 0.0699$	$P < .0001$
Change vs baseline – test between two groups Two-Sample T-Test	$P = 0.0787$	
PSA		
Baseline value	2.8 ± 2.3	3.6 ± 3.5
Value visit 2	2.9 ± 2.1	3.1 ± 2.4
Change from baseline	0.1 ± 2.5	−0.5 ± 3.7
Test of change from baseline	0.5837	0.5036
Change vs baseline – test between two groups Two-Sample T-Test	$P = 0.3613$	

anti-inflammatory medication and is therefore meant to act mainly on symptoms of the lower urinary tract defined as storage symptoms [24]. Secondly, IPSS echoes the patient's symptoms in the last 4 weeks and does not reflect the 1-day status at visit 2. Therefore, a complete remission of the lower urinary tract inflammation at visit 2 may not be related to an evident improvement in IPSS. Moreover, despite the fact that IPSS is a validated questionnaire, it reflects the patient's feelings and is surely less objective than the other tests performed [25]. As a last comment, we prevented adding bias to this study by not prescribing any alpha-blockers; this choice was made based on the evidence that a lower urinary tract inflammatory disease has to be treated to improve the patients' symptoms [26]. Consequently, IPSS is a tool more suitable for evaluating the long-term outcome of a medical or surgical treatment rather than for the first control after a course of therapy with an anti-inflammatory medication [27].

Given that a significant number of patients took both BDP and SR, we decided to perform a post-hoc analysis in order to exclude any confounding results consequent to the association therapy; none of the comparisons between groups of all the parameters evaluated (voiding frequency, uroflowmetry, perineal pain, IPSS and PSA) were found to be statistically significant. These results confirm the positive effects of BDP suppositories in the treatment of lower urinary tract inflammation. As this is the very first study of its kind, the effectiveness of BDP in lower urinary tract inflammation should be confirmed in a randomized, double-blinded, prospective study.

Conclusion

Beclomethasone dipropionate proved to be a safe and tolerable drug for treating lower urinary tract inflammations as no adverse events or adverse reactions were reported during the course of the study. All the main parameters (voiding frequency, uroflowmetry, urine stream, perineal pain) improved, except for an increase in IPSS. No significant differences were observed between patients treated with only beclomethasone dipropionate and those also treated with serenoa repens. Although randomized, controlled studies are required to substantiate these findings, our preliminary clinical observations support the use of beclomethasone dipropionate rectal suppositories in male patients affected by lower urinary tract inflammation.

Abbreviations
BDP, Beclomethasone dipropionate; DRE, Digital rectal examination; IPSS, International Prostate Symptom Score; PSA, Prostate Specific Antigen; PVR, Post voided residual; SR, Serenoa repens.

Acknowledgements
The authors would like to thank SOFAR S.p.A for their funding of data analysis and the writing of the manuscript.

Funding
From SOFAR S.p.A for data analysis and the writing of the manuscript.

Authors' contributions
GB has made the study design and the critical review. GB, MP, NB and GT have been involved in data interpretation, performed the statistical analysis and drafting the manuscript. GL has been involved in data collection. MS and AM have reviewed the references. GT and GL have been involved in tables drawn. GG and AM have reviewed the manuscript. All authors read and approved the final manuscript.

Competing interests
Dr. Bozzini reports personal fees from SOFAR S.p.A. for data analysis and the writing of this paper. He also reports grants and non-financial support not related to the submitted work. Topster® is also a product of SOFAR.

Author details
[1]Departmentt of Urology, Humanitas Mater Domini, Via Gerenzano 2, I - 21053 Castellanza, Varese, Italy. [2]Humanitas University, Milan, Italy. [3]Department of Urology, Humanitas Research Hospital, Milan, Italy.

References

1. Rees J, Abrahams M, Doble A, Cooper A. Prostatitis Expert Reference Group (PERG). Diagnosis and treatment of chronic bacterial prostatitis and chronic prostatitis/chronic pelvic pain syndrome: a consensus guideline. BJU Int. 2015 Feb 24; doi:10.1111/bju.13101.
2. Gurunadha Rao Tunuguntla HS, Evans CP. Management of prostatitis. Prostate Cancer and Prostatic Dis. 2002;5(3):172–9.
3. Collins MM, Stafford RS, O'Leary MP, Barry MJ. How common is prostatitis? A national survey of physician visits. J Urol. 1998;159:1224–8.
4. Artibani W, Pesce F, Prezioso D, Scarpa RM, Zattoni F, Tubaro A, Rizzi CA, Santini AM, Simoni L. FLOW study group. Italian validation of the urogenital distress inventory and its application in LUTS patients. Eur Urol. 2006;50(6):1323–9.
5. Bartoletti R, Cai T, Mondaini N, et al. Prevalence, incidence estimation, risk factors and characterization of chronic prostatitis/chronic pelvic pain syndrome in urological hospital outpatients in Italy: results of a multicenter case–control observational study. J Urol. 2007;178(6):2411–5.
6. Wagenlehner Florian ME et al. Prostatitis and Male Pelvic Pain Syndrome. Dtsch Arztebl Int. 2009;106(11):175–83.
7. Öztekin I et al. Therapeutic Effects of Oligonol, Acupuncture, and Quantum Light Therapy in Chronic Nonbacterial Prostatitis. Evid Based Complement Alternat Med. 2015;2015:687196.
8. Yang MG, Zhao XK, Wu ZP, et al. Corticoid combined with an antibiotic for chronic nonbacterial prostatitis. Zhonghua Nan Ke Xue. 2009;15(3):237–40.
9. Talbot M, Bates S. Variability of the symptoms of chronic abacterial prostatitis/chronic pelvic pain syndrome during intermittent therapy with rectal prednisolone foam for ulcerative colitis. Int J STD AIDS. 2001;12(11):752–3.
10. Fascì Spurio F et al. Low Bioavailability and Traditional Systemic Steroids in IBD: Can the Former Take Over the Latter? Gastrointestin Liver Dis. 2013;22(1):65–71.
11. Campieri M. New steroids and new salicylates in inflammatory bowel disease: a critical appraisal. Gut. 2002;50(Suppl III):iii43–6.
12. Kumana CR, Seaton T, Meghji M, Castelli M, Benson R, Sivakumaran T. Beclomethasone dipropionate enemas for treating inflammatory bowel disease without producing Cushing's syndrome or hypothalamic pituitary adrenal suppression. Lancet. 1982;1(8272):579–83.
13. Cohen RD1, Dalal SR. Systematic Review: Rectal Therapies for the Treatment of Distal Forms of Ulcerative Colitis. Inflamm Bowel Dis. 2015 May 27. [Epub ahead of print].
14. Barry MJ, Fowler Jr FJ, O'Leary MP, Bruskewitz RC, Holtgrewe HL, Mebust WK, Cockett AT. The American Urological Association symptom index for benign prostatic hyperplasia. The Measurement Committee of the American Urological Association. Journal of Urology. 1992;148(5):1549–57.
15. Naber KG, Bergman B, Bishop MC, Bjerklund-Johansen TE, Botto H, Lobel B, Jinenez Cruz F, Selvaggi FP. EAU guidelines for the management of urinary and male genital tract infections. Eur Urol. 2001;40(5):576–88.
16. Grabe M, Bartoletti R, Bjerklund Johansen TE, Cai T, Çek M, Köves B, Naber KG, Pickard RS, Tenke P, Wagenlehner F, Wullt B. Guidelines on Urological Infections. http://uroweb.org/guideline/urological-infections/. Accessed 04 Aug 2015.
17. Bernichtein S et al. Anti-Inflammatory properties of Lipidosterolic extract of Serenoa repens (Permixon®) in a mouse model of prostate hyperplasia. Prostate. 2015;75(7):706–22.
18. Debruyne F, Boyle P, Calais Da Silva F, Gillenwater JG, Hamdy FC, Perrin P, Teillac P, Vela-Navarrete R, Raynaud JP, Schulman CC. Evaluation of the clinical benefit of permixon and tamsulosin in severe BPH patients-PERMAL study subset analysis. Eur Urol. 2004;45(6):773–9. discussion 779–80.
19. Debruyne F, Koch G, Boyle P, Da Silva FC, Gillenwater JG, Hamdy FC, Perrin P, Teillac P, Vela-Navarrete R, Raynaud JP. Comparison of a phytotherapeutic agent (Permixon) with an alpha-blocker (Tamsulosin) in the treatment of benign prostatic hyperplasia: a 1-year randomized international study. Eur Urol. 2002;41(5):497–506. discussion 506–7.
20. Latil A, Pétrissans MT, Rouquet J, Robert G, de la Taille A. Effects of hexanic extract of serenoa repens (permixon(®) 160 mg) on inflammation biomarkers in the treatment of lower urinary tract symptoms related to benign prostatic hyperplasia. Prostate. 2015;75(16):1857–67.
21. Magri V, Marras E, Restelli A, Wagenlehner FM, Perletti G. Multimodal therapy for category III chronic prostatitis/chronic pelvic pain syndrome in UPOINTS phenotyped patients. Exp Ther Med. 2015;9(3):658–66.
22. Morgia G et al. Serenoa repens, lycopene and selenium versus tamsulosin for the treatment of LUTS/BPH. An Italian multicenter double-blinded randomized study between single or combination therapy (PROCOMB trial). Prostate. 2014;74(15):1471–80.
23. Lee HN, Kim TH, Lee SJ, Cho WY, Shim BS. Effects of prostatic inflammation on LUTS and alpha blocker treatment outcomes. Int Braz J Urol. 2014;40(3):356–66.
24. Haylen BT, de Ridder D, Freeman RM, Swift SE, Berghmans B, Lee J, Monga A, Petri E, Rizk DE, Sand PK, Schaer GN. IUGA/ICS Joint Report On The Terminology For Female Pelvic Floor Dysfunction: Standardisation and Terminology Committees IUGA and ICS, Joint IUGA/ICS Working Group on Female Terminology. Neurourol Urodyn. 2010;29(1):4–20.
25. Matsukawa Y, Hattori K, Sassa N, Yamamoto T, Gotoh M. What are the factors contributing to failure in improvement of subjective symptoms following silodosin administration in patients with benign prostatic hyperplasia? Investigation using a pressure-flow study. Neurourol Urodyn. 2013;32(3):266–70.
26. Park SG, Chung BH, Lee SW, Park JK, Park K, Cheon J, Lee KS, Kim HJ, Seong DH, Oh SJ, Kim SW, Lee JY, Choo SH, Choi JB. Alpha-blocker treatment response in men with lower urinary tract symptoms based on sympathetic activity: prospective multicenter open-Labeled observational study. Int Neurourol J. 2015;19(2):107–12.
27. Fujimura T et al. Assessment of lower urinary tract symptoms in men by international prostate symptom score and core lower urinary tract symptom score. BJU Int. 2012;109(10):1512–6.

Role for intravesical prostatic protrusion in lower urinary tract symptom: a fluid structural interaction analysis study

Junming Zheng[1], Jiangang Pan[1], Yi Qin[1], Jiale Huang[2], Yun Luo[3], Xin Gao[3] and Xing Zhou[1*]

Abstract

Background: Numerous studies indicated that Intravesical prostatic protrusion is relevant to prognosis of LUTS, however, the confounding effect that is brought about by prostate volume, urethra anterior curvature angle and other factors makes it hard to evaluate the role of intravesical prostatic protrusion in clinical observation.

Methods: We proposed a fluid structural interaction analysis approach. 3D models were constructed based on MRI images, and prostatic urethra diameters were calibrated with urodynamic data. Comparisons of urine flow dynamics were made between models with various degree of intravesical prostatic protrusion, while the intravesical pressure, anterior urethra curvature angle and diameter of prostatic urethra were same among all models to rule out their confounding effects.

Results: Simulation result showed that the decrement of diameter and increment of variation in cross-sectional area for prostatic urethra were related to the degree of intravesical prostatic protrusion. Such deformation would lead to deterioration of flow efficiency and could compromise the effect of bladder outlet obstruction alleviation treatment.

Conclusions: These results provided further evidence for intravesical prostatic protrusion being an independent risk factor for bladder outlet obstruction severity and demonstrated that intravesical prostatic protrusion would be a promising marker in clinical decision making.

Background

Intravesical prostatic protrusion (IPP) is the extent to which the prostate protrudes into the bladder, defined as distance from protruded prostate to the base of bladder, and can be measured in midline sagittal plane of the prostate [1]. Population based data indicated that 10 % of male between 40 to 79 years old had an IPP of 10 mm or greater [2]. IPP is considered as a prognostic factor for LUTS [3, 4]. And the fact that IPP can be evaluated with non-invasive trans-abdominal ultra-sound made it a promising candidate for initial assessment of LUTS patient [5]. But the mechanism underlying the relationship between IPP and bladder outlet obstruction is still unclear. One key issue the confounding effect caused

by prostate volume variation and urethra curvature angle. Because they are both risk factors for LUTS severity and are closely related with IPP, it is difficult to control these confounding factors with observational study. Computational modeling on the other hand, is a promising alternate, and would shed a light on understanding the role for IPP in bladder outlet obstruction.

Hydraulic energy is the driven force in voiding process. It is lost due to resistance of urethra. Accurate reconstruction of anatomical feature for lower urinary tract is crucial for calculation of hydraulic energy loss. Computational fluid dynamic (CFD) study was proved to be advantageous in such aspect [6–8]. However, rigid wall boundary assumption in previous studies ruled out the interaction between urine flow and urethra wall movement, especially prostatic urethra wall. To overcome this limitation and investigate the role for IPP in bladder outlet obstruction, we carried out a fluid structural interaction analysis in models reconstructed from MRI data

* Correspondence: ZhouxingZh@126.com
[1]Department of Urology, The Second Affiliated Hospital of Guangzhou Medical University, 250 Changgang road, Guangzhou 510260, China
Full list of author information is available at the end of the article

with various degree of IPP, then compared the difference in flow efficiency among these models.

Methods

The model and boundary conditions

A retrospective revision of the clinical data for all patients, presenting with lower urinary tract symptoms secondary to benign prostate hyperplasia (LUTS/BPH), who also completed MRI scan of pelvic region and pressure flow study before surgery, in the time period from January 2000 to December 2014 was carried out. Diagnosis of LUTS/BPH was established if criteria of the 5th International Consensus Committee on BPH [9] was met. The data from MRI scanning (Discovery MR750, GE Healthcare) are needed for model reconstruction, and the pressure flow study are needed for calibration of arbitrary determined parameters of the model. Patients with a history of neurogenic bladder, previous pelvic surgery or urinary cancer were excluded, detrusor insufficiency was also ruled out. Ten male patients were included for the study after providing informed consent. Approval for the study was granted by the ethics committee of Second Affiliated Hospital of Guangzhou Medical University.

Organ contouring for prostate, bladder and surrounding connective tissue was done in Mimics (Materialise, Leuven Belgium) by studying axial T2 MRI images of each patient. This was conducted by one senior urologist and confirmed by another radiologist. Degree of IPP was measured in mid-sagittal plane. First a line was drawn from the anterior to posterior intersections of the bladder base and prostate, then the distance between the protruded prostate to this line is defined as IPP (Fig. 1a, f), and categorized as grade I(<5 mm), grade II(5 ~ 10 mm) and grade III(>10 mm) [10]. Then three-dimensional models were constructed from contouring region of each slice (Fig. 1e), and optimized (Fig. 1f) with SolidWorks (DS Solidworks, Massachusetts, USA).

Since prostatic urethra can't be clearly identified in MRI images [11], model was reconstructed with arbitrary parameters. The urethra model was divided into three parts. The proximal part (Fig. 2a) was a translational zone from bladder to urethra, 10 mm in length with a diameter decreasing from the width of normal bladder neck(8 mm) to prostatic urethra width [6]. The distal part (Fig. 2a) was another 10 mm long translational zone between distal prostatic and anterior urethra. The urethra in-between started at bladder neck, curved anteriorly at veru montanum and ended near at the prostatic apex [11]. These key points were marked specifically during organ contouring to define a fitting spline that would be closest to the prostatic urethra course (Fig. 1a-d). Then this part of urethra was modeled as a cylindrical structure running along the spline.

The diameter for anterior urethra($d_{urethra}$) was set to 5 and 4 mm for meatus, corresponding to the average cross-sectional area of around 20 mm^2 for anterior urethra [12, 13]. Diameter for prostatic urethra during voiding process was a parameter paramount for accurate simulation. The value should be between 1 mm and the diameter of anterior urethra [14]. Five candidate diameters (1, 1.5, 2, 3 and 4 mm) were proposed for initial diameter of prostatic urethra ($d_{prostate}$). Result of Abrams-Griffiths nomogram in our pilot study showed that these 5 candidate diameter covers the pressure-flow relationship from obstructed to unobstructed scenario (Additional file 1: Figure S1). This coincided with previous result [15]. In this way, we could preserve the anatomic feature of anterior urethra curvature, and find the optimum diameter which would represent the obstruction level in prostatic urethra at the same time.

Fluid structural interaction analysis in ANSYS (ANSYS, Inc. Canonsburg, USA) was employed to study the deformation of prostate and its influence on urine flow. Boundary conditions were configured as follows (Fig. 1f): (1) Superior wall of bladder was set as inlet with preset total pressure; (2) Meatus of the urethra was set as outlet with 1 atm (101,325 Pa) static pressure; (3) Fluid-structural interface region included the bladder wall which lay over the protruded prostate, the surrounding connective tissue, the bladder neck and prostatic urethra; (4) Fixed support was added to the lateral wall of prostate and the surrounding connective tissue, representing the supportive structure around the prostate, along with fascia and pelvic supportive structures. The properties of the fluid were set as water. Pilot studies indicated that for all models in our simulation, the reynolds number, defined as $Re = \rho vd/\eta$ (ρ is the density of fluid, η is the dynamic viscosity of fluid, v and d are the velocity and hydraulic diameter of flow, respectively), range from 7000 to 13,000 (Additional file 2: Table S1), which were greater than 4000. So κ-ε turbulence model was used for CFD analysis. For the structural analysis, prostate was assumed to be linear elastic [16] (Poisson ratio:0.4, Young's modulus: 21kPa). The same assumption was applied to connective tissue (Poisson ratio:0.4, Young's modulus:15kPa).

Simulation planning

By adopting five candidate diameter of prostatic urethra to all ten patients, 50 candidate models were reconstructed. Intravesical pressure (P_{ves}) measured at maximal urine flow rate (V_m) was used as total pressure for inlet, then flow rate (V_c) was calculated with fluid structural analysis model. Bladder volume was set to be more than 200 ml in all models. Calculated flow rate (V_c) and measured flow rate (V_m) were compared to select the optimal $d_{prostate}$.

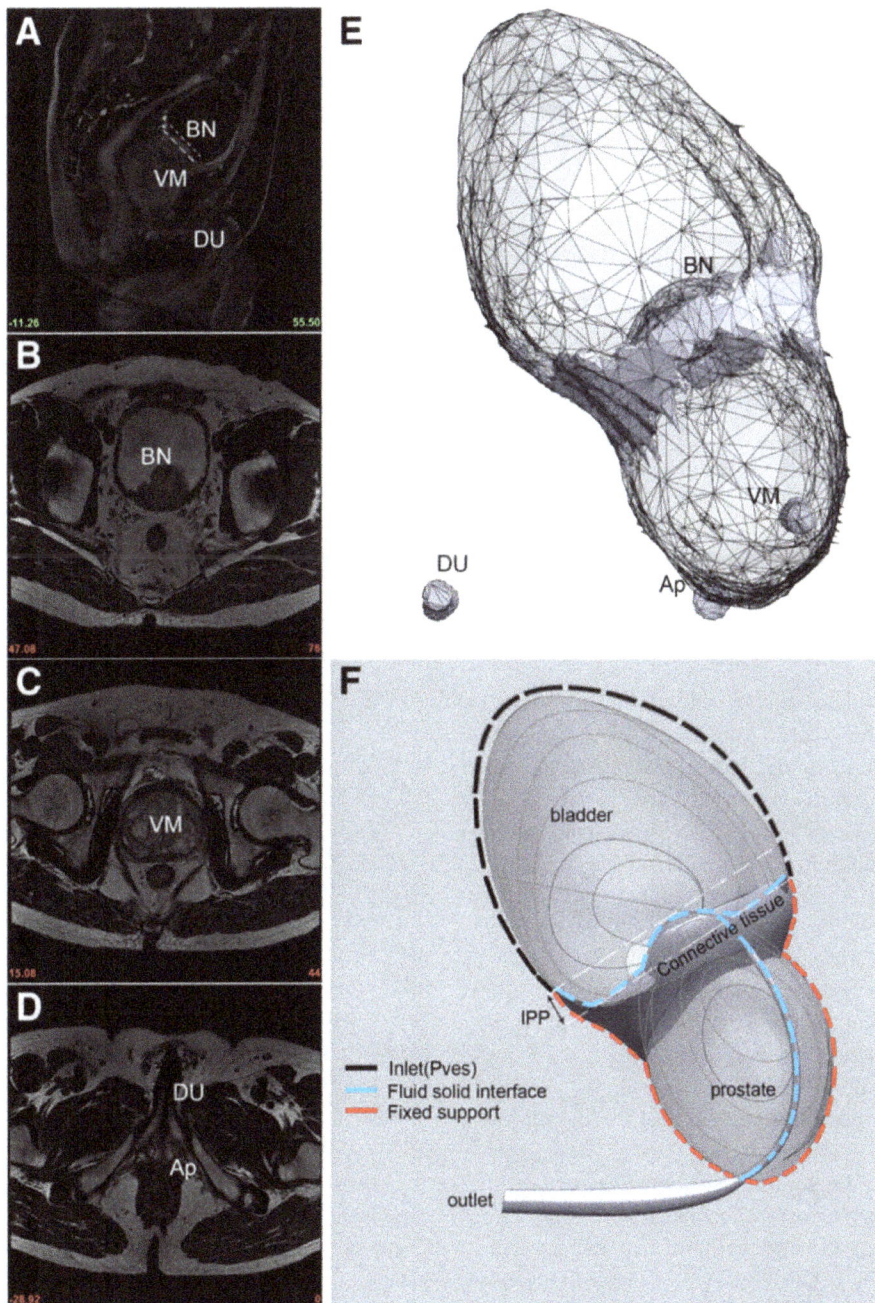

Fig. 1 Prostate and bladder model construction MR images of lower urinary tract were collected (**a** sagittal plane, **b-d** axial plane, **b** bladder neck, **c**: veru montanum, **d** prostatic apex), and 3D model were reconstructed from organ contouring (**e**), and optimized (**f**). Measurement for IPP was shown in dash line in A and F. VM: veru montanum, BN: bladder neck, Ap: prostate apex, U: anterior urethra

One model from a patient with grade 2 IPP was selected by random, and marked as model 2. Another two models with different grades of IPP were created by adjusting the shape of the protruded part. These two models were marked as model 1 (grade 1 IPP model) and model 3 (grade 3 IPP model). Shape of the bladder neck, prostatic urethra diameter and anterior urethra curvature angle were same among three models (Additional file 3:

Figure S2). Same boundary conditions were applied to all models. For each model, Fluid structural interaction(FSI) analysis were conducted under three different inlet pressure(7840.8, 17081.1, 13721.4 Pa), results of prostatic deformation and flow efficiency were compared among three models. Then, to simulate the obstruction alleviated scenario, initial diameter of prostatic urethra was increased to 2 and 3 mm, respectively. Then urine flow

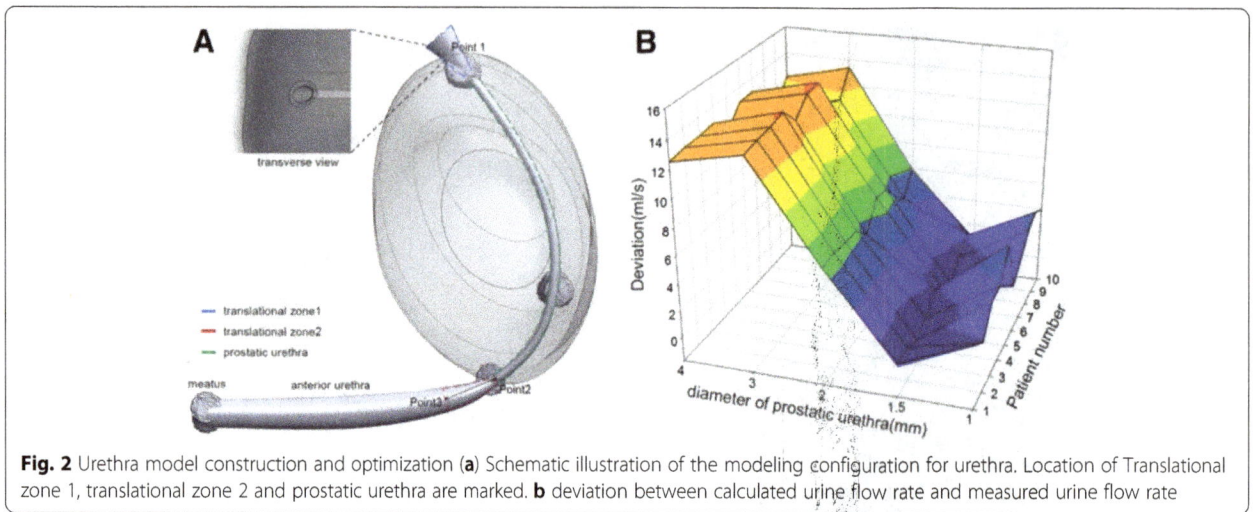

Fig. 2 Urethra model construction and optimization (**a**) Schematic illustration of the modeling configuration for urethra. Location of Translational zone 1, translational zone 2 and prostatic urethra are marked. **b** deviation between calculated urine flow rate and measured urine flow rate

rate was recalculated under the intravesical pressure of 80cmH2O (7480.8 Pa).

Results

The demographic data of ten patients was listed in Table 1. Pressure flow data (Additional file 4: Table S2) showed that mean maximal urine flow rate(Q_{max}) was 9.5 ml (7 ~ 12 ml), detrusor pressure at Q_{max} ($P_{det,Qmax}$) was 56.7 cmH2O (42 ~ 70 cmH2O), voided volume was 188.5 ml (153 ~ 245 ml). This result indicated that all patients can be categorized as obstructed according to Blaivas' criteria [17]. For each patient, a model was constructed using MRI images, and urine flow rate was calculated. The deviation between calculated and measured flow rate in each candidate model were charted in a 3D mesh. Minimal deviation was acquired when $d_{prostate}$ = 1.5 mm, and maximal deviation was found when $d_{prostate}$ = 3 mm (Fig. 2b). Initial diameter of prostatic urethra for model 1, model 2 and model 3 were set to be 1.5 mm.

During voiding, we found that deformation of the prostate would lead to urethra constriction (Fig. 3a-c), and its magnitude increased with intravesical pressure. The constriction of urethra was most prominent near bladder neck, then loosened gradually and returned to its initial diameter at prostatic apex. Under each intravesical pressure, urethra diameter of different models was

Table 1 Patient demographics

measure	Mean	Minimal-maximal
Sample size	10	
Age	64.1	59–70
Prostate volume(ml)	92.3	53.5–115.3
Intravesical protrusion(mm)	8.67	3.2–12.3
Maximal flow rate(ml/s)	9.5	7–12
Pves at maximal flow rate(Pa)	10,046	8722.89–11271.15

compared. Such comparison leads to an interesting discovery. In region near bladder neck, the widest urethra was found in model 1 (**grade 1 IPP model**), followed by model 2 and model 3(grade 3 IPP model), but this order was reversed in distal prostatic urethra. Such pattern of constriction indicated that the variation of cross sectional area for urethra was most prominent in model 3, and lowest in model 1 (Fig. 3d-f).

Total pressure, defined as $P = \frac{\rho}{2}\bar{v}^2 + \bar{p}$, was a combination of static pressure and dynamic pressure, often used to evaluate flow efficiency. As urine flow runs from bladder to urethra meatus, total pressure decreased due to urethra resistance. In our simulation, such pressure loss was most prominent in model 3 (Fig. 4a-c), most of which occurred in the constricted urethra near bladder neck. In the other two models, less total pressure was loss around the bladder neck. For these two models, the majority of total pressure loss took place in distal prostatic urethra (Fig. 4d-f).

Vorticity, defined as curl of velocity [18]: $\omega = \nabla \times \vec{v}$, was used to study the pattern of flow energy dissipation. Consistent with pattern in total pressure loss, highest magnitude of vorticity for model 3 was found in bladder neck region while the highest vorticity magnitude for model 1 located in veru montanum and prostatic apex (Fig. 4g).

Flow velocity reached its peak as urine run through bladder neck, and then it decreased gradually (Fig. 5a-c). Histograms for flow velocity distribution in sagittal plane were compared among models (Fig. 5d-f). For each model, two peaks were found, corresponding to flow velocity in prostatic urethra and anterior urethra, respectively. Comparison among models indicated that flow velocity in majority part of model 1 was higher than the other two models.

Urine flow rate at the urethra meatus in model 1 was greater than the other two models, and increasing

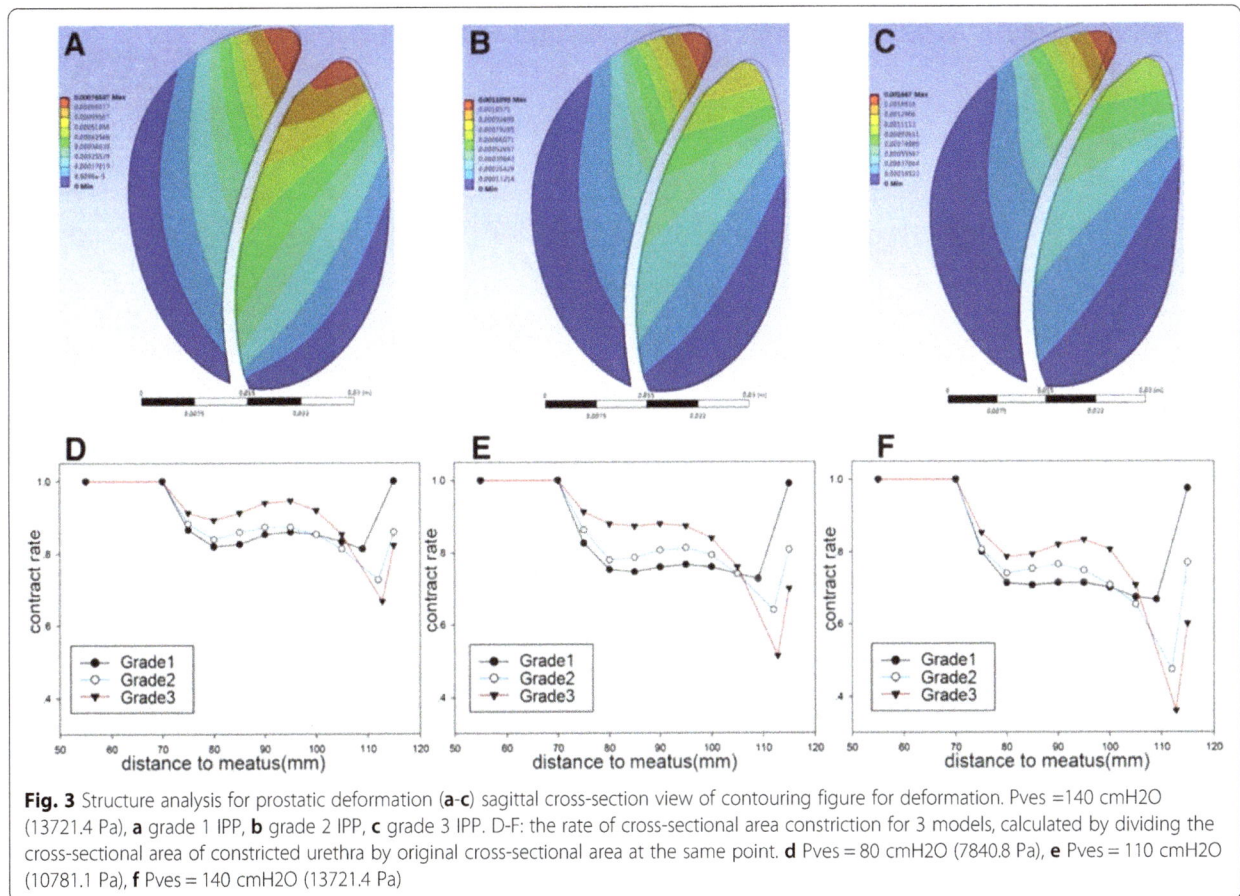

Fig. 3 Structure analysis for prostatic deformation (a-c) sagittal cross-section view of contouring figure for deformation. Pves =140 cmH2O (13721.4 Pa), **a** grade 1 IPP, **b** grade 2 IPP, **c** grade 3 IPP. D-F: the rate of cross-sectional area constriction for 3 models, calculated by dividing the cross-sectional area of constricted urethra by original cross-sectional area at the same point. **d** Pves = 80 cmH2O (7840.8 Pa), **e** Pves = 110 cmH2O (10781.1 Pa), **f** Pves = 140 cmH2O (13721.4 Pa)

intravesical pressure would further widen this gap (Fig. 5g). Then, to simulate obstruction alleviated scenario, prostatic urethra diameter was increased to 2 and 3 mm for the three models. Urine flow rate was calculated in the diameter increased models under the pressure of 80 cmH2O (7840.8 Pa). We found that urine flow rate in all models increased as initial urethra diameter widen, but at different rates. The gap in flow rate between model 1 and model 3 went up to 4 ml/s when the diameter was 2 mm. Then it went down to 1 ml/s when diameter was 3 mm (Fig. 5h).

Discussion

In patient with LUTS symptom, the confounding effect between prostate volumes, anterior urethra curvature angle, detrusor muscle contractility and intravesical prostatic protrusion (IPP) make it hard to understand IPP's role with clinical observation. Invasive methods such as pressure flow study are generally not applicable to routine clinical practice. Computational fluid dynamic(CFD) was already proved to be an effective method in investigating flow dynamic in studies regarding airway flow [19], circulation [20] and urine transport [21]. It is an attractive alternative to elucidate the role for IPP in LUTS manifestation.

This is the first study to investigate voiding behavior of lower urinary tract with fluid structural interaction analysis (FSI) and provide a scope for better understanding of prostate deformation. Our results showed that intravesical pressure above 7840.8 Pa was enough to cause prominent deformation of the prostate in model 3, which would lead to constriction of prostatic urethra. Clinical studies showed that maximum intravesical pressure in LUTS patient is usually between 8820.9 to 14701.5 Pa [22, 23]. So it was obvious that for LUTS patient with severe intravesical prostatic protrusion, intravesical pressure during voiding would cause the prostatic deformation which would lead to severe constriction of prostatic urethra.

Structural analysis showed that the most severe constriction in bladder neck and greatest variation of cross-sectional area for urethra were found in model 3. The anatomy feature of fascia surrounding the prostate might shed light on this. Prostate was attached anteriorly by pubo-prostatic ligaments, laterally by endopelvic-fascia, and posteriorly by Denonvilliers' fascia [24]. As these supportive structures go superiorly, they fuse with other fascia, leaving the protruded portion of the prostate susceptible to radial component of intravesical pressure. And this may be the underlying cause for the difference in deformation between three models.

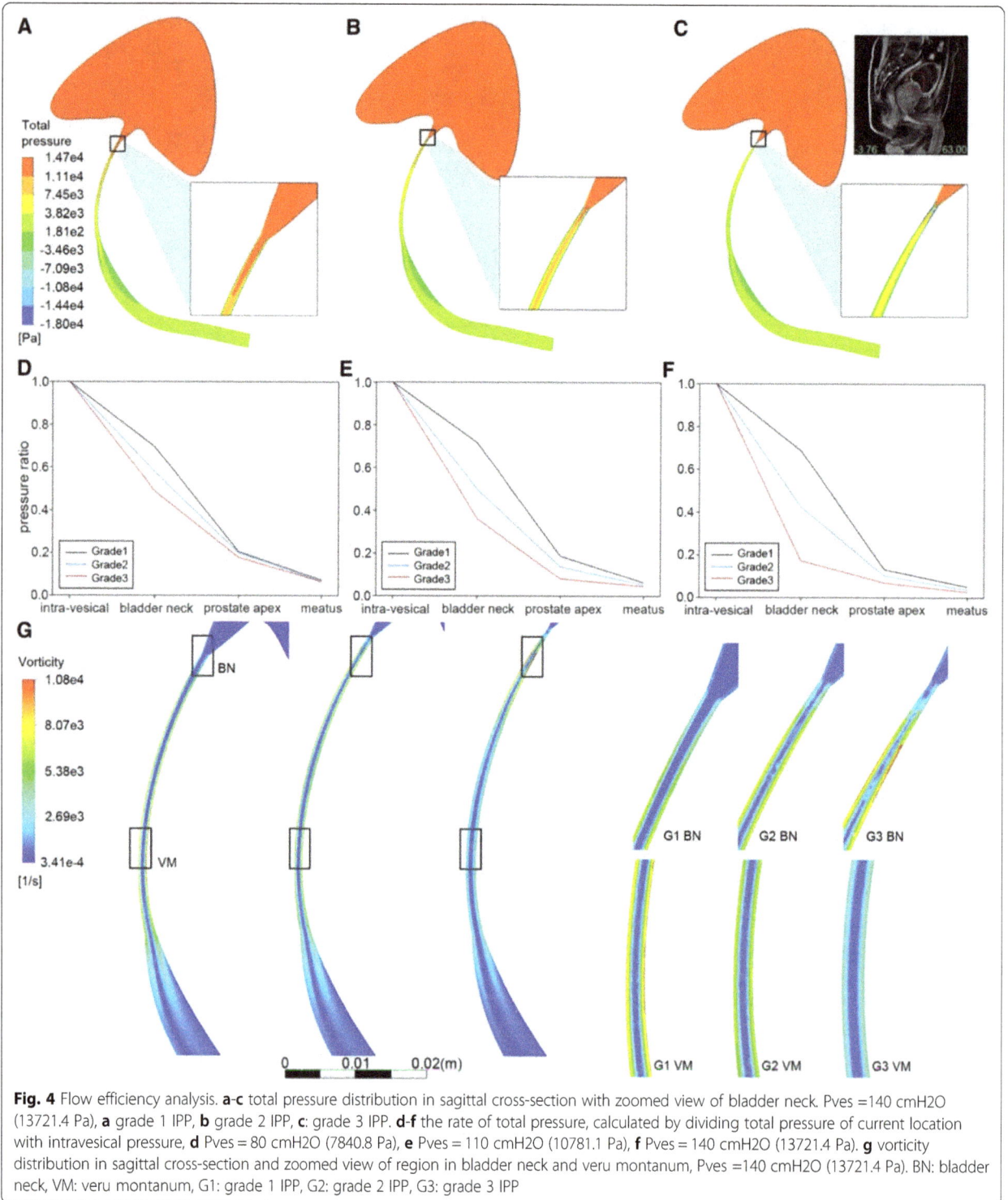

Fig. 4 Flow efficiency analysis. **a-c** total pressure distribution in sagittal cross-section with zoomed view of bladder neck. Pves =140 cmH2O (13721.4 Pa), **a** grade 1 IPP, **b** grade 2 IPP, **c**: grade 3 IPP. **d-f** the rate of total pressure, calculated by dividing total pressure of current location with intravesical pressure, **d** Pves = 80 cmH2O (7840.8 Pa), **e** Pves = 110 cmH2O (10781.1 Pa), **f** Pves = 140 cmH2O (13721.4 Pa). **g** vorticity distribution in sagittal cross-section and zoomed view of region in bladder neck and veru montanum, Pves =140 cmH2O (13721.4 Pa). BN: bladder neck, VM: veru montanum, G1: grade 1 IPP, G2: grade 2 IPP, G3: grade 3 IPP

The variation for urethral cross-sectional area in model 3 was the main reason for its flow energy dissipation [25]. Such variation was most prominent near the bladder neck, which coincided with the distribution of pressure loss and vorticity magnitude. As degree of intravesical protrusion decreased, location for major pressure loss shifted towards distal part of prostatic urethra, and the amount of total pressure drop also decreased. Since factors other than intravesical prostatic protrusion were same among three models, our results indicated that intravesical prostatic protrusion could affect the flow efficiency independently.

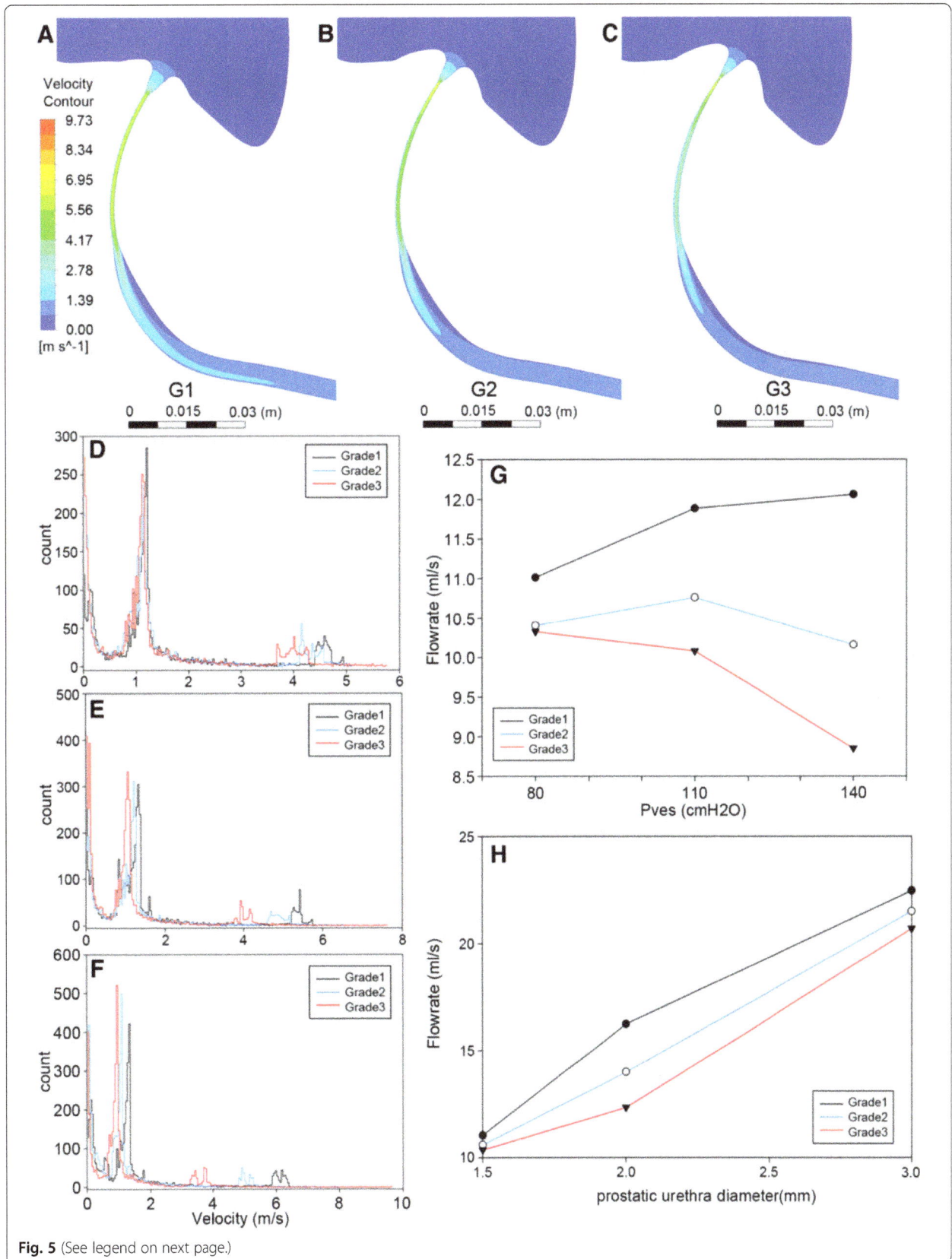

Fig. 5 (See legend on next page.)

(See figure on previous page.)
Fig. 5 Flow velocity and flow rate analysis. **a-c** sagittal cross-section view of contouring figure for flow velocity, Pves =140 cmH2O, **a** grade 1 IPP, **b** grade 2 IPP, **c** grade 3 IPP. **d-f** histogram of flow velocity for three models. **d** Pves = 80 cmH2O (7840.8 Pa), **e** Pves = 110 cmH2O (10781.1 Pa), **f** Pves = 140 cmH2O (13721.4 Pa). **g** flow rate for all models under each particular intravesical pressure in our simulation. **h** flow rate for models with increased initial urethra diameter, calculated under the intravesical pressure of 80 cm (7840.8 Pa)

A non-linear relationship between intravesical pressure and maximum urine flow rate (Q_{max}) was found in our simulation. While flow rate in model 1 increased along with intravesical pressure, it decreased in model 3. This was clinical relevant since patient with LUTS often tend to strain to pass urine. The results in our study demonstrated that for patients with grade 3 intravesical prostatic protrusion (IPP), this could further aggravate the symptom of weak urine stream, while the increased intra-abdominal pressure predispose patients to complications including hernia and hemorrhoids [26, 27].

The simulation result for obstruction alleviated scenario also suggested that treatment outcome differs between patients with different grade of intravesical prostatic protrusion. Although a major relieve of obstruction could greatly increase the flow efficiency for all models, the raise in flow rate for model 3 was only half of that for model 1 when the relief of obstruction was relatively minor. This coincide with the finding that alpha blocker treatment is more effective in patients with mild IPP than in those with moderate or severe IPP [28].

Although our work presents some interesting finding, there are some limitations. All models were constructed and adjusted based on data acquired from Asian patients retrospectively which need confirmation in a larger population involving African and Caucasian patients. The future scope of our research is to confirm the relationship between FSI results and treatment response through a larger multicenter study.

Conclusions

3D model of lower urinary tract was constructed from MRI images and adjusted according to urodynamic data. Fluid-structural interaction analysis was implemented. Results demonstrated that intravesical prostatic protrusion (IPP) predisposed the prostate to the deformation caused by intravesical pressure. The constriction of prostatic urethra and increased variation of cross-sectional area around bladder neck would lead to deterioration of urine flow efficiency, and compromise the effect of obstruction alleviation treatment. This study provided further evidence suggesting that IPP influence bladder outlet obstruction independently, and the flow efficiency deterioration was more resistant to obstruction alleviation treatment as the degree of IPP increased.

Additional files

Additional file 1: Figure S1. The relationship between pressure and flow rate for five sets of prostatic urethra diameters.

Additional file 2: Table S1. Reynolds number of each patient was calculated for all five candidate urethra diameters.

Additional file 3: Figure S2. A: Cross section in sagittal plane showing the original model (model 2) and the other two models (model 1 and model 3) share the same urethral path, B: 3 models have the same initial shape for bladder neck.

Additional file 4: Table S2. Result for pressure flow studies.

Abbreviations
IPP: Intravesical prostatic protrusion; LUTS: Lower urinary tract symptom; LUTS/BPH: Lower urinary tract symptom secondary to benign prostatic hyperplasia; FSI: Fluid structural interaction analysis; CFD: Computational fluid dynamic; MRI: Magnetic Resonance Imaging; atm: The standard atmosphere; Q_{max}: Maximal urine flow rate; $P_{det,Qmax}$: Detrusor pressure at maximal urine flow rate; P_{ves}: Intravesical pressure; 3D: Three dimensional.

Competing interests
The authors declare that they have no competing interests.

Authors' contributions
In this study, XZ designed the research study; JZ wrote the paper; JZ and JH performed the model reconstruction and FSI analysis; WX and JP help in organ contouring and result revision. YQ, YL and XG gather medical data. All authors read and approved the final manuscript.

Acknowledgments
The authors would like to thank Qiaozhen Zhang for help in patient medical record collection. This study was supported by Guangdong Science and Technology Planning Project (2013B021800199) and project (2011B031800030).

Author details
[1]Department of Urology, The Second Affiliated Hospital of Guangzhou Medical University, 250 Changgang road, Guangzhou 510260, China. [2]School of Mechanical and Automotive Engineering, South China University of Technology, Guangzhou, China. [3]Department of Urology, Third Affiliated Hospital of Sun Yat-sen University, Guangzhou 510630, China.

References
1. Lee LS, Sim HG, Lim KB, Wang D, Foo KT. Intravesical prostatic protrusion predicts clinical progression of benign prostatic enlargement in patients receiving medical treatment. Int J Urol. 2010;17(1):69–74.
2. Lieber MM, Jacobson DJ, McGree ME, Sauver JLS, Girman CJ, Jacobsen SJ. Intravesical prostatic protrusion in men in Olmsted County, Minnesota. J Urol. 2009;182(6):2819–24.
3. Cumpanas AA, Botoca M, Minciu R, Bucuras V. Intravesical prostatic protrusion can be a predicting factor for the treatment outcome in patients with lower urinary tract symptoms due to benign prostatic obstruction treated with tamsulosin. Urology. 2013;81(4):859–63.
4. Mariappan P, Brown DJ, McNeill AS. Intravesical prostatic protrusion is better than prostate volume in predicting the outcome of trial without catheter in

white men presenting with acute urinary retention: a prospective clinical study. J Urol. 2007;178(2):573–7.

5. Mangera A, Chapple C. Modern evaluation of lower urinary tract symptoms in 2014. Curr Opin Urol. 2014;24(1):15–20.

6. Tojo M, Yasuda K, Yamanishi T, Hattori T, Nagashima K, Shimazaki J. Relationship between bladder neck diameter and hydraulic energy at maximum flow. J Urol. 1994;152(1):144–9.

7. Yamanishi T, Yasuda K, Sakakibara R, Hattori T, Tojo M. The effectiveness of terazosin, an α1-blocker, on bladder neck obstruction as assessed by urodynamic hydraulic energy. BJU Int. 2000;85(3):249–53.

8. Sakuyama G, Ishii T, Yamanishi T, Igarashi T. MP-09.01 Hydrodynamic Aspects of Intravesical Protrusion of the Prostate in Patients with Voiding Dysfunction. Urology. 2011;78(3):S94.

9. Roehrborn CG. Focus on lower urinary tract symptoms: nomenclature, diagnosis, and treatment options: highlights from the 5th international consultation on benign prostatic hyperplasia june 25–27, 2000, paris, france. Rev Urol. 2001;3(3):139–45.

10. Reis LO, Barreiro GC, Baracat J, Prudente A, D'Ancona CA. Intravesical protrusion of the prostate as a predictive method of bladder outlet obstruction. Int Braz J Urol. 2008;34(5):627–37.

11. Villeirs GM, Verstraete KL, De Neve WJ, De Meerleer GO. Magnetic resonance imaging anatomy of the prostate and periprostatic area: a guide for radiotherapists. Radiother Oncol. 2005;76(1):99–106.

12. Wise Jr H, Many M, Birtwell W, Eyrick T, Maguire M. Measurement of urethral resistance. Invest Urol. 1968;5(6):539–51.

13. Griffiths DJ. Urethral obstruction. In: Urodynamics. Bristol: Adam Hilger Ltd; 1980. p. 97–108.

14. Ishii T, Kambara Y, Yamanishi T, Naya Y, Igarashi T. Urine Flow Dynamics through Prostatic Urethra with Tubular Organ Modeling using Endoscopic Imagery. IEE J Transl Eng Health Med. 2014;2:1–9.

15. Pel JJ, van Mastrigt R. Development of a CFD urethral model to study flow-generated vortices under different conditions of prostatic obstruction. Physiol Meas. 2007;28(1):13.

16. Chai X, van Herk M, van de Kamer JB, Hulshof MC, Remeijer P, Lotz HT, et al. Finite element based bladder modeling for image-guided radiotherapy of bladder cancer. Med Phys. 2011;38(1):142–50.

17. Blaivas JG. Obstructive uropathy in the male. Urol Clin North Am. 1996;23(3):373–84.

18. Fox RW, McDonald AT. Introduction to fluid mechanics. 4th ed. New York: John Wiley and Sons; 1992.

19. Zhao M, Barber T, Cistulli PA, Sutherland K, Rosengarten G. Simulation of upper airway occlusion without and with mandibular advancement in obstructive sleep apnea using fluid-structure interaction. J Biomech. 2013;46(15):2586–92.

20. Faludi R, Szulik M, D'hooge J, Herijgers P, Rademakers F, Pedrizzetti G, et al. Left ventricular flow patterns in healthy subjects and patients with prosthetic mitral valves: an in vivo study using echocardiographic particle image velocimetry. J Thorac Cardiovasc Surg. 2010;139(6):1501–10.

21. Hosseini G, Williams JJ, Avital EJ, Munjiza A, Xu D, Green JA, editors. Computational simulation of urinary system. San Francisco, USA: Proc World Congress Eng Comput Sci; 2012.

22. Hung C, Lin A, Chen K, Chang L. The subjective assessment and pressure-flow study of outcome of surgical treatment for patients with prostatism and high voiding pressure. Chin Med J (Engl). 1995;56(3):186–91.

23. Lee M, Lee S, Hur N, Kim S, Choi B. Correlation between intravesical pressure and prostatic obstruction grade using computational fluid dynamics in benign prostatic hyperplasia. Proc Inst Mech Eng H. 2011;225(9):920–8.

24. Raychaudhuri B, Cahill D. Pelvic fasciae in urology. Ann R Coll Surg Engl. 2008;90(8):633.

25. Ascuitto R, Kydon D, Ross-Ascuitto N. Pressure loss from flow energy dissipation: relevance to Fontan-type modifications. Pediatr Cardiol. 2001;22(2):110–5.

26. Light HG, Routledge JA. Intra-abdominal pressure: Factor in hernia disease. Arch Surg. 1965;90(1):115–7. doi:10.1001/archsurg.1965.01320070117025.

27. Fox A, Tietze PH, Ramakrishnan K. Anorectal conditions: hemorrhoids. FP essentials. 2014;419:11–9.

28. Park HY, Lee JY, Park SY, Lee SW, Kim YT, Choi HY, et al. Efficacy of alpha blocker treatment according to the degree of intravesical prostatic protrusion detected by transrectal ultrasonography in patients with benign prostatic hyperplasia. Korean J Urol. 2012;53(2):92–7. doi:10.4111/kju.2012.53.2.92.

Wilms tumor with inferior vena cava duplication

Feng Guo[1†], Tianyou Li[1†], Wei Liu[1], Gang Wang[1], Rui Ma[2] and Rongde Wu[1*]

Abstract

Background: Wilms tumor is the most common renal tumor of childhood. Duplication of the inferior vena cava is an uncommon anomaly. In the present study, we present a case of Wilms tumor with the inferior vena cava duplication, which has not been reported previously.

Case presentation: A 14-month-old female presented with an enlarging abdominal mass. Computed tomography imaging demonstrated a large mass in the right kidney, duplication of the inferior vena cava below the renal veins and compression of the right inferior vena cava caused by the enormous mass. A right radical nephrectomy was performed. Final pathology was consistent with Wilms tumor. Postoperative adjuvant chemotherapy was executed. Computed tomography imaging at 3 months postoperatively showed the right inferior vena cava played a dominant role and the left inferior vena cava was not detected clearly. During the follow-up of 18 months, no local recurrence or metastasis has been observed.

Conclusion: It is important to recognize the case of Wilms tumor with the inferior vena cava duplication to avoid injury of retroperitoneal venous anomalies and life-threatening hemorrhage during surgery through preoperative computed tomography.

Keywords: Wilms tumor, Inferior vena cava duplication, Computed tomography

Background

Wilms tumor (WT) is the most common renal tumor in childhood. Duplication of the inferior vena cava (IVC) is an uncommon anomaly. Although it is asymptomatic and often detected incidentally by imaging, IVC duplication may represent a hazard for bleeding during surgery, such as nephrectomy. In the present study, we present a case of WT with IVC duplication, which has not been reported previously.

Case presentation

A 14-month-old female was referred to our hospital with a history of an enlarging abdominal mass noted by her parents for 3 days. Physical examination revealed an abdominal mass with clear and smooth margins extending from the right upper quadrant to the right hemipelvis. Routine blood tests were normal apart from mild anaemia and urine analysis did not show hematuria. Ultrasonography of the abdomen revealed a unilateral $10.8 \times 7.2 \times 9.2$ cm solid tumor in the right kidney, whereas the contralateral kidney was normal. Computed tomography (CT) revealed a large lesion arising from the inferior aspect of the right kidney, occupying the right flank and extending across the midline. Enhanced CT detected duplication of IVC below the renal veins and compression and displacement of the right IVC caused by the enormous tumor (Fig. 1). An additional movie file shows this in more detail [see Additional file 1].

Neither intravascular extension nor invasion to adjacent organs and regional lymph nodes was detected by CT. Chest radiography was reported normal.

With the presumptive diagnosis of WT, a right-sided radical nephrectomy was performed. Final pathology was consistent with favorable histology, stromal-predominant (60%) WT. The renal vessel and IVC were tumor free. The renal hilar and para-aortic lymph nodes were also free from tumor and the final pathological stage was Stage I. According to the regimen of the National Wilms' Tumor

* Correspondence: wrd2190@126.com

†Feng Guo and Tianyou Li contributed equally to this work.

[1]Department of Pediatric Surgery, Shandong Provincial Hospital Affiliated to Shandong University, 324 Jingwu Road, Jinan 250021, Shandong Province, People's Republic of China

Full list of author information is available at the end of the article

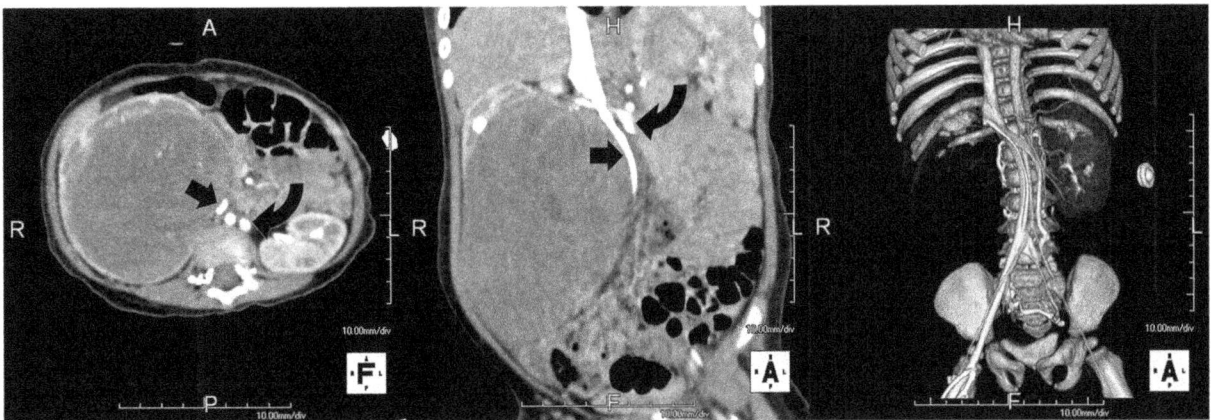

Fig. 1 Axial, coronal and three-dimensional reconstruction computed tomography scan with contrast showing a large mass in the right kidney, duplication of the inferior vena cava below the renal veins and compression and displacement of the right inferior vena cava. Straight arrow denotes the right inferior vena cava, and curved arrow the left inferior vena cava

Study Group 5, the patient received postoperative chemotherapy with dactinomycin and vincristine. CT imaging at 3 months postoperatively showed no evidence of residual or recurrent disease. Interestingly, the right IVC played a dominant role and the left IVC seemed to disappear in postoperative enhanced CT (Fig. 2). An additional movie file shows this in more detail [see Additional file 2]. During the follow-up of 18 months, no local recurrence or metastasis has been observed.

Discussion

WT is the most common tumor of the urinary tract under the age of 15 [1]. Up to now, WT with IVC duplication has not been reported. The development of the IVC is a complex embryological process between weeks 6 and 10 of gestation, including the development, regression, anastomoses, and replacement of embryonic veins [2]. Double IVC is a rare anomaly, and occurs in 1.5% (range 0.2–3%) [3–5]. According to the caliber of the duplicated IVC and the preaortic trunk, IVC duplication

has been classified into three types [4]. The classification may not be appropriate for the present case considering the notable changes of the caliber of the duplicated IVC before and after the operation. The compression of the right IVC caused by tumor resulted in the dominant venous drainage of the left IVC. After the tumornephrectomy, the right IVC gradually took over the venous drainage. Then the left IVC might start to regress and could not be detected at 3 months postoperative CT image. To our knowledge, this is the first detection of the postnatal regression of left IVC, which indicates that vena caval development might proceed not limited to the embryonic period.

Although IVC duplication is usually asymptomatic, it might have significant clinical implications. As an uncommon anomaly, the duplication of IVC can be misdiagnosed as a pathological lesion such as ureteric dilatation or lymphadenopathy on CT images. The left side of a double IVC might be interpreted erroneously as enlarged retroperitoneal lymph nodes [2, 6–8], which

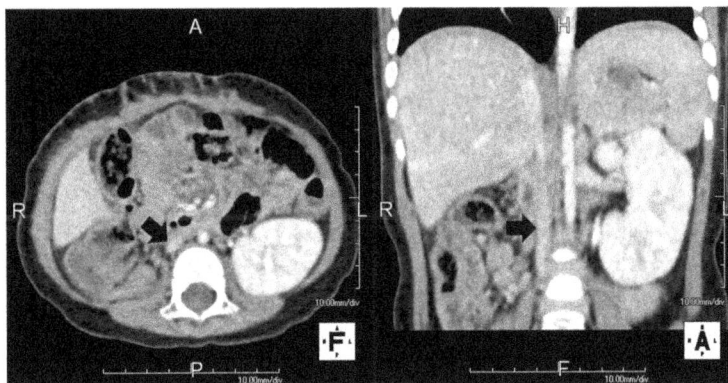

Fig. 2 Axial and coronal computed tomography scan with contrast 3 months after operation showing the right inferior vena cava played a dominant role and the left inferior vena cava was not detected clearly. Straight arrow denotes the right inferior vena cava

might induce preoperative overstaging by radiographic imaging in WT. Serious overstaging due to erroneous interpretation of the CT appearance of a double IVC has been reported in testicular tumor [6, 7].

A radical nephrectomy with lymph node sampling is the "gold standard" surgical protocol for unilateral WT [9–11]. However, retroperitoneal surgery such as nephrectomy might injure the anomalous venous structures that are in fact typically thin walled, dilated and tortuous [12]. Thus, it is vital to recognize the abnormal vasculature such as IVC duplication and avoid a life-threatening hemorrhage in retroperitoneal surgery or intervention [4, 13–16].

In addition to an en bloc resection of the tumor, lymph node sampling is another significant goal in WT surgery [17]. However, patients with anomalous venous anatomy might have unusual patterns of lymph node metastases, for the reason that the lymphatic drainage generally follows the vascular architecture [18]. Thus, lymph node sampling or dissection in a patient with a venous anomaly might be adjusted accordingly [7].

WT involves IVC invasion in 4–8% of cases [19], and caval extension of WT has been an important surgical challenge. Although tumor thrombus of renal vein or IVC was not found in the present case, extension of renal cell carcinoma into duplications of IVC and the retroaortic renal veins has been reported [18, 20–22].

CT is the most reliable technique for detecting tumor and retroperitoneal venous anomalies. Three-dimensional CT angiography can be used for detecting the duplication of IVC before surgery or other interventional procedures of the retroperitoneum are undertaken [23]. In WT, preoperative CT is also an important diagnostic tool and adjunct in assessing lymph node involvement to provide accurate treatment recommendations [24].

In our case, a plain chest X-ray was performed for the evaluation of pulmonary metastases and the report was normal. Considering the disadvantage of radiation exposure, a routine pulmonary CT that was still controversial [25] was not performed.

Conclusion

WT with IVC duplication is extremely rare. Preoperative CT can detect potential venous anomalies in retroperitoneum. Appropriate care can be taken to avoid injury of retroperitoneal venous anomalies and life-threatening hemorrhage during surgery.

Abbreviations

CT: Computed tomography; IVC: Inferior vena cava; WT: Wilms tumor

Funding

This work was supported by grants from the National Natural Science Foundation of China(No.81501844), Shandong Provincial Natural Science Foundation(No.BS2015YY009) and Jinan Science & Technology Development Program, China(No.201602170).

Authors' contributions

RW and FG made contributions to conception and design. FG and TL collected the patient details and wrote the paper. FG and WL made contributions to patient management. RM made contributions to computed tomography diagnosis and imaging. TL, GW and WL critically revised the article. All authors read and approved the final manuscript.

Competing interests

The authors declare that they have no competing interests.

Author details

[1]Department of Pediatric Surgery, Shandong Provincial Hospital Affiliated to Shandong University, 324 Jingwu Road, Jinan 250021, Shandong Province, People's Republic of China. [2]Shandong Medical Imaging Research Institute, Medical School of Shandong University, Jinan, Shandong Province, People's Republic of China.

References

1.   Birch JM, Breslow N. Epidemiologic features of Wilms tumor. Hematol Oncol Clin North Am. 1995;9(6):1157–78.
2.   Bass JE, Redwine MD, Kramer LA, Huynh PT, Harris JH Jr. Spectrum of congenital anomalies of the inferior vena cava: cross-sectional imaging findings. Radiographics. 2000;20(3):639–52.
3.   Chen H, Emura S, Nagasaki S, Kubo KY. Double inferior vena cava with interiliac vein: a case report and literature review. Okajimas Folia Anat Jpn. 2012;88(4):147–51.
4.   Natsis K, Apostolidis S, Noussios G, Papathanasiou E, Kyriazidou A, Vyzas V. Duplication of the inferior vena cava: anatomy, embryology and classification proposal. Anat Sci Int. 2010;85(1):56–60.
5.   Jhansi P. Duplication of the inferior vena cava–report of a rare congenital variation. Int J Anat Var (IJAV). 2012;5:141–3.
6.   Cohen SI, Hochsztein P, Cambio J, Sussett J. Duplicated inferior vena cava misinterpreted by computerized tomography as metastatic retroperitoneal testicular tumor. J Urol. 1982;128(2):389–91.
7.   Klimberg I, Wajsman Z. Duplicated inferior vena cava simulating retroperitoneal lymphadenopathy in a patient with embryonal cell carcinoma of the testicle. J Urol. 1986;136(3):678–9.
8.   Evans JC, Earis J, Curtis J. Thrombosed double inferior vena cava mimicking paraaortic lymphadenopathy. Br J Radiol. 2001;74(878):192–4.
9.   Ritchey ML, Kelalis PP, Breslow N, Etzioni R, Evans I, Haase GM, D'Angio GJ. Surgical complications after nephrectomy for Wilms' tumor. Surg Gynecol Obstet. 1992;175(6):507–14.
10. Ritchey ML, Shamberger RC, Haase G, Horwitz J, Bergemann T, Breslow NE. Surgical complications after primary nephrectomy for Wilms' tumor: report from the National Wilms' tumor study group. J Am Coll Surg. 2001;192(1): 63–8 quiz 146.
11. Fuchs J, Kienecker K, Furtwangler R, Warmann SW, Burger D, Thurhoff JW, Hager J, Graf N. Surgical aspects in the treatment of patients with unilateral wilms tumor: a report from the SIOP 93-01/German Society of Pediatric Oncology and Hematology. Ann Surg. 2009;249(4):666–71.
12. Downey RS, Sicard GA, Anderson CB. Major retroperitoneal venous anomalies: surgical considerations. Surgery. 1990;107(4):359–65.
13. Bartle EJ, Pearce WH, Sun JH, Rutherford RB. Infrarenal venous anomalies and aortic surgery: avoiding vascular injury. J Vasc Surg. 1987;6(6):590–3.
14. Karkos CD, Bruce IA, Thomson GJ, Lambert ME. Retroaortic left renal vein and its implications in abdominal aortic surgery. Ann Vasc Surg. 2001;15(6):703–8.

15. Christakis PG, Cimsit B, Kulkarni S. Complication arising from a duplicated inferior vena cava following laparoscopic living donor nephrectomy: a case report. Transplant Proc. 2012;44(5):1450–2.

16. Stefanczyk L, Majos M, Majos A, Polguj M. Duplication of the inferior vena cava and retroaortic left renal vein in a patient with large abdominal aortic aneurysm. Vasc Med. 2014;19(2):144–5.

17. Kieran K, Anderson JR, Dome JS, Ehrlich PF, Ritchey ML, Shamberger RC, Perlman EJ, Green DM, Davidoff AM. Lymph node involvement in Wilms tumor: results from National Wilms Tumor Studies 4 and 5. J Pediatr Surg. 2012;47(4):700–6.

18. Habuchi T, Okagaki T, Arai K, Miyakawa M. Renal cell carcinoma extending into left side of double inferior vena cava. Urology. 1993;41(2):181–4.

19. Khanna G, Rosen N, Anderson JR, Ehrlich PF, Dome JS, Gow KW, Perlman E, Barnhart D, Karolczuk K, Grundy P. Evaluation of diagnostic performance of CT for detection of tumor thrombus in children with Wilms tumor: a report from the Children's oncology group. Pediatr Blood Cancer. 2012;58(4):551–5.

20. Handel DB, Heaston DK, Korobkin M, Silverman PM, Dunnick NR. Circumaortic left renal vein with tumor thrombus: CT diagnosis with angiographic and pathologic correlation. AJR Am J Roentgenol. 1983; 141(1):97–8.

21. Pinsk R, Nemcek AA Jr, Fitzgerald SW. Tumor thrombus in a retroaortic left renal vein and incidental right circumcaval ureter. Urol Radiol. 1992; 13(3):166–9.

22. Kumar S, Panigrahy B, Ravimohan SM, Pandya S, Mandal AK, Singh SK. Rare case of renal cell carcinoma with double inferior vena cava with venous thrombosis. Urology. 2008;72(2):461 e7–10.

23. Mathews R, Smith PA, Fishman EK, Marshall FF. Anomalies of the inferior vena cava and renal veins: embryologic and surgical considerations. Urology. 1999;53(5):873–80.

24. Lubahn JD, Cost NG, Kwon J, Powell JA, Yang M, Granberg CF, Wickiser JE, Rakheja D, Gargollo PC, Baker LA, et al. Correlation between preoperative staging computerized tomography and pathological findings after nodal sampling in children with Wilms tumor. J Urol. 2012;188(4 Suppl):1500–4.

25. Owens CM, Veys PA, Pritchard J, Levitt G, Imeson J, Dicks-Mireaux C. Role of chest computed tomography at diagnosis in the management of Wilms' tumor: a study by the United Kingdom Children's Cancer study group. J Clin Oncol. 2002;20(12):2768–73.

Spontaneous ureteric rupture, a reality or a faux pas?

Gaurav Aggarwal* and Samiran Das Adhikary

Abstract

Background: Rupture of the urinary collecting system with or without any perinephric extravasation is an extremely rare occurrence and usually known to occur following an obstructive pathology.

Spontaneous or non-traumatic rupture, in the absence of any distal obstruction, though reported in literature, is not yet a proven entity and needs to be distinguished from physiological forniceal rupture, to validate its occurrence. Our case illustrates that spontaneous ureteric rupture does exist and requires a high level of vigil for prompt diagnosis and early simple management.

Case presentation: A 65 year old non diabetic gentleman presented with a 2 day history of right sided severe abdominal pain with no history of any prior trauma, surgery, urinary retention or calculus disease. His ultrasound whole-abdomen was suggestive of increased liver echogenicity, but his contrast enhanced CT scan (CECT) documented a ureteric rupture, with leakage of contrast from the upper ureters, well away from the renal pelvis He was promptly managed with cysto-ureteroscopy, retrograde pyelography (RGP) and double-J (DJ) stenting. His post operative course was uneventful and he was discharged on the second post operative day, without event. An RGP at 6 weeks of follow up showed no contrast extravasation from the ureter and his DJ stent was removed without event.

Conclusion: Spontaneous ureteric rupture, in the absence of any inciting cause, is an entity which exists and is easily manageable, once diagnosed timely. Thus, the need to maintain a high index of vigil, in order to identify this clinically entity at the earnest, institute prompt treatment and hence ensure that a "spontaneous" rupture, doesn't become a "faux pas" in the true sense of the word.

Keywords: Ureteric rupture, Spontaneous, DJ stenting, Case report

Background

Urinary collecting system rupture with or without perinephric extravasation is an extremely rare occurrence and usually thought to occur following an obstructive pathology.

Spontaneous or non-traumatic rupture [1, 2], though reported in literature, is not yet a proven entity and needs to be distinguished from physiological forniceal rupture, to validate its occurrence.

Our case illustrates that spontaneous ureteric rupture exists and requires a high level of vigil for prompt diagnosis and simple management.

* Correspondence: drgaurav1981@rediffmail.com
Department of Urology, Apollo Hospital, Bhubaneshwar 751005, Odisha, India

Case Presentation

A 65 year old non diabetic, non-alcoholic gentleman presented with a 2 day history of right sided severe abdominal pain with no prior trauma, surgery, urinary retention or calculus disease.

Clinically, he was vitally stable, apart from mild tachycardia (pulse rate 92 beats/min). On local examination, there was no abdominal or costo-vertebral tenderness and rest of his abdomen was unremarkable, however his pain was seemingly out of proportion to these examination findings. His serum urea/creatinine, liver function tests, serum amylase/lipase as well as all other biochemical tests were within normal limits.

His ultrasound whole-abdomen was suggestive of increased liver echogenicity, with no evidence of any abnormality to the kidneys, ureters, bladder as well as no intra or retroperitoneal fluid collection, and he was being evaluated along the lines of a liver abscess.

However, a CECT scan when done, reported a ureteric rupture with leakage of contrast from the upper ureter, well away from the renal pelvis, at the level of the 2nd lumbar vertebra (Fig. 1).

He was promptly taken up for cysto-ureteroscopy, retrograde pyelography (RGP) and DJ stenting. Intraoperative RGP demonstrated the upper ureteric rupture at a fair distance from the pelvis without cystoscopic evidence of any calculus or obstructive uropathy (Fig. 2).

He was managed via cystoscopy and placement of a DJ Stent (5Fr, No 26). His post operative course was uneventful and he was discharged on the second post operative day, without event.

At 6 weeks of follow up, there was no contrast extravasation as confirmed via an RGP done during stent removal (Fig. 3).

The patient was discharged without event and advised to remain on 6 monthly follow ups, with imaging to be done as per his subsequent symptoms.

Discussion

Ureteric rupture is in itself an infrequently encountered entity and a spontaneous rupture is even rarer [1].

Rupture of the ureter is usually expected to occur following trauma, which may be blunt, penetrating or even iatrogenic [1, 2]. Spontaneous or non-traumatic rupture, if at all, is considered to be secondary to some downstream obstruction by a calculus, papilla, stricture or via extrinsic compression [1, 2].

The symptom at presentation, mainly sudden, severe lower abdominal pain is usually not in sync with the clinical signs and may mimic an episode of acute appendicitis or diverticulitis [2].

Thus, the diagnosis frequently gets delayed leading to long term patient morbidity [2]. Initially, an excretory urography was considered as the imaging modality of choice, however, in the current era, a contrast enhanced CT scan (CECT) forms the mainstay for imaging with intraoperative retrograde urography (RGU) being the gold standard [1–3].

Koga et al. (11 cases) [4] and Stravodimos et al. (5 cases) [5] remain the largest series till date, having reported spontaneous peripelvic collections, of which only 4 of the cases in the work by Stravodimos et al. were not found to have any cause, or could be said as "spontaneous" ruptures.

On account of these few and interspersed reports and lack of specific guidelines, management strategies vary among surgeons, from endoscopic stenting to even open surgical repair [3–5]. There have been reports in literature documenting even percutaneous drainage, as well as conservative management with just antibiotics till clinical deterioration, but all of them suggest that a prompt intervention definitely reduces long term morbidity [6].

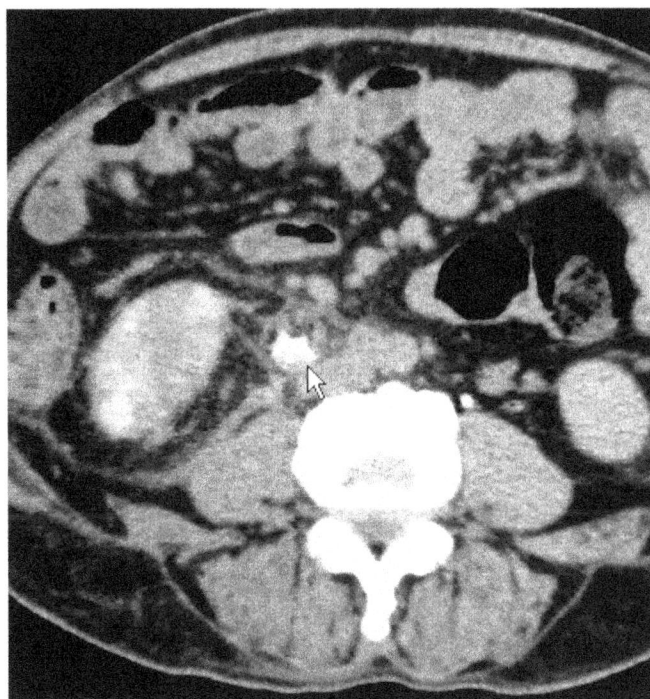

Fig. 1 CECT with arrow demonstrating contrast leak from the upper ureter, well away from the fornix

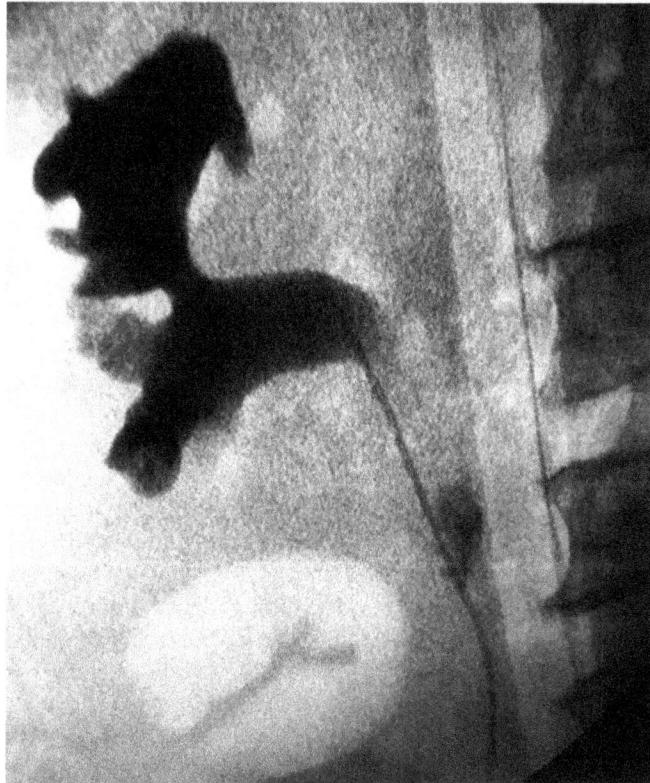

Fig. 2 Intra-operative RGP, demonstrating contrast extravasation from upper ureter

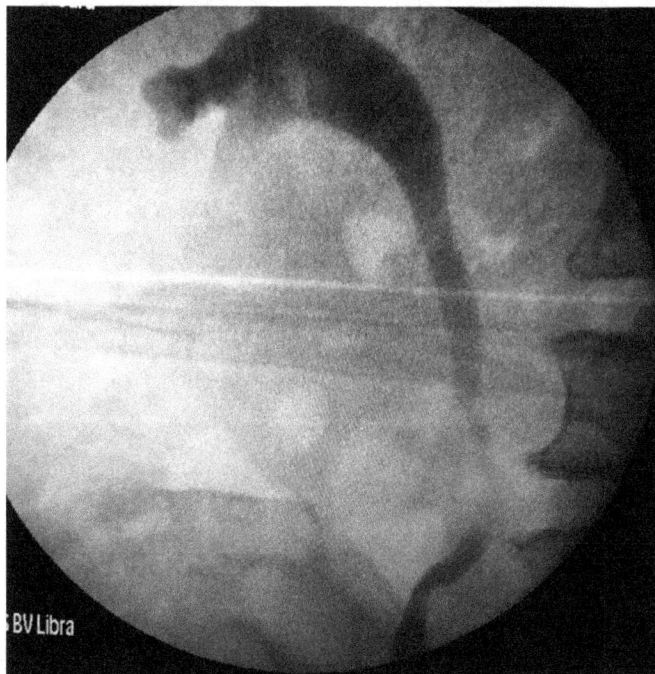

Fig. 3 A follow up RGP at the time of stent removal, demonstrating the completely healed ureter (no contrast extravasation)

Prognosis remains excellent, once diagnosed early, and managed promptly, with immediate relief. On the contrary, a delay in instituting treatment may lead to serious consequences such as a perinephric or retroperitoneal collection, abscess formation and subsequently urosepsis [6].

Thus, our case illustrates that timely diagnosis and prompt management in the acute setting via simple DJ stenting is sufficient to allow complete healing and prevent long term complications.

Conclusion

Spontaneous ureteric rupture, in the absence of any inciting cause, is an existing entity, easily manageable, once diagnosed timely.

As is said, *"what the mind knows is what the eyes see"*. This statement typically exemplifies the need to keep this clinical entity in mind, so as to prevent a *"spontaneous"* rupture from becoming a *"faux pas"* in the true sense of the word.

Abbreviations
CECT, Contrast Enhanced CT Scan; RGP, Retrograde Pyelography; DJ Stenting, Double J stenting.

Funding
Nil.

Authors' contribution
Both authors have drafted the manuscript and were actively involved in management of the patient.

Competing interests
The authors declare that they have no competing interests.

Consent for publication
The patient has given consent for this case to be published.

References
1. Kaplan LM, Farrer JH, Lupu AN. Spontaneous rupture of ureter. Urology. 1987;29:313–6.
2. Pampana E, Altobelli S, Morini M et al. Spontaneous Ureteral Rupture Diagnosis and Treatment. Case Reports in Radiology. http://dx.doi.org/10.1155/2013/851859.
3. Seung-Kwon Choi Solmin L, Sunchan K, et al. A Rare Case of Upper Ureter Rupture: Ureteral Perforation Caused by Urinary Retention Korean. J Urol. 2012;53(2):131–3.
4. Koga S, Arakaki Y, Matsuoka M, et al. Spontaneous peripelvic extravasation of urine. Int Urol Nephrol. 1992;24:465–9.
5. Stravodimos K, Adamakis I, Koutalellis G, et al. Spontaneous perforation of the ureter: clinical presentation and endourologic management. J Endourol. 2008;22:479–84.
6. Fken A, Akbas T, Arpaci T. Spontaneous rupture of the ureters. Singapore Med J. 2015;56(2):e29–31. doi: 10.11622/smedj.2015029.

30

Bioelectrical activity of the pelvic floor muscles during synchronous whole-body vibration

Magdalena Stania[1]*, Daria Chmielewska[1], Krystyna Kwaśna[1], Agnieszka Smykla[1], Jakub Taradaj[1] and Grzegorz Juras[2]

Abstract

Background: More and more frequently stress urinary incontinence affects young healthy women. Hence, early implementation of effective preventive strategies in nulliparous continent women is essential, including pelvic floor muscle training. An initial evaluation based on the bioelectrical activity of the pelvic floor muscles (PFM) during whole-body vibration (WBV) would help to devise the best individualized training for prevention of stress urinary incontinence in woman. We hypothesized that synchronous WBV enhances bioelectrical activity of the PFM which depends on vibration frequency and peak-to-peak vibration displacement.

Methods: The sample consisted of 36 nulliparous continent women randomly allocated to three comparative groups. Group I and II subjects participated in synchronous whole-body vibrations on a vibration platform; the frequency and peak-to-peak displacement of vibration were set individually for each group. Control participants performed exercises similar to those used in the study groups but without the concurrent application of vibrations. Pelvic floor surface electromyography (sEMG) activity was recorded using a vaginal probe during three experimental trials limited to 30s, 60s and 90s. The mean amplitude and variability of the signal were normalized to the Maximal Voluntary Contraction – MVC.

Results: Friedman's two-way ANOVA revealed a statistically significant difference in the mean normalized amplitudes (%MVC) of the sEMG signal from the PFM during 60s- and 90s-trials between the group exposed to high-intensity WBV and control participants ($p < 0.05$). Longer trial duration was associated with a statistically significant decrease in the variability of sEMG signal amplitude in the study and control groups ($p < 0.05$).

Conclusions: Synchronous high-intensity WBV (40 Hz, 4 mm) of long duration (60s, 90s) significantly enhances the activation of the PFM in young continent women. Prolonged maintenance of a static position significantly decreases the variability of sEMG signal amplitude independent of whole-body vibrations. Single whole-body vibrations in nulliparous continent women does not cause pelvic floor muscle fatigue.

Keywords: Electromyography, Healthy volunteers, Pelvic floor, Vibration

* Correspondence: m.stania@awf.katowice.pl
[1]Department of Physiotherapy Basics, Jerzy Kukuczka Academy of Physical Education, Mikołowska 72a, 40-065 Katowice, Poland
Full list of author information is available at the end of the article

Background

Whole-body vibration training (WBV) provides valuable assistance in sports training and physiotherapy. Exercises on a vibration platform have been used in the treatment of patients with non-specific chronic low back pain [1], Parkinson's disease [2], multiple sclerosis [3], hemiplegia [4] and in children with cerebral palsy [5]. Some researchers also report on the use of mechanical vibration for neuromuscular stimulation of weakened pelvic floor muscles (PFM) in women with stress urinary incontinence [6, 7].

Mechanical vibration of a human skeletal muscle induces a tonic reflex contraction which is termed a tonic vibration reflex (TVR). TVR is a result of repeated, fast and short extension of a musculotendinous unit [8]. Stimulation of the endings of myelinated Ia fibres resulting from a change in the length of neuromuscular spindles causes activation of α-motoneurons in the spinal cord; consequently, the muscle contracts. Additionally, mechanical oscillations mask short-latency phasic spinal reflexes by increasing presynaptic inhibition [8].

Muscle activity is frequently analysed using surface electromyography (sEMG). EMG records and quantifies the electrical activity generated by muscle fibers. Depolarisation and repolarisation of the surface membrane of muscle fibers is the source of the electrical potential changes detected. Auchincloss et al. [9] demonstrated between-trial reliability of EMG data recorded from the PFM using two different vaginal probes with the subjects performing two tasks (Maximal Voluntary Contraction MVC and coughing). Some authors [10, 11] emphasize the need for the elimination of vibration-induced motion artifacts from raw EMG data using digital band-stop filters. Ritzmann et al. [12], on the other hand, argue that the effect of motion artifacts on EMG recording is insignificant; the periodic spikes in EMG signal during whole-body vibration are not motion artifacts, but rather stretch reflex.

Whole-body vibrations induce an increase in myoelectric activity [13, 14]. Bioelectrical muscle activity depends on several factors and among these vibration frequency and peak-to-peak vibration displacement [13], initial position in a given exercise and related initial muscle extension [14], anatomical location of the investigated muscle [15], vibration type (sinusoidal vs stochastic vibration) [6, 14] and additional load [14].

The pelvic floor muscles have typical striated fibers, specific function and characteristic location; they are characterized by synchronous and harmonic contractions [16] and prolonged tension (except for micturition and defecation) [17]. Women with stress urinary incontinence frequently exhibit weakening of the pelvic floor muscles [18]. The aim of therapeutic interventions in women with stress urinary incontinence and weakened pelvic floor muscles is to enhance muscular power so that they would be able to quickly and intensively contract these muscles to prevent involuntary urine loss in case intra-abdominal pressure should increase rapidly [6].

More and more frequently stress urinary incontinence affects young healthy women [19]. Hence, early implementation of effective preventive strategies in nulliparous continent women is essential, including pelvic floor muscle training. There is scientific basis for hypothesizing about beneficial effects of mechanical vibration on the pelvic floor muscles in continent as well as incontinent subjects [6, 7, 20]. However, such hypotheses require verification.

Previous studies had demonstrated differential effect of the sinusoidal and stochastic whole-body vibration, with the superiority of stochastic vibration especially pronounced in subjects with impaired PFMs function [6]. However, Luginbuehl et al. [7] found no significant change in the PFM activity during continuous or intermittent stochastic resonance whole-body vibration.

Literature review yields numerous reports on the effect of vibration on maximum strength and power enhancement [21]; however, the findings of these studies are not unequivocal. The discrepancies probably result from divergence in whole-body vibration training protocols. There is no evidence based on neurophysiological investigations regarding the values of vibration parameters which would produce the optimum effect in the neuromuscular system.

An increase in the activity of striated muscle during WBV [13, 14] indicates that similar effects might be expected for the pelvic floor muscles.

The aim of this study was to evaluate bioelectrical activity of the pelvic floor muscles during synchronous low- and high-intensity whole-body vibration in three trials. Another aim was to assess pelvic floor muscle fatigue during 90s whole-body vibration. The study participants were young continent women. An evaluation based on the performance and bioelectrical activity of the pelvic floor muscles during whole-body vibration would help to devise the best individualized training for prevention of stress urinary incontinence in woman. It would also facilitate the understanding of the effect of whole-body vibration on muscle performance.

Methods

Subjects

This was a randomized, controlled, 3 parallel-group study among thirty-six nulliparous continent women. Physical characteristics of the study participants are presented in Table 1. Young healthy adults who were not professional athletes were recruited. Exclusion criteria included a history of disequilibrium, acute inflammatory conditions

Table 1 Characteristics of the study participants

Group	Parameters of vibrations	Age [years] mean ± SD	Body mass [kg] mean ± SD	Height [cm] mean ± SD
I	2 mm/20 Hz	22.4 ± 1.6	63.5 ± 5.3	168.9 ± 2.3
II	4 mm/40 Hz	21.8 ± 1.7	64.4 ± 6.2	167 ± 3.1
III (control)	no vibrations	22.7 ± 1	63.6 ± 6.7	167.8 ± 3.7

and infections, epilepsy, cardiovascular diseases, acute phase of osteoarthritis, stress urinary incontinence, pregnancy, childbirth(s), pelvic surgery, diabetes, hypertension, neurological abnormalities, urinary tract infection, elevated temperature, spinal pain and Body Mass Index over 30 kg/m^2. Candidates were presented with a comprehensive description of the aim and methods of the study. After obtaining their informed consent, a personal history was taken from each participant. Demographic data included age, height, weight, Body Mass Index, employment status. The experiment was carried out in the Department of Physiotherapy Basics and the Department of Human Motor Behavior at the Jerzy Kukuczka Academy of Physical Education in Katowice, Poland. The study was approved by the Bioethics Committee at the Academy of Physical Education in Katowice, Poland.

Result distribution in a randomly selected sample was unimodal; skewness and flatness were lower than 2.5. Therefore center stratification and dispersion measure were best assessed with the arithmetic mean and standard deviation. We assumed the probability of a type I error a = 0.05, target power of 1-beta = 0.80 and a 25 % minimum significant difference between the means of parameters studied. The resultant minimum sample size was 10 patients. The target sample size was 36; 6 additional participants were to be recruited to account for dropouts (due to artifact signals of sEMG). The actual sample size was 33. The study participants were randomly assigned to 3 groups (Group I – 12; Group II – 10, and Group III – 11). Simple randomization technique was used in the experiment. The main coordinator who allocated the participants to groups had opaque, sealed envelopes, each containing a piece of paper marked with either group I, II or III. The physician selected and opened an envelope in the presence of a physiotherapist to see the symbol and then directed the participant to the corresponding group.

sEMG recordings of three women (two from group II and one from group III) were excluded from analysis due to artifact signals. Group I and II subjects participated in synchronous whole-body vibrations on a vibration platform; the frequency and peak-to-peak displacement of vibration were set individually for each group, i.e. 2 mm/20 Hz for group I and 4 mm/40 Hz for group II. In order to show a wider range of possible muscle reactions, specific combinations of

low and high intensity parameters, available with the used platform, were applied. Control participants (group III) performed exercises similar to those used in the study groups but without the concurrent application of vibrations. The control participants assumed the same static position, which was standing with their knees and hips joints flexed to 35° while their arms were stretched horizontally in front to hold the railing. Hence, their position was the same as that assumed by group I and II subjects exercising on the vibration platform. Three static exercise trials of 30s, 60s and 90s were performed in a randomized order.

The study design is presented in Fig. 1. No important difference in any characteristic was found at baseline between the groups.

sEMG measurements

The first participant was enrolled in the study on the 6th of May 2014, the last one on the 14th of November 2014. The measurements were taken in the morning hours to minimize the impact of fatigue. The subjects were asked not to take up intensive physical exercises 24 h before the measurement. Temperature in the examination room was 24 °C. The measurements were performed under standard testing conditions, the same for all subjects.

sEMG was recorded using Myo Trace 400 (Noraxon U.S.A. Inc.) with a preamplifier (band pass filter 20 Hz–500 Hz, Common Mode Rejection Ratio of >100 dB at 60 Hz, input impedance >100 MΩ, amplifier gain 500). A 16-bit analog to digital (A/D) converter with an anti-aliasing filter set to 500 Hz frequency was also used.

Pelvic floor sEMG activity was recorded using a small diameter vaginal probe with two metal sensors (Everyway Medical Instruments Co). The probe was inserted using a small amount of antiallergic lubricant with the sensors positioned laterally in the vagina. Vaginal electrode placement was checked during breaks between the consecutive measurement sessions. After cleansing the skin site with an alcohol swab, the reference surface electrode was placed over the right anterior superior iliac spine (round self-adhesive electrode; silver/silver chloride) in accordance with SENIAM recommendations (Surface ElectroMyoGraphy for the Non- Invasive Assessment of Muscles) [22]. sEMG cables were fixed on the skin with tape in order to avoid artifacts.

Prior to the measurements, the participants were asked to urinate a full void. All sEMG recordings were performed by the same examiner.

Whole-body vibration

Synchronous whole-body vibration was carried out on a vibration platform (Fitvibe 600, Gymna Uniphy N.V.). Test participants were in a static position during the

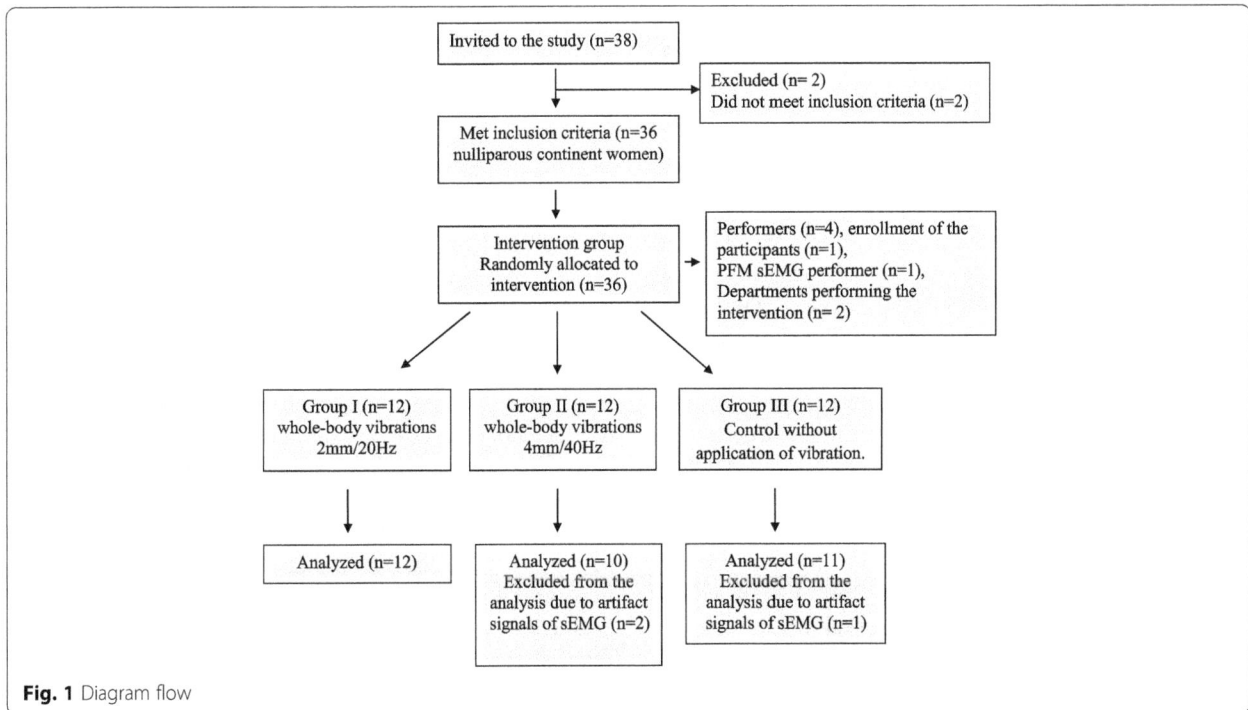

Fig. 1 Diagram flow

exercises. Briefly, each subject was asked to stand on the platform, loading their feet uniformly, with the knee and hip joints bent at 35° and the upper extremities stretched horizontally forwards, holding on to a railing. The ranges of flexion of the hip and knee joints were measured with a goniometer to ensure the subjects maintained the required position. The above mentioned position is quite safe as knee flexion reduces the amount of vibration that reaches the head [10]. No unintended effects were observed during WBV in group I and II.

Testing procedure

The experiment consisted of two phases: 1/ the maximal voluntary contractions (MVC) procedure to recruit pelvic floor muscles and 2/ three static exercise trials (30s, 60s, 90s) performed in a randomized order to determine PFM activity during (groups I, II) or without (group III) WBV.

During the first phase, each participant was instructed to perform MVC of the pelvic floor muscles as forcefully as possible for about 5 s. Three attempts were made with 60-s rests between each contraction to reduce the effect of muscle fatigue. During MVCs verbal encouragement was provided. MVCs were used as reference values.

The MVC procedure to recruit pelvic floor muscles: supine lying [23]; the hip and knee were positioned at 30° and 90° of flexion, respectively. The positions were controlled with the goniometer.

During the second phase, all group I and II participants were exposed to WBV during three exercise trials applied at random order. Vibration exposure during a single trial was limited to 30s, 60s and 90s (up to 5 s were allowed for the vibration platform to reach its preset peak-to-peak displacement and frequency). A 10-min rest period was used between trials in order to eliminate any potential fatigue; the subjects were blinded to WBV frequency and peak-to-peak displacement. sEMG signal from the pelvic floor muscles was recorded during static position maintained on a vibrating platform. During the 30-s, 60-s and 90-s sEMG recording the following parameters were measured: mean amplitude (% MVC) and variability of the signal (the variability of data around the mean value of the selected period of the analysis, expressed as %MVC).

The mean amplitude as well as the mean and median frequency of the sEMG signal [24] were additionally measured to determine the effect of fatigue during the 90-s sEMG recordings. The analysis was performed for two subperiods, ie., from the 6th to 10th seconds and from the 86th to the 90th seconds. The initial subperiod (5 s) in which the vibration platform had not reached its preset peak-to-peak displacement and frequency was excluded from analysis. Percentage changes in the mean and median frequency and mean amplitude were calculated using the formula for the difference of two subperiods. Five 1-s intervals of both subperiods yielded five values of the variables under analysis.

The raw sEMG data were full wave rectified. Root mean square values were calculated using a 100 ms sliding window. The raw sEMG signal was used for the analysis of a 90-s contraction parameters (mean and median frequency of the sEMG signal).

Statistical analysis

The Shapiro-Wilk test was used to check the data for normal distribution, while variance homogeneity was assessed using the Levene test. Since several parameters failed to meet the assumption regarding the normal distribution of variables and variance homogeneity, non-parametric tests were used. Friedman's two-way ANOVA for ranks was applied when the same parameter had been measured several times (k > =2) under different conditions on the same subjects. The Bonferroni post-hoc test, which reveals which means are significantly different from each other, was also performed. Inter-trial changes in the amplitude of the sEMG signal from the pelvic floor muscles were analysed using the Kruskal-Wallis ANOVA with the Tukey post hoc test.

Values are expressed as mean +/- SD. The level of statistical significance for all analyses was set at $p < 0.05$.

Results

Mean amplitude

A comparison of mean normalized amplitudes between 30s, 60s and 90s trials did not reveal significant differences in any of the groups ($p > 0.05$) (Fig. 2).

Friedman's two-way ANOVA revealed a statistically significant difference in the mean normalized amplitudes of the sEMG signal from the pelvic floor muscles during 60s- and 90s-trials between the group exposed to high-intensity WBV and control participants ($p < 0.05$) (Table 2). The mean amplitude of the sEMG signal during all trials was higher compared to the control; however, the difference did not reach statistical significance ($p > 0.05$). During all trials, the activity of the pelvic floor muscles was higher in the group who received 40Hz/4mm vibrations than in the study participants with 20Hz/2mm vibrations but again, the differences did not reach the level of statistical significance ($p > 0.05$).

Variability of amplitude

Longer trial duration was associated with a statistically significant decrease in the variability of sEMG signal amplitude in the study and control groups ($p < 0.05$) (Fig. 3).

Kruskal-Wallis ANOVA did not reveal statistically significant differences between the groups with respect to the normalized variability of pelvic floor muscle sEMG signal amplitude ($p > 0.05$) (Table 3).

Sustained 90-s contraction

In the 90s trial, absolute values (differences between the final and initial subperiods) of the median and mean frequency and mean normalized amplitude of pelvic floor muscle sEMG signal were negative, indicating a decrease in these parameters. However, intergroup differences were not statistically significant ($p > 0.05$) (Table 4). The Tukey post hoc test also did not reveal statistically significant differences.

Discussion

Surface electromyography is among the modalities to investigate the function of the pelvic floor muscles in real time [25]. sEMG was used to evaluate pelvic floor muscles' activity in nulliparous, asymptomatic women by body position during voluntary contractions of the PFMs [26]. The reliability of repeated surface electromyography of the pelvic floor muscles was confirmed in young continent women based on the analysis of the resting, mean and peak amplitudes, time before peak and area [27].

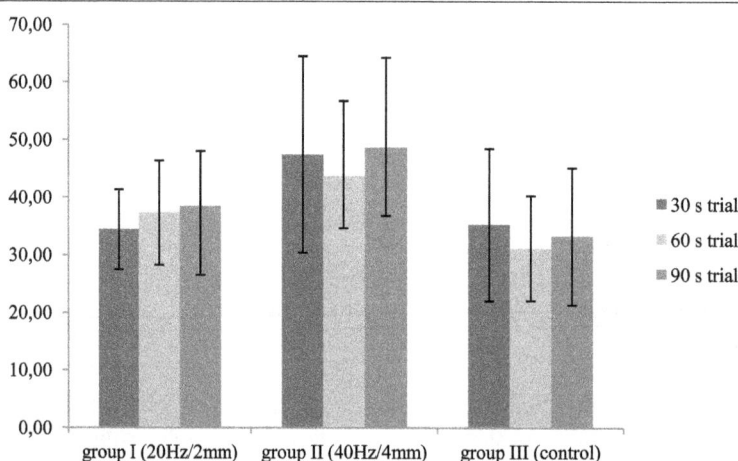

Fig. 2 Inter-trial comparison of mean normalized amplitude of the sEMG signal from the pelvic floor muscles (%MVC) in the study and control groups

Table 2 Comparison of mean normalized amplitude of the sEMG signal from the pelvic floor muscles (%MVC) between the groups

Mean amplitude (% MVC)								
Trial			30s trial		60s trial		90s trial	
Group	n		Mean (%)	SD	Mean (%)	SD	Mean (%)	SD
I (20Hz/2mm)	12		34.41	6.96	37.33	9.02	38.41	9.61
II (40Hz/4mm)	10		47.43	17.04	43.70	13.03	48.67	15.56
III (control)	11		35.23	13.22	31.13	9.09	33.22	11.91
p^a(I/II/III)			0.16		0.056		0.06	
p (I/II)			0.079		0.37		0.18	
p (I/III)			0.99		0.36		0.6	
p (II/III)			0.11		0.031		0.026	

p^a - Friedman's ANOVA
p - Tukey post hoc test

Literature reports fail to provide consistent guidelines regarding whole-body vibration parameters. Torvinen et al. [28] emphasized the significance of appropriate frequency and amplitude selection. Using a variety of vibration protocols, the investigators demonstrated beneficial effects with respect to muscle strength and jump height after just one intervention type. The importance of appropriate parameter selection has been confirmed in the present experiment. The mean of the normalized sEMG activity of the pelvic floor muscles was significantly higher during high-intensity whole-body vibration (40 Hz, 4 mm) in the 60- and 90-sec tests compared to the control ($p < 0.05$). Low-intensity whole-body vibration did not result in significant changes in the mean sEMG amplitude of the pelvic floor muscles between the study and control groups ($p > 0.05$). Similar results were published by Lauper et al. [6]. Low-intensity whole body sinusoidal vibrations (5Hz/2mm, 5Hz/4mm,15Hz/2mm) applied in standing with slightly flexed

knee joint did not enhance the activity of the pelvic floor muscles compared to standing with no vibration. A significant increase in the normalized EMG signal amplitude from the pelvic floor muscles was still observed at the combination of 15Hz/4mm.

Based on literature review, Luo et al. [21] recommend that in order to activate the muscle most effectively, vibration frequency should be in the range of 30–50 Hz. This is consistent with our results; vibrations of 40 Hz resulted in an increase in the mean activity of the pelvic floor muscles.

Increased muscle activation during whole-body vibration is mainly attributed to the tonic vibration reflex [29]. Stretching of musculotendinous units during exercise on a vibration platform causes frequency-dependent stimulation of neuromuscular spindles and, consequently, changes in the EMG signal [12]. An increase in muscle activity observed in EMG recordings results from the recruitment of a large number of

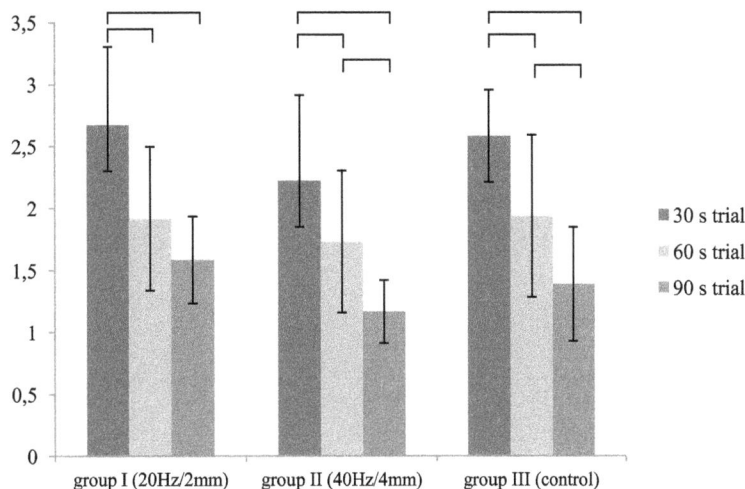

Fig. 3 Inter-trial comparison of the normalized variability of pelvic floor muscle sEMG signal amplitude (%MVC) in the study and control groups. Horizontal bars with vertical dashes indicate statistically significant differences between duration of the trial at the same peak-to-peak displacement and frequency of vibration ($p < 0.05$)

Table 3 Normalized variability of pelvic floor muscle sEMG signal amplitude in the study and control groups

Variability of amplitude (% MVC)

Trial		30s trial		60s trial		90s trial	
Group	n	Mean (%)	SD	Mean (%)	SD	Mean (%)	SD
I (20Hz/2mm)	12	2.67	0.63	1.92	0.58	1.59	0.35
II (40Hz/4mm)	10	2.22	0.69	1.73	0.57	1.17	0.25
III (control)	11	2.58	0.37	1.94	0.66	1.39	0.46
p^a(I/II/III)		0.23		0.87		0.055	
p (I/II)		0.21		0.77		0.043	
p (I/III)		0.93		0.99		0.43	
p (II/III)		0.36		0.73		0.39	

p^a - Friedman's ANOVA
p - Tukey post hoc test

motor units and high firing rates of thereof. According to Krol et al. [13], increased signal of the rmsEMG obtained while higher amplitude of vibration was applied (ie., 4 mm vs 2 mm) might be associated with faster and greater stretching of the muscle. The increase in muscle activity with increasing frequency of vibration at the same amplitude may be associated with higher rates of stretching.

Neuromuscular response to mechanical vibration also depends on the anatomical location of the muscle. Exercises performed on a vibration platform in the standing position cause an increase in bioelectrical activity, and especially in the muscles that have a distal location in the lower limb [14]. In the course of the transmission of mechanical vibrations in human tissues, the intensity of the vibration is reduced due to the damping properties which are defined as any effect that tends to decrease the amplitude of oscillation [30]. The damping effect has been attributed to joint kinematics (in particular, ankle and knee joints), muscle tuning mechanism, the sensitivity of skin receptors, viscoelastic elements and passive soft tissue and bony constraints, eg. bones, cartilage and synovial fluid [30]. Pollock et al. [31] demonstrated that vibration of 30 Hz/5.5 mm applied during standing with knee flexion (15.1°+/−4.8°) resulted in only 2.7 % of WBV acceleration being transmitted from the big toe to the head, which could be attributed to the damping effect. Above the knee at frequencies > 15 Hz, acceleration decreased with distance from the platform. It may be, that the big distance between the pelvic floor muscles and the platform as well as low vibration parameters (20 Hz, 2 mm) caused the absence of changes in the mean activity of the pelvic floor muscles during low-intensity WBV in our experiment.

Stress urinary incontinence affects women during and after menopause [32], after vaginal delivery [33], hysterectomy [34], sportswomen [35], but also - more and more frequently - young healthy women [19]. Hence, early implementation of effective preventive strategies is essential, including pelvic floor muscle training. A significantly higher activation of the pelvic floor muscles during vibration of 40 Hz and peak-to-peak displacement of 4 mm in a group of young women seems to provide an argument for the use of some elements of high-intensity vibration training in the prevention of stress urinary incontinence.

However, the knowledge on the use of vibration training in the treatment of this condition remains unsatisfactory. Sønksen et al. [20] carried out a pilot study to investigate the effect of perineal transcutaneous mechanical nerve stimulation (frequency 100 Hz and amplitude 2 mm) on the severity of stress urinary incontinence symptoms. Perineal transcutaneous nerve stimulation performed weekly for 6 weeks reduced the daily number of incontinence episodes and pad use. Seventy-three per cent of the patients reported complete resolution of

Table 4 Comparison of relative changes of mean and median frequency of the sEMG signal and mean amplitude of the PFMs between the groups

Group	n	Median Frequency [Hz]		Mean Amplitude [%MVC]		Mean Frequency [Hz]	
		Mean	SD	Mean	SD	Mean	SD
I	12	−5.15	7.42	0.69	4.7	−3.47	7.2
II	11	−2.77	6.07	0.66	0.8	−4.22	5.79
III	10	−3.67	4.85	−0.18	3.18	−4.26	7.83
	p^a(I...III)	0.86		0.45		0.99	

p^a - Kruskal-Wallis ANOVA

stress incontinence symptoms. Lauper et al. [6] examined differences in pelvic floor muscle activation depending on the type of whole-body vibrations, ie., sinusoidal vibration and stochastic resonance vibration. The latter led to a significantly higher activation than maximum voluntary contraction, especially in post partum women with weakened pelvic floor muscles. However, in the study of Luginbuehl et al. [7] there was no significant change in PFM activity over time during stochastic resonance in women with self-reported stress urinary incontinence.

Briefly, each subject was asked to stand on the platform, loading their feet uniformly, with the knee and hip joints bent at 35° and the upper extremities stretched horizontally forwards, holding on to a railing.

With an increase in trial duration, both the study and control groups exhibited a significant decrease in the variability of sEMG signal amplitude from the pelvic floor muscles ($p < 0.05$). Body alignment for static exercise, with the knees flexed to 35° and upper limbs stretched out forwards, is a rarely assumed, unnatural and uncomfortable position. Balance control during body sway from the vertical position requires precise neuromuscular coordination and the involvement of various structures of the central and peripheral nervous systems [36]. It may be that a 30 s trial was not enough for the controller (nervous system) and responder (locomotor system) to coordinate and stabilize their actions in a nontypical body position. Since our findings revealed a decrease in the variability of sEMG signal amplitude with longer trials, we believe that an analysis of bioelectrical activity of muscles during whole-body vibration should be based on longer vibration times.

In order to assess measurement variability, Grape et al. [27] calculated the standard error of measurement. The variability between two sEMG sessions carried out on the same day with 30 min apart was smaller compared to the third performer 26–30 days later. However, due to the lack of normalization, a comparison between Grape et al.'s and our results is not possible.

EMG-fatigue slopes provide a non-invasive and standardized method to estimate neuromuscular fatigability of skeletal muscles. Mean and median frequency and the amplitude of EMG signal are among the parameters of the complete power range used in the assessment of muscle fatigue [24]. A 450-s contraction of the biceps brachii at 25 % MVC resulted in a decrease of median and mean frequency and an increase in mean amplitude thus confirming the development of muscle fatigue [24]. In our young and continent participants, 90 s vibration did not cause pelvic floor muscle fatigue. A single 90 s vibration session in young healthy women was probably not sufficient to cause pelvic floor muscle fatigue. Nevertheless, the question requires further investigations.

An analysis of raw pelvic floor EMG data revealed significantly lower values of absolute mean amplitude and mean and median frequency in women with weakened pelvic floor muscles compared to healthy participants [6]. The authors believe that such results are due to decreased muscle fiber recruitment and synchronization and low muscle strength and power in postpartum women. Luginbuehl et al. [7] demonstrated no significant change in the value of amplitude and median frequency of the EMG during stochastic resonance whole body vibration. According to the authors, it can be due to a no more than moderate to submaximal PFM activity during stochastic resonance whole body vibration.

Pelvic floor muscle fatigue has been investigated by several other authors [19, 37–40]. It was also evaluated based on changes in vaginal pressure during MVC measurement [19], perineal ultrasound to assess bladder neck motility [39], time-to-fatigue test with a relative force of 80 % [40] and Borg Scale of Perceived Exertion [38].

The neuromuscular systems alters the recruitment strategies and motor unit firing frequencies during prolonged fatiguing contractions [41]. A single 90 s vibration session in young healthy women was probably not sufficient to cause pelvic floor muscle fatigue in this experiment.

Our study has several limitations including a relatively small number of study participants. Also, we could not compare the results with incontinent women as no comparison group had been formed. Finally, we did not measure the actually generated vibration parameters and skidding of the feet as recommended by the International Society of Musculoskeletal and Neuronal Interactions [42].

Conclusions

Our findings seem to indicate that high-intensity whole-body vibrations (frequency 40Hz, peak-to-peak displacement 4 mm) of long duration (60s, 90s) increase the mean amplitude of sEMG signal from the pelvic floor muscles in young continent women. Single 90s whole-body vibrations in young healthy women does not cause pelvic floor muscle fatigue.

The findings of the present study may have implications for clinical practice and for public health policy in terms of preventive strategies of stress incontinence in women. A significant decrease in sEMG amplitude variability suggests that research should involve long exposure to whole-body vibrations.

However, we would like to emphasize the need for further multidirectional studies on changes in pelvic floor muscle activation during whole-body vibration in women with a history of stress urinary incontinence.

Abbreviations
PFM: Pelvic floor muscles; WBV: Whole-body vibration; sEMG: Surface electromyography; MVC: Maximal Voluntary Contraction.

Competing interests
The authors declare that they have no competing interests.

Authors' contributions
MS participated in the conception and design of the study, data collection, data analysis and manuscript writing. DC participated in data collection, data analysis and manuscript writing. KK participated in project design and development. AS participated in data collection. JT participated in the conception and design of the study. GJ participated in the conception of the study and manuscript editing. All authors read, edited and approved the final version of manuscript.

Acknowledgements
The authors are thankful to Professor Andrzej Małecki MD, PhD, DSc (Jerzy Kukuczka Academy of Physical Education in Katowice – Poland) and Grzegorz Sobota, MSc PhD (Jerzy Kukuczka Academy of Physical Education in Katowice – Poland) for providing moral and scientific support for the accomplishment of this research. No authors received any external funding for the present study.
This study was supported by The Academy of Physical Education in Katowice, Poland.

Author details
[1]Department of Physiotherapy Basics, Jerzy Kukuczka Academy of Physical Education, Mikołowska 72a, 40-065 Katowice, Poland. [2]Department of Human Motor Behavior, Jerzy Kukuczka Academy of Physical Education, Mikołowska 72a, 40-065 Katowice, Poland.

References
1. Del Pozo-Cruz B, Mocholí M, Adsuar J, Parraca J, Muro I, Gusi N. Effects of whole body vibration therapy on main outcome measures for chronic non-specific low back pain: a single blind randomized controlled trial. J Rehabil Med. 2011;43:689–94.
2. Pinto N, Monteiro M, Meyer P, Santos-Filho S, Azevedo-Santos F, Bernardo R, et al. The effects of whole-body-vibration exercises in Parkinson's disease: a short review. J Med Med Sci. 2010;2(1):594–600.
3. Hilgers C, Mündermann A, Riehle H, Dettmers C. Effects of whole-body vibration training on physical function in patients with multiple sclerosis. NeuroRehabilitation. 2013;32(3):655–63.
4. Tihanyi T, Horváth M, Fazekas G, Hortobágyi T, Tihanyi J. One session of whole body vibration increases voluntary muscle strength transiently in patients with stroke. Clin Rehabil. 2007;21(9):782–93.
5. Ruck J, Chabot G, Rauch F. Vibration treatment in cerebral palsy: a randomized controlled pilot study. J Musculoskelet Neuronal Interact. 2010;10(1):77–83.
6. Lauper M, Kuhn A, Gerber R, Luginbühl H, Radlinger L. Pelvic floor stimulation: what are the good vibrations? Neurourol Urodyn. 2009;5:405–10.
7. Luginbuehl H, Lehmann C, Gerber R, Kuhn A, Hilfiker R, Baeyens JP, et al. Continuous versus intermittent stochastic resonance whole body vibration and its effect on pelvic floor muscle activity. Neurourol Urodyn. 2012;31(5):683–7.
8. Eklund G, Hagbarth K. Normal variability of tonic vibration reflex in man. Exp Neurol. 1966;16:80–92.
9. Auchincloss C, McLean L. The reliability of surface EMG recorded from the pelvic floor muscles. J Neurosci Methods. 2009;182:85–96.
10. Abercromby A, Amonette W, Layne C, McFarlin B, Hinman M, Paloski W. Variation in neuromuscular responses during acute whole-body vibration exercise. Med Sci Sports Exerc. 2007;39(9):1642–50.
11. Fratini A, Cesarelli M, Bifulco P, Romano M. Relevance of motion artifact in electromyography recordings during vibration treatment. J Electromyogr Kinesiol. 2009;19(4):710–8.
12. Ritzmann R, Kramer A, Gruber M, Gollhofer A, Taube W. EMG activity during whole body vibration: motion artifacts or stretch reflexes? Eur J Appl Physiol. 2010;110(1):143–51.
13. Krol P, Piecha M, Slomka K, Sobota G, Polak A, Juras G. The effect of whole-body vibration frequency and amplitude on the myoelectric activity of vastus medialis and vastus lateralis. J Sports Sci Med. 2011;10:169–74.
14. Ritzmann R, Gollhofer A, Kramer A. The influence of vibration type, frequency, body position and additional load on the neuromuscular activity during whole body vibration. Eur J Appl Physiol. 2013;113(1):1–11.
15. Hazell T, Jakobi J, Kenno K. The effects of whole-body vibration on upper - and lower - body EMG during static and dynamic contractions. Appl Physiol Nutr Metab. 2007;32(6):1156–63.
16. Enck P, Vodušek D. Electromyography of pelvic floor muscles. J Electromyogr Kinesiol. 2006;16(6):568–77.
17. Resende A, Petrcelli C, Bernardes B, Alexandre S, Nakamura M. ZanettiM. Electromyographic evaluation of pelvic floor muscles in pregnant and nonpregnant women. Int Urogynecol J. 2012;23(8):1041–5.
18. Ashton-Miller J, DeLancey J. Functional anatomy of the female pelvic floor. Ann N Y Acad Sci. 2007;1101:266–96.
19. Ree M, Nygaard I, Bø K. Muscular fatigue in the pelvic floor muscles after strenuous physical activity. Acta Obstet Gynecol Scand. 2007;86(7):870–6.
20. Sønksen J, Ohl D, Bonde B, Laessøe L, McGuire E. Transcutaneous mechanical nerve stimulation using perineal vibration: a novel method for the treatment of female stress urinary incontinence. J Urol. 2007;178(5):2025–8.
21. Luo J, McNamara B, Moran K. The use of vibration training to enhance muscle strength and power. Sports Med. 2005;35(1):23–41.
22. Hermens H, Freriks B, Merletti R, Stegeman D, Blok J, Rau G, et al. European recommendations for surface electromyography. Results of the SENIAM project. 8th ed. Enschede: Roessingh Research and Development; 1999.
23. Madill S, McLean L. Quantification of abdominal and pelvic floor muscle synergies in response to voluntary pelvic floor muscle contractions. J Electromyogr Kinesiol. 2008;18(6):955–64.
24. Tarata M. Mechanomyography versus elctromyography in monitoring the muscular fatique. Biomed Eng Online. 2003;2:3.
25. Bø K. Urinary incontinence, pelvic floor dysfunction, exercise and sport. Sports Med. 2004;34(7):451–64.
26. Chmielewska D, Stania M, Sobota G, Kwaśna K, Błaszczak E, Taradaj J, et al. Impact of different body positions on bioelectrical activity of the pelvic floor muscles in nulliparous continent women. Biomed Res Int. 2015;2015:905897.
27. Grape H, Dedering A, Jonasson A. Retest reliability of surface electromyography on the pelvic floor muscles. Neurourol Urodyn. 2009;28:395–9.
28. Torvinen S, Kannu P, Sievänen H, Järvinen TA, Pasanen M, Kontulainen S, et al. Effect of a vibration exposure on muscular performance and body balance. Randomized cross-over study. Clin Physiol Funct Imaging. 2002;22(2):145–52.
29. Zaidell L, Mileva K, Sumners D, Bowtell J. Experimental evidence of the tonic vibration reflex during whole-body vibration of the loaded and unloaded leg. PLoS ONE. 2013;8(12):e85247.
30. Wakeling J, Nigg B, Rozitis A. Muscle activity damps the soft tissue resonance that occurs in response to pulsed and continuous vibrations. J Appl Physiol. 2002;93(3):1093–103.
31. Pollock R, Woledge R, Mills K, Martin F, Newham D. Muscle activity and acceleration during whole body vibration: effect of frequency and amplitude. Clin Biomech. 2010;25(8):840–6.
32. Devreese A, Staes F, Janssens L, Penninckx F, Vereecken R, De Weerdt W. Incontinent women have altered pelvic floor muscle contraction patterns. J Urol. 2007;178(2):558–62.
33. Boyles S, Li H, Mori T, Osterweil P, Guise J. Effect of mode of delivery on the incidence of urinary incontinence in primiparous women. Obstet Gynecol. 2009;113(1):134–41.
34. Lakeman M, Van Der Vaart C, Van Der Steeg J, Roovers J. Predicting the development of stress urinary incontinence 3 years after hysterectomy. Int Urogynecol J. 2011;22(9):1179–84.
35. Da Roza T, Poli de Araujo M, Viana R, Viana S, Natal Jorge N, Bø K, et al. Pelvic floor muscle training to improve urinary incontinence in young, nulliparous sport students: a pilot study. Int Urogynecol J. 2012;23:1069–73.
36. Winter D, Patla A, Prince F, Ishac M, Gielo-Perczak K. Stiffness control of balance in quiet standing. J Neurophysiol. 1998;80:1211–21.

37. Schabrun S, Stafford R, Hodges P. Anal sphincter fatigue: is the mechanism peripheral or central? Neurourol Urodyn. 2011;30(8):1550–6.

38. Burti J, Hacad C, Zambon J, Polessi E, Almeida F. Is there any difference in pelvic floor muscles performance between continent and incontinent women? Neurourol Urodyn. 2015;34(6):544-8.

39. Peschers U, Vodušek D, Fanger G, Schaer G, DeLancey J, Schuessler B. Pelvic muscle activity in nulliparous volunteers. Neurourol Urodyn. 2001;20(3):269–75.

40. Verelst M, Leivseth G. Are fatigue and disturbances in pre-programmed activity of pelvic floor muscles associated with female stress urinary incontinence? Neurourol Urodyn. 2004;23(20):143–7.

41. Gandevia S. Spinal and supraspinal factors in human muscle fatigue. Physiol Rev. 2001;81(4):1725–89.

42. Rauch F, Sievanen H, Boonen S, Cardinale M, Degens H, Felsenberg D, et al. Reporting whole-body vibration intervention studies: recommendations of the International Society of Musculoskeletal and Neuronal Interactions. J Musculoskelet Neuronal Interact. 2010;10(3):193–8.

31

A rare diaphragmatic ureteral herniation case report: endoscopic and open reconstructive management

Frank C. Lin[1*], Jamie S. Lin[2], Samuel Kim[3] and Jonathan R. Walker[1]

Abstract

Background: Ureteral herniations are a rare occurrence, generally found incidentally on cross sectional imaging or during surgical intervention for unrelated processes. Several locations of ureteral herniations can occur including the inguinal, femoral, sciatic, obturator, and thoracic regions. While few reports of ureteral hernias are reported in the literature overall, the vast majority of those reported are inguinoscrotal herniations found during evaluation and treatment of inguinal hernias. Pelvic outlet ureteral herniations intrinsically are more common secondary to their dependent locations. Intrathoracic ureteral herniations through diaphragmatic defects are an exceptionally rare subset of ureteral herniations and have only been described sparingly. Fewer than ten case reports of diaphramatic ureteral herniations have been reported and none have described both cystoscopic management and open reconstruction.

Case presentation: We report the case of a 81 year old female with flank pain who was found to have idiopathic diaphragmatic hernia with incarcerated proximal ureter. She had no prior injury or surgery that explained her clinical presentation. She was initially observed and then managed conservatively with ureteral stent exchanges. Ultimately she underwent open surgical repair of her diaphragmatic hernia, reduction, resection and anastomosis of redundant proximal incarcerated ureteral segment, and nephropexy for a hypermobile right renal unit. This case report illustrates the pre- and post-operative imaging studies of a very rare intrathoracic ureteral herniation as well as surgical approach to repair.

Conclusion: A herniated ureter is a potential source of serious renal and ureteral complications. The thoracic herniation of ureter is the rarest of the ureteral herniations. When discovered, they should be managed to preserve renal function and prevent strangulation of the affected segment of ureter. This case report documents the treatment of a thoracic ureteral herniation with observation, conservative endoscopic management, and finally open surgical reconstruction.

Keywords: Ureter, Ureteral hernia, Diaphramatic hernia, Ureteral reconstruction, Renal obstruction, Case report

Background

Ureteral herniations are a rare occurrence normally found incidentally on imaging or during surgical hernia correction and can be a cause of ureteral obstruction [1]. These herniations can occur in several locations including the inguinal, femoral, sciatic, obturator, and thoracic regions [2]. Diaphragmatic herniations, however, are the rarest form of ureteral herniations with fewer than ten cases reported since 1958 [3]. They have been identified in the retrocrural area [4] and through congenital Bochdalek hernias [5–7].

Prior cases of obstructing diaphragmatic ureteral hernias have been managed with ureteral stent placement or open reduction, but none have described situations requiring open hernia reduction and ureteral reconstruction [8]. Here, we present a unique case of a right-sided posterior diaphragmatic hernia containing an incarcerated right proximal ureter with subsequent hydroureteronephrosis, and what we believe to be the first documented open-

* Correspondence: flin@email.arizona.edu
[1]Division of Urology, Department of Surgery, University of Arizona, 1501 N. Campbell Ave, Tucson, AZ 85724, USA
Full list of author information is available at the end of the article

reduction and reconstruction of a thoracic ureteral herniation.

Case presentation

The patient was an 81-year-old Caucasian woman with a history of persistent right-sided flank pain with no associated symptoms including dysuria, hematuria, frequency, or urinary retention. She had no history of prior abdominal surgery, trauma, or congenital defects. Given the unclear etiology, we obtained cross-sectional imaging which demonstrated a right-sided Bochdalek diaphragmatic hernia incarcerating her proximal ureteral segment (Fig. 1). Initially, she was managed conservatively with surveillance monitoring since her pain was tolerable and her renal function was preserved. Although her kidney function remained unchanged, follow-up imaging at the next visit surprisingly demonstrated an interval increase in hydroureteronephrosis (Fig. 2). Additionally, the entrapped ureteral portion had progressed with now obvious hydronephrosis of the renal pelvis. A Tc-99m MAG-3 nuclear medicine renal scan with furosemide confirmed our suspicion – she had moderate obstruction of the right kidney. This study also demonstrated an asymmetric split function with 64% left and 36% right in the setting of a stable baseline creatinine (0.7mg/dL).

In attempt to reduce the entrapped ureter and unobstruct the right kidney, a double-pigtail ureteral stent was endoscopically placed. We were able to reduce the herniation with the use of a super stiff wire and a standard soft stent was placed in the usual retrograde fashion. During her stent exchanges, it became apparent that the herniated ureteral segment was enlarging as the curl of the double-J stent retracted into the distal ureter requiring ureteroscopy to visualize and engage. Longer stents were used to ensure that the distal curl remained in the bladder lumen despite recurrent herniation. Stiffer stents were also used however these maneuvers eventually were no longer able to straighten and reduce the ureter, leaving it entrapped in the thoracic cavity. After several stent exchanges were completed, the patient became symptomatic with ureteral stent discomfort including flank pain, urinary frequency and urgency. Due to concern that her diaphragmatic defect was enlarging, we discussed definitive surgical options with her; nephrectomy versus resection and anastomoses of her right ureter with diaphragmatic hernia repair. She ultimately opted to preserve her right kidney and proceed with open-resection reduction and repair.

We approached her open surgical repair through a standard supra-11 incision carried down through her flank muscles where we entered the retroperitoneal space. First, we freed her affected kidney from the surrounding tissue and then identified the incarcerated ureteral segment using our previously placed stent. The redundant ureter was mobilized out of the diaphragmatic defect and returned to the retroperitoneal abdominal cavity. We closed her diaphragmatic defect using interrupted 0 silk sutures, and then excised the redundant proximal ureteral segment where we spatulated and reapproximated the proximal and distal ends. Last, we replaced the patient's ureteral stent and completed the anastomosis over a 7-French x 26 cm double-J ureteral stent. Due to the dissection of the renal hilum and perinephric tissue, the kidney appeared to have more mobility. To help maintain proper drainage and reduce tension on the anastomosis, we performed a nephropexy, securing the posterior aspect of the kidney to the flank muscles with a 0 silk. From there, we performed the standard two-layered incision closure.

The patient had an uncomplicated post-operative course and was discharged home after regaining bowel function and returning to her baseline physical activity on post-operative day three. There were no complications during surgery or recovery. Two months later, we removed her ureteral stent and obtained follow-up imaging which demonstrated repair of the diaphragmatic defect without hernia recurrence (Fig. 3). We also repeated the Tc-99m MAG-3 nuclear medicine renal scan, which now demonstrated normal clearance of the previously obstructed right kidney. Post operative creatinine

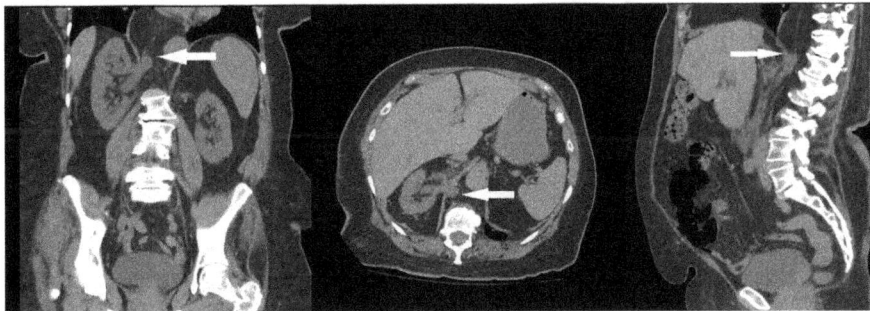

Fig. 1 Patient's initial computed tomography (CT) at presentation demonstrating small loop of ureter within right-sided diaphragmatic hernia. Coronal, Axial, Sagittal views with white arrow showing segment of herniated ureter

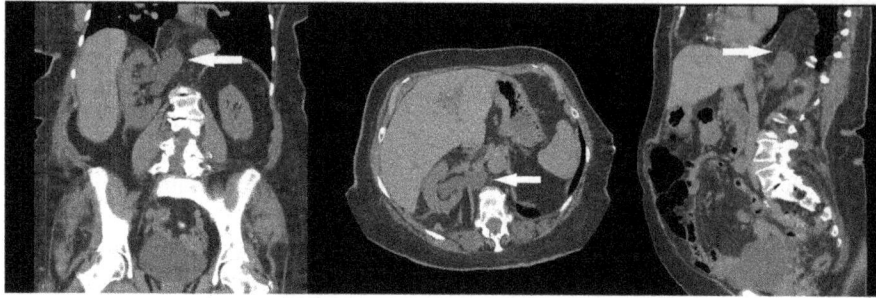

Fig. 2 Follow up computed tomography (CT) 18 months later demonstrating increased hydroureteronephrosis and increased segment of entrapped ureter. Coronal, Axial, Sagittal views with white arrow showing segment of herniated ureter

was 0.7 mg/dL with no obstruction detected. Split cortical function was 54% left and 46% right; an improvement the patient's preoperative findings.

Discussion

Ureteral herniation is a rare anatomic entity. In 1975, Pollack et al. reported that there had been 120 reports of ureteral hernias at the time of their case series publication [9]. While the exact case number is unknown, recent publications have documented fewer than 200 cases [10, 11]. These herniations, have been described in several anatomic regions including inguinal, femoral, sciatic, obturator, and thoracic regions. Out of these listed, inguinal ureteral hernias are the most common, occurring approximately 42–64% of the time, and have the greatest risk of inadvertent injury due to the herniorrhaphies associated with that area [9, 12]. Conversely, literature review revealed fewer than 10 documented thoracic ureteral herniation cases and none were from sequelae to iatrogenic injuries. This subset likely represents the rarest form of ureteral herniations.

Thoracic ureteral hernias were first documented by Swithinbank in 1958 [3]. This case involved a right-sided diaphragmatic ureteral herniation in a 60 year-old female who was found to be symptomatic with right-sided flank pain. She ultimately underwent open-reduction of the ureteral hernia with repair of diaphragmatic defect; however, no reconstruction was performed and the redundant ureter was left in the retroperitoneal space. The paucity of these occurrences is thought to be secondary to their non-dependent anatomic location. From case reports, elderly patients appear to be at highest risk. While the etiology of this is unknown, this could largely be attributed to study bias in that cross sectional imaging is more frequently performed in the elderly population. Further metaanalysis of prior case reports and series may help elucidate a more clear pattern. Previous reports have also discussed thoracic variants, but ours is the first to detail open-reduction and reconstruction after progression of herniation and obstruction.

In general, ureteral hernias are an incidental finding. If symptomatic, they can present with flank pain, gross hematuria, renal dysfunction, nephrolithiasis, and urosepsis [11, 13]. While these symptoms are non-specific, and the likelihood of diagnosing a herniated ureter is low, the consequences of misdiagnosis can result in permanent ureteral injury, loss of renal function, and/or urosepsis. Diagnostic studies such as computer tomography, magnetic resonance imaging, intravenous and retrograde pyelography can be helpful in diagnosing this entity.

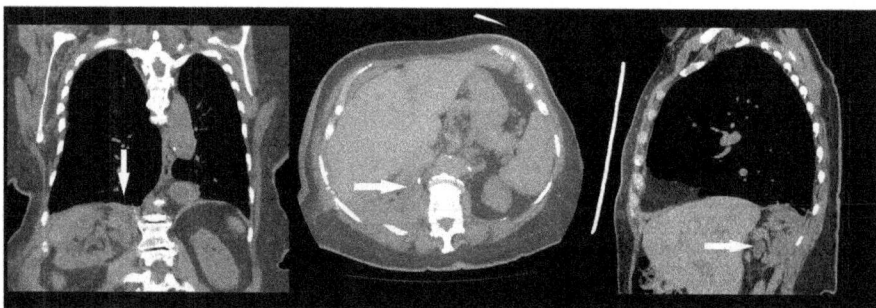

Fig. 3 Post-surgical computed tomography (CT) demonstrating repair of diaphragmatic hernia and segmental resection of ureter. Coronal, Axial, Sagittal views with white arrow showing resolution of hydroureteronephrosis and repair of diaphragmatic hernia. Note the changes in the position of the right kidney from nephroxy and no redundant ureter is evident

Ureteral hernias are managed conservatively unless there is an urgency to treat (e.g. obstruction, urosepsis, or intractable flank pain). These patients can generally be followed in clinic with both labs and imaging to monitor for progression. Isolated lab tests may be inadequate in detecting obstruction in the setting of a normal functioning contralateral kidney, as it may not reflect true kidney function as our patient demonstrated. If intervention is warranted, endoscopic stent placement is the routine management therapy. However, if endoscopy is unsuccessful in reducing the herniation, then open-reduction surgery may be a viable option for renal preservation, as we demonstrated. Care should be taken to avoid injuring the ureter with the end-goal of relieving the ureteric obstruction and ensuring that impairment of renal function is minimized. Each case should be evaluated on its own merit and follow-up imaging and diagnostics studies should be obtained to ensure successful reduction.

Conclusion

Thoracic ureteral herniations are extremely uncommon, and imaging and functional studies are necessary for monitoring possible progression of the anatomic defect. Here, we demonstrate for the first time, a successful open-reduction and reconstructive surgery for an elderly women found to have an idiopathic thoracic ureteral herniation. We suggest that this approach may be an alternative option for patients that cannot be managed with routine endoscopic management.

Acknowledgments
The authors thank the patient for allowing us to publish this case report.

.

Authors' contributions
FL carried out the surgery, participated in the follow up care, performed literature review, and drafted the manuscript. JL performed literature review, and drafted the manuscript. SK participated in the surgery, participated in the follow up care, edited the manuscript. JW carried out the surgery, participated in the follow up care, and edited the manuscript. All authors read and approved the final manuscript.

Competing interests
The authors declare that they have no competing interests.

Author details
[1]Division of Urology, Department of Surgery, University of Arizona, 1501 N. Campbell Ave, Tucson, AZ 85724, USA. [2]Renal-Electrolyte and Hypertension Division, Department of Medicine, University of Pennsylvania, Perelman School of Medicine, 3400 Civic Blvd, Philadelphia, PA 19104, USA. [3]Division of Cardiothoracic Surgery, Department of Surgery, University of Arizona, 1501 N. Campbell Ave, Tucson, AZ 85724, USA.

References
1. Allam ES, Johnson DY, Grewal SG, Johnson FE. Inguinoscrotal herniation of the ureter: Description of five cases. Int J Surg Case Rep. 2015;14:160–3.
2. Catalano O, Nunziata A, Cusati B, Siani A. Retrocrural loop of the ureter: CT findings. AJR Am J Roentgenol. 1998;170(5):1293–4.
3. Swithinbank AH. Intrathoracic deviation of a ureteric loop. Br J Surg. 1958; 45(192):379–81.
4. Almeida L, Carvalhaes F, Bitencourt A, Moreira F. Ureteral Hernia Mimicking Retrocrural Lymphadenopathy in 18F-FDG PET/CT. Clin Nucl Med. 2015; 40(8):e415–6.
5. Chawla K, Mond DJ. Progressive Bochdalek hernia with unusual ureteral herniation. Comput Med Imaging Graph. 1994;18(1):53–8.
6. Dru CJ, Josephson DY. Bochdalek-type Diaphragmatic Hernia Leading to High-grade Kidney Obstruction. Urology. 2016;97:e17–8.
7. Song YS, Hassani C, Nardi PM. Bochdalek hernia with obstructive uropathy. Urology. 1338;77(6).
8. Salari K, Yura Emily M, Harisinghani M, Eisner Brian H. Evaluation and Treatment of a Ureterosciatic Hernia Causing Hydronephrosis and Renal Colic. Journal of Endourology Case Reports. 2015;1(1):1–2.
9. Pollack HM, Popky GL, Blumberg ML. Hernias of the ureter - An anatomic-roentgenographic study. Radiology. 1975;117(2):275–81.
10. Sukumar S, Kumar PG, Thomas A. Thoracic curlicue: A case of ureteral herniation. Indian J Urol. 2010;26(1):131–2.
11. Yanagi K, Kan A, Sejima T, Takenaka A. Treatment of ureterosciatic hernia with a ureteral stent. Case Rep Nephrol Dial. 2015;5(1):83–6.
12. Hwang CM, Miller FH, Dalton DP, Hartz WH. Accidental ureteral ligation during an inguinal hernia repair of patient with crossed fused renal ectopia. Clin Imaging. 2002;26(5):306–8.
13. Hatzidakis A, Kozana A, Glaritis D, Mamoulakis C. Right-sided Bochdalek hernia causing septic ureteric obstruction. Percutaneous treatment with placement of a nephroureteral double pigtail. BMJ Case Rep. 2014;31:2014.

32

Spontaneous renal allograft rupture complicated by urinary leakage

Evaldo Favi[1*], Samuele Iesari[2], Alessandro Cina[3] and Franco Citterio[4]

Abstract

Background: For more than forty years, graftectomy has been the standard treatment of spontaneous renal transplant rupture. However, recent evidences suggest that graft salvage strategies can be safely pursued, even in difficult cases.

Case presentation: We report on a thirty-nine-year-old woman who received a deceased donor kidney transplant and experienced spontaneous allograft rupture due to acute rejection. The rupture was further complicated by urinary leakage. The kidney and the ureter were successfully repaired. Eight years after transplantation, graft function is still excellent.

Conclusion: Due to the lack of transplantable organs and the long time usually spent on the waiting list, graftectomy should be only considered in case of refractory haemodynamic instability or compromised graft viability.

Keywords: Renal allograft rupture, Urinary leakage, Acute rejection, Graft repair

Background

Spontaneous renal allograft rupture is a rare but life threatening complication of kidney transplantation. Graftectomy is the safest option. However, if the patient can be stabilised, graft repair should be always considered because of the long waiting list and the low chance of receiving a second transplant.

To the best of our knowledge, this is the first report on a patient who had her transplant saved after experiencing acute rejection, spontaneous graft rupture and urinary leakage.

Case presentation

A thirty-nine-year-old woman with end stage renal disease secondary to eclampsia was admitted to our institution for her primary deceased donor kidney transplantation on January 2006. Pre-transplant comorbidities included hypertension, dyslipidemia and secondary

* Correspondence: evaldofavi@gmail.com
[1]Transplant Unit, Renal Department, Royal London Hospital, Whitechapel Road, London E1 1BB, UK
Full list of author information is available at the end of the article

hyperparathyroism. The donor was a twenty-six-year-old male who died from acute obstruction of the foramina of Monroe. Cold ischemia time was ten hours. The kidney was medium-sized, had one artery, one vein and one ureter. The donor and the recipient were blood group compatible and six HLA antigens mismatched. The highest recipient Panel Reactivity Antibody was 15 % and the direct microcytotoxicity crossmatch was negative. Macroscopically, the kidney looked normal. It was extraperitoneally transplanted in the left iliac fossa, as standard procedure. After declamping, the organ reperfused immediately. The graft ureter was anastomosed to the bladder according to the single stitch technique. The patient was enrolled in a phase III randomized, multicenter, clinical trial and received basiliximab (Simulect®, Novartis Pharmaceuticals Corporation), cyclosporine (Sandimmune Neoral®, Novartis Pharmaceuticals Corporation), everolimus (Certican®, Novartis Pharmaceuticals Corporation) and steroids.

The early post-operative course was complicated by delayed graft function requiring haemodialysis. According to the protocol, her baseline immunosuppression was not changed. Daily ultrasound evaluation showed a well-sized graft with no fluid collections, no hydrone-phrosis, and good intra-parenchymal flow. Haematologic and coagulation profiles were normal.

On post-operative day four, the recipient suddenly complained of abdominal pain and the urinary output dropped. Blood pressure, pulse rate and haemoglobin concentration remained stable. Four hours later, the abdominal pain increased and the area over the graft became distended and tender. Hypotension rapidly developed, the pulse rate increased and the patient became anuric. Aggressive resuscitation was promptly initiated. An urgent Doppler ultrasound scan was performed. It showed a large hypoechoic collection surrounding the graft with good flow in the renal artery and a patent renal vein. Subsequent contrast-enhanced CT scan revealed a ruptured graft and a massive retroperitoneal haematoma with active bleeding from the transplanted kidney (Fig. 1). The patient was immediately brought to theatre and explored. A large peri-graft haematoma was evacuated. The kidney was swollen but pink and the arterial pulse was good. A 5 cm long and 1.5 cm deep laceration was found along the middle portion of the convex border of graft, actively bleeding. After en block clamping of the renal vessels, the transplant was fully inspected. Haemostasis was achieved using a haemostatic matrix (Floseal® Hemostatic Matrix, Baxter International Inc.) and by apposition of several mattress polyglactin 910 (Vicryl™, Ethicon Inc.) sutures tied over flaps of absorbable hemostats (Surgicel® Original Absorbable Hemostat, Ethicon Inc.). To prevent extension of the rupture, a polyglactin 910 mesh (Vicryl™ Woven Mesh, Ethicon Inc.) was wrapped around the graft. The procedure took 140 min and renal clamping was 45 min. The total intra-operative blood loss (including the haematoma) was 500 mL and two units of packed red blood cells were transfused. Considering the severity

of the bleeding, the complex repair, and the risk of further damage to the kidney, a graft biopsy was not taken at the time of the operation. However, the clinical picture was highly suggestive of acute rejection and we therefore decided to administer a course of rabbit anti-thymocyte globulins (Thymoglobulin®, Genzyme Inc.). Cyclosporine and everolimus were also switched to tacrolimus (Prograf®, Astellas Pharma Inc.) and mycophenolate mofetil (CellCept®, Genentech USA Inc.). After the operation, the patient remained anuric requiring haemodialysis for twenty-one days. Renal function improved and serum creatinine concentration fell to 2 mg/dL.

On post-operative day fifty-two, clear fluid started to seep from the wound. Urgent CT scan showed a large (5 × 2.3 cm) fluid collection in continuity with the area of the previous rupture (Fig. 2). Urinary leakage was confirmed by chemical analysis of the fluid. A nephrostomy tube and a trans-abdominal drain were inserted to control the leak and evacuate the collection. Two days later, the patient became febrile and the urinary output dropped. A nephrostogram was performed. It demonstrated another urinary leak at the site of the ureteral anastomosis (Fig. 3). Following an unsuccessful simultaneous cystoscopy and fluoroscopy guided ureteral stent placement, a surgical exploration was planned. The abdomen was entered through a midline incision and the graft was inspected. The distal part of the transplanted ureter, partially necrotized, was resected and the proximal stump was anastomosed to the bladder according to the Lich-Gregoire technique. A double-J pyeloureteral stent was placed to protect the anastomosis. The procedure took 143 min. The post-operative course was uneventful. Renal function gradually recovered, serum creatinine fell to 1.7 mg/dL and the patient was eventually discharged.

Eight years after transplantation, the patient is doing well and her serum creatinine is 1 mg/dL.

Discussion

Spontaneous renal allograft rupture is defined as a laceration of the renal capsule when there are no other identifiable injuries noted at the time of the organ retrieval [1]. Its incidence has been reported as between 0.3 and 9.6 %, depending on the series [2–4]. This complication usually occurs within the first two weeks after transplantation although late ruptures have been reported [5].

Several causes have been proposed [1–3, 5–7]. Acute rejection is the most important, accounting for 60 to 80 % of cases. Less frequent etiologies include renal vein thrombosis, acute tubular necrosis, ureteral obstruction, renal biopsy, trauma, local ischaemia, septic infarction

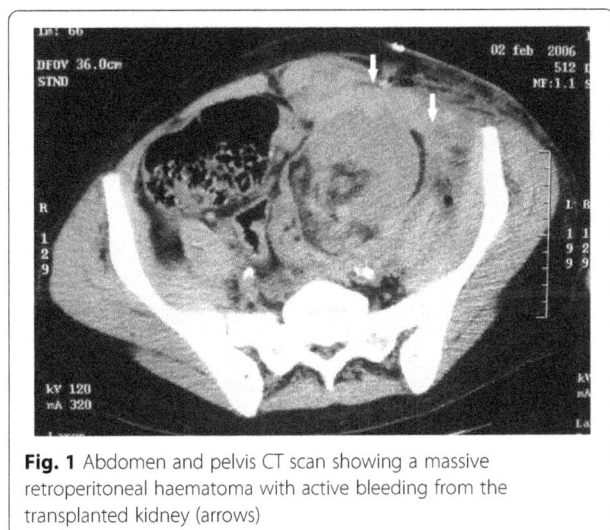

Fig. 1 Abdomen and pelvis CT scan showing a massive retroperitoneal haematoma with active bleeding from the transplanted kidney (arrows)

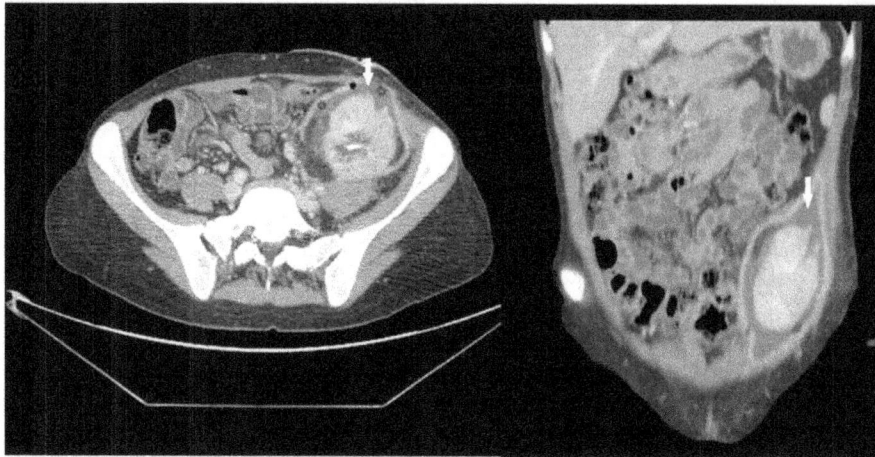

Fig. 2 Abdomen and pelvis CT scan showing a large urine collection around the graft, in continuity with the area of the previous rupture (arrows). (left) axial reconstruction; (right) coronal reconstruction

and cancer. The rupture most frequently occurs longitudinally, along the convex border of the kidney. Clinical presentation is often typical, with severe graft dysfunction and acute blood loss. Immediate ultrasound evaluation can rapidly and safely confirm the diagnosis with 87 % sensitivity and 100 % specificity [8].

In case of haemodynamic instability, immediate surgical exploration is mandatory. Initial reports of conservative management of graft rupture showed poor results, with less than 30 % success rate. Failure to control acute bleeding, inability to reverse acute rejection, post-surgical development of multiple organ failure and uncontrollable coagulopathy were the main causes of the high rate of graft nephrectomies observed. In the last

decades, improved surgical technique and post-operative care have significantly reduced transplant-related mortality and morbidity. Complex operations are now safely performed with good results. Current reports demonstrate that ruptured grafts can be saved with a success rate as high as 80 %. Moreover, recipients undergoing successful repair have long-term outcomes similar to the general transplant population. Recurrent rupture, the most dangerous complication of graft repair, only occurs in 5 % of patients and does not significantly jeopardise the prognosis (see Table 1 for details). Fibrin glue and collagen foam can be used to facilitate haemostasis without endangering the transplant through unnecessary manipulation of oedematous and fragile tissues [9]. Renal corsetage with various materials, including polyglactin 910 mesh, lyophilized dura, grafts of peritoneum, pieces of external oblique aponeurosis and polypropylene mesh has also been reported [10]. In this setting, external compression is particularly helpful because it supports haemostasis and at the same time prevents further extension of the rupture.

Conclusions

When spontaneous renal transplant rupture occurs, nephrectomy is justified only in case of refractory haemodynamic instability or compromised kidney viability. When irreversible graft damage can be ruled out and the patient can be readily resuscitated, transplant salvage should always be attempted.

Consent

Written informed consent for publication of this Case report and any accompanying images has been obtained from the patient. A copy of the written consent is available for review by the Editor of this journal.

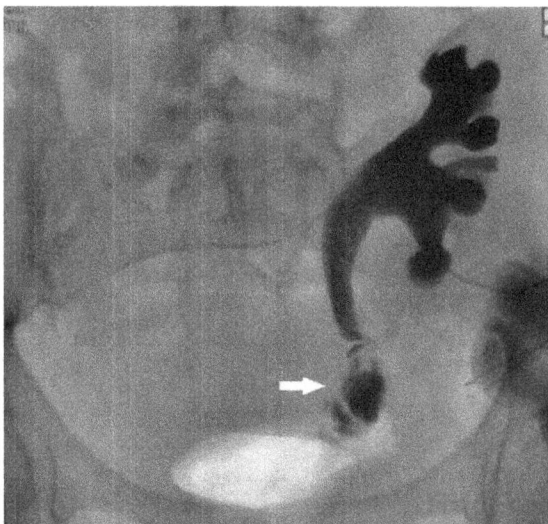

Fig. 3 Nephrostogram demonstrating urinary leakage at the site of the ureteral reimplantation (arrow)

Table 1 Management and outcomes of spontaneous renal allograft rupture (SRAR) over time

Authors year	SRAR/KTx (#)	Incidence (%)	p.o. day mean	p.o. day median	p.o. day range	FU MAX Months	Graftectomy (# / %)	Repair (# / %)	Death (# / %)
Murray 1968 [11]	4/110	3.6	3 ± 2	2.5	1 – 6	33	1 / 33 %	3 / 77 %	0
Salaman 1969 [12]	3/74	4.1	-	-	-	-	2 / 66.6 %	1 / 33.3 %	-
Siedek 1969 [13]	1/21	4.8	9	9	-	-	1 / 100 %	0	0
Flanigan 1971 [14]	2/46	4.3	-	-	≤8	-	2 / 100 %	0	0
Haimov 1971 [15]	1/30	3.3	2	2	2	4	0	1 / 100 %	0
Lord 1972 [16]	1/280	0.4	14	-	-	0.5	1 / 100 %	0	1 / 100 %
Minale 1972 [17]	6/100	6	4.5 ± 1	4	3 - 7	60	0	6 / 100 %	0
Ghose 1973 [18]	6/71	8.4	-	-	-	-	3 / 50 %	3 / 50 %	-
Fjeldborg 1974 [19]	7/200	3.5	-	-	-	-	2 / 28.6 %	5 / 71.4 %	-
Kootstra 1974 [20]	2/39	5.1	27 ± 27	27	8 - 46	-	1 / 50 %	0	1 / 100 %
Homan 1977 [21]	21/246	8.5	-	-	2 - 49	8	2 / 9.5 %	19 / 90.5 %	0
Van Cangh 1977 [22]	9/325	2.8	-	-	-	-	6 / 66.6 %	3 / 33.3 %	-
Brekke 1978 [23]	16/448	3.6	-	-	-	-	10 / 62.5 %	6 / 37.5 %	-
Montes 1978 [24]	13/419	3.1	-	-	-	-	5 / 38.5 %	8 / 61.5 %	-
Susan 1978 [25]	4/474	0.8	10.5 ± 5	10.5	5–16	15	0	4 100 %	0
Dryburgh 1979 [26]	9/93	9.7	-	-	1–18	22	7 / 78 %	2 / 22 %	2 / 22 %
Prompt 1979 [27]	8/327	2.4	7 ± 3.5	8.5	2–11	0.8	6 / 75 %	2 / 25 %	0
Oesterwitz 1980 [28]	22/364	6	5 ± 3	4.5	1–14	60	10 / 45 %	12 / 55 %	0
Van Der Vliet 1980 [29]	1/211	0.5	-	-	-	-	1 / 100 %	0	-
Goldman 1981 [30]	7/350	2	-	-	3–7	58	3 / 43 %	4 / 57 %	0
Nghiem 1981 [31]	7/585	1.2	18 ± 20	8	3–58	96	2 / 29 %	5 / 71 %	0
Thukral 1982 [32]	3/100	3	7 ± 1	8	6–8	60	0	3 / 100 %	0
Serrallach 1985 [33]	5/66	7.6	7 ± 3	8	4–10	15	0	5 / 100 %	0
Chopin 1989 [34]	4/85	4.7	17 ± 13	15	5–32	12	1 / 25 %	3 / 75 %	0
Said 1994 [10]	3/75	4	7 ± 3.5	7	4–11	10	2 / 67 %	1 / 33 %	0
Yadav 1994 [35]	15/237	6.3	-	-	-	120	4 / 27 %	11 / 73 %	-
Heimbach 1995 [4]	8/238	3.4	11	-	8–17	94	1 / 12.5 %	7 / 87.5 %	0
Azar 1996 [3]	12/331	3.6	10	9	4–21	-	12 / 100 %	0	1 / 8 %
Zadrozny 1997 [36]	8/112	7.1	-	-	-	-	5 / 62.5 %	3 / 37.5 %	0
Pontones Moreno 1998 [37]	21/868	2.4	-	-	-	-	4 / 19 %	17 / 81 %	0
Szenohradszky 1999 [7]	53/628	8.4	-	-	-	-	37 / 70 %	16 / 30 %	-

Table 1 Management and outcomes of spontaneous renal allograft rupture (SRAR) over time *(Continued)*

Millwala 2000 [38]	4/145	2.7	–	–	–	6	2 / 50 %	2 / 50 %	1 / 25 %
Ramos 2000 [39]	11/934	1.2	–	5	2–13	–	10 / 90.9 %	1 / 9.1 %	0
Hochleitner 2001 [2]	14/1811	0.8	9.5	111 ± 6	3–23	111	5 / 36 %	9 / 64 %	0
Guleria 2003 [40]	3/172	1.7	7	6 ± 1	5–7	–	0	3 / 100 %	0
Finley 2003 [5]	22/4418	0.5	7	299 ± 793	0–2825	214	8 / 36 %	14 / 64 %	0
He 2003 [41]	38/1000	3.8	–	–	–	60	2 / 5.3 %	31 / 81.6 %	0
Busi 2004 [42]	4/778	0.5	6.5	77.5 ± 4	4–13	0.5	3 / 75 %	1 / 25 %	0
Risaliti 2004 [43]	2/297	0.7	–	–	–	–	–	–	–
Sanchez de la Nieta 2004 [44]	10/657	1.5	–	7.5	1–10	–	5 / 50 %	5 / 50 %	0
Shahrokh 2005 [45]	6/1682	0.4	–	6	4–13	60	3 / 50 %	3 / 50 %	0
Martinez Mansur 2006 [46]	11/492	2.8	–	–	–	–	7 / 63.6 %	4 / 36.4 %	–
Overall	407/19939	2	–	–	0–2825	53	176 / 44.2 %	223 / 54.8 %	7 / 1.8 %

Abbreviation
CT: Computed tomography.

Competing interests
The authors declare that they have no competing interests.

Authors' contributions
EF collected data, reviewed the literature and drafted the manuscript. SI reviewed the literature, drafted the manuscript and formatted the text for submission. AC collected, analyzed and interpreted data. FC revised the project. All authors read and approved the final manuscript.

Acknowledgments
We thank Lauren Sarah Harris (MS, Barts and The London School of Medicine - London, UK) who kindly provided language revision.

Author details
[1]Transplant Unit, Renal Department, Royal London Hospital, Whitechapel Road, London E1 1BB, UK. [2]General Surgery, Department of Biotechnological and Applied Clinical Sciences, University of L'Aquila, Via Pompeo Spennati, 67100 L'Aquila, Italy. [3]Department of Bioimaging, Università Cattolica del "Sacro Cuore", Policlinico Universitario "Agostino Gemelli", Largo Agostino Gemelli 8, 00168 Rome, Italy. [4]Renal Transplant Unit, Department of Surgery, Università Cattolica del "Sacro Cuore", Policlinico Universitario "Agostino Gemelli", Largo Agostino Gemelli 8, 00168 Rome, Italy.

References
1. Richardson AJ, Higgins RM, Jaskowski AJ, Murie JA, Dunnill MS, Ting A, et al. Spontaneous rupture of renal allografts: the importance of renal vein thrombosis in the cyclosporine era. Br J Surg. 1991;77:558–60.
2. Hochleitner BW, Kafka R, Spechtenhauser B, Bösmüller C, Steurer W, Königsrainer A, et al. Renal allograft rupture is associated with rejection or acute tubular necrosis, but not with renal vein thrombosis. Nephrol Dial Transplant. 2001;16:124–7.
3. Azar GJ, Zarifian A, Frentz GD, Tesi RJ, Etheredge EE. Renal allograft rupture: a clinical review. Clin Transplant. 1996;10:635–8.
4. Heimbach D, Miersch WD, Buszello H, Schoeneich G, Kleht HU. Is the transplant-preserving management of renal allograft rupture justified? Br J Urol. 1995;75:729–32.
5. Finley DS, Roberts JP. Frequent salvage of ruptured renal allografts: a large single center experience. Clin Transplant. 2003;17:126–9.
6. Chan YH, Wong KM, Lee KC, Li CS. Spontaneous renal allograft rupture attributed to acute tubular necrosis. Am J Kidney Dis. 1999;34:355–8.
7. Szenohradszky P, Smehak G, Szederkenyi E, Marofka F, Csajbok E, Morvay Z, et al. Renal allograft rupture: a clinicopathologic study of 37 nephrectomy cases in a series of 628 consecutive renal transplants. Transplant Proc. 1999;31:2107–11.
8. Soler R, Perez-Fontan FJ, Lago M, Moncalian J, Perez-Fontan M. Renal allograft rupture: diagnostic role of ultrasound. Nephrol Dial Transplant. 1992;7:871–4.
9. Hanke P, Fassbinder W, Brox G. Treatment of spontaneous kidney allograft rupture by means of fibrin sealant and collagen fleece: experimental and clinical studies. Transplant Proc. 1986;18:1029–33.
10. Said R, Duarte R, Chaballout A, Boghdadly SE, Nezamuddin N, Mattoo T. Spontaneous rupture of renal allograft. Urology. 1994;43:554–5.
11. Murray JE, Wilson RE, Tilney NL, Merrill JP, Cooper WC, Birtch AG, et al. Five years' experience in renal transplantation with immunosuppressive drugs: survival, function, complications, and the role of lymphocyte depletion by thoracic duct fistula. Ann Surg. 1968;168:416–35.
12. Salaman JR, Calne RY, Pena J, Sells RA, White HJ, Yoffa D. Surgical aspects of clinical renal transplantation. Br J Surg. 1969;56:413–7.
13. Siedek M. Observations in rejections of kidney transplants. Langenbecks Arch Surg. 1969;325:714–9.
14. Flanigan WJ, Caldwell FT, Williams GD, Brewer TE, Glenn WE, Headstream JW, et al. Clinical patterns of renal allograft rejection. Ann Surg. 1971;173:733–47.
15. Haimov M, Glabman S, Burrows L. Spontaneous rupture of the allografted kidney. Arch Surg. 1971;103:510–2.
16. Lord RS, Effeney DJ, Hayes JM, Tracy GD. Renal allograft rupture: cause, clinical features and management. Ann Surg. 1973;177:268–73.
17. Minale C, Linder E, Largiader F. Spontaneous rupture of a transplanted kidney. Dtsch Med Wochenschr. 1972;97:459–61.
18. Ghose MK, Kest LM, Cohen SM, Roza O, Berman LB, Lidsky I, et al. Spontaneous rupture of renal allotransplants. J Urol. 1973;109:790–5.
19. Fjeldborg O, Kim CH. Spontaneous rupture of renal transplant. Scand J Urol Nephrol. 1974;8:31–6.
20. Kootstra G, Meijer S, Elema JD. "Spontaneous" rupture of homografted kidneys. Arch Surg. 1974;108:107–12.
21. Homan WP, Cheigh JS, Kim SJ, Mouradian J, Tapia L, Riggio RR, et al. Renal allograft fracture: clinicopathological study of 21 cases. Ann Surg. 1977;186:700–3.
22. Van Cangh PJ, Ehrlich RM, Smith RB. Renal rupture after transplantation. Urology. 1977;9:8–10.
23. Brekke I, Flatmark A, Laane B, Mellbye O. Renal allograft rupture. Scand J Urol Nephrol. 1978;12:265–70.
24. Montes F, McMaster P, Calne RY, Evans DB. Rupture of the allografted kidney–is repair possible? Proc Eur Dial Transplant Assoc. 1978;15:378–83.
25. Susan LP, Braun WE, Banowsky LH, Straffon RA, Valenzuela R. Ruptured human renal allograft. Pathogenesis and management Urology. 1978;11:53–7.
26. Dryburgh P, Porter KA, Krom RA, Uchida K, West JC, Weil 3rd R, et al. Should the ruptured renal allograft be removed? Arch Surg. 1979;114:850–2.
27. Prompt CA, Johnson WH, Ehrlich RM, Lee DB, Smith RB, Schultze RG. Nontraumatic rupture of renal allografts. Urology. 1979;13:145–8.
28. Oesterwitz H, Tulatz A, Scholz D, May G. Spontaneous rupture of cadaver kidney allotransplants: how successful is a repair? Report of 22 cases and review of the literature. Eur Urol. 1980;6:284–8.
29. van der Vliet JA, Kootstra G, Tegzess AM, Meijer S, Krom RA, Slooff MJ, et al. Management of rupture in allografted kidneys. Neth J Surg. 1980;32:45–8.
30. Goldman M, De Pauw L, Kinnaert P, Vereerstraeten P, Van Geertruyden J, Toussaint C. Renal allograft rupture: possible causes and results of surgical conservative management. Transplantation. 1981;32:153–6.
31. Nghiem DD, Goldman MH, Mendez-Picon G, Rao KG, Woodlief RM, Fields WR, et al. Noninvasive assessment of the transplanted kidney: ultrasound vs. computerized tomography. Am Surg. 1981;47:492–4.
32. Thukral R, Mir AR, Jacobson MP. Renal allograft rupture: a report of three cases and review of the literature. Am J Nephrol. 1982;2:15–27.
33. Serrallach N, Gutierrez J, Serrate R, Aguilo F, Munoz J, Franco E, et al. Renal allograft rupture: surgical treatment by renal corsetage with lyophilized human dura. J Urol. 1985;133:452–5.
34. Chopin DK, Abbou CC, Lottmann HB, Popov Z, Lang PR, Buisson CL, et al. Conservative treatment of renal allograft rupture with polyglactin 910 mesh and gelatin resorcin formaldehyde glue. J Urol. 1989;142:363–5.
35. Yadav RV, Sinha R. Graft repair: the treatment of choice for renal allograft rupture. J Urol. 1994;151:1498–9.
36. Zadrozny D, Pirski MI, Draczkowski T, Gacyk W. The treatment of renal allograft rupture. Transplant Proc. 1997;29:156.
37. Pontones Moreno JL, Rodrigo Aliaga M, Monserrat Monfort JJ, Guillen Navarro M, Sanchez Plumed J, Jimenez Cruz JF. Post-transplantation renal rupture. Actas Urol Esp. 1998;22:840–5. discussion 6.
38. Millwala FN, Abraham G, Shroff S, Soundarajan P, Rao R, Kuruvilla S. Spontaneous renal allograft rupture in a cohort of renal transplant recipients: a tertiary care experience. Transplant Proc. 2000;32:1912–3.
39. Ramos M, Martins L, Dias L, Henriques AC, Soares J, Queiros J, et al. Renal allograft rupture: a clinicopathologic review. Transplant Proc. 2000;32:2597–8.
40. Guleria S, Khazanchi RK, Dinda AK, Aggarwal S, Gupta S, Bhowmik D, et al. Spontaneous renal allograft rupture: is graft nephrectomy an option? Transplant Proc. 2003;35:339.
41. He B, Rao MM, Han X, Li X, Guan D, Gao J. Surgical repair of spontaneous renal allograft rupture: a new procedure. ANZ J Surg. 2003;73:381–3.
42. Busi N, Capocasale E, Mazzoni MP, Benozzi L, Valle RD, Cambi V, et al. Spontaneous renal allograft rupture without acute rejection. Acta Biomed. 2004;75:131–3.
43. Risaliti A, Sainz-Barriga M, Baccarani U, Adani GL, Montanaro D, Gropuzzo M, et al. Surgical complications after kidney transplantation. G Ital Nefrol. 2004;21 Suppl 26:S43–7.

44. Sanchez de la Nieta MD, Sanchez-Fructuoso AI, Alcazar R, Perez-Contin MJ, Prats D, Grimalt J, et al. Higher graft salvage rate in renal allograft rupture associated with acute tubular necrosis. Transplant Proc. 2004;36:3016–8.

45. Shahrokh H, Rasouli H, Zargar MA, Karimi K, Zargar K. Spontaneous kidney allograft rupture. Transplant Proc. 2005;37:3079–80.

46. Martinez Mansur R, Piana M, Codone J, Elizalde F, Diez M, Duro J, et al. The rupture of the renal graft. Arch Esp Urol. 2006;59:489–92.

33

Congenital mid-ureteral stricture: a case report of two patients

Hamdan Alhazmi*⊕ and Abdullah Fouda Neel

Abstract

Background: Congenital hydronephrosis is a common foetal anomaly. There are numerous causes of hydronephrosis. The diagnosis of ureteral anomalies remains challenging. Congenital mid-ureteral stricture (CMS) is less common than proximal and distal strictures. In most cases involving CMS, this condition is diagnosed intra-operatively. The gold standard treatment is resection of the stenosed segment and ureteroureterostomy.

Case presentation: We report two patients with CMS which presented as antenatal hydronephrosis with postnatal workup showed a picture of pelviuretric junction obstruction which required surgical correction. Intraoperative retrograde pyelography (RGP) confirmed the diagnosis of mid ureteral stricture which make us to change the planned surgical intervention from pyeloplasty to excision of the ureteral stricture and ureteroureterostomy as definitive management.

Conclusion: CMS should be considered whenever proximal mega-ureter is an associated finding. Despite advanced radiological modalities, RGP remains the mainstay approach for diagnosing ureteral anomalies.

Keywords: Mid-ureteral stricture, Children, Antenatal hydronephrosis, Ureter

Background

Congenital ureteral stricture is a rare cause of paediatric hydronephrosis [1]. Congenital mid-ureteral stricture (CMS) is associated with severe hydronephrosis and proximal ureteral dilatation [2, 3]. However, this condition is typically diagnosed intra-operatively [3]. Here, we report two cases of CMS that were managed at our institute.

Case presentation

Case 1

At the age of one week, a male child presented with right antenatal hydronephrosis. His postnatal ultrasound showed Society for Fetal Urology (SFU) grade 4 hydronephrosis without clear hydroureter for the right kidney; the left kidney appeared to be normal (Fig. 1-a). A voiding cysto-urethrogram (VCUG) produced normal findings. Subsequently, a mercaptoacetyltriglycine (MAG3) renal scan at four weeks of age revealed a hydronephrotic obstructed right kidney (DRF = 46%) with poor washout

in response to furosemide (T1/2 = 24 min). Accordingly, the patient was admitted electively and underwent right RGP (Fig. 1-b). Right mid-ureteral stricture was detected. The stenosed segment was resected (1.5*0.5 cm), and oblique ureteroureterostomy was performed. A pathological review revealed focal chronic ureteral inflammation with narrow lumen (1 mm). The most recent ultrasound, which was performed 18 months postoperatively, showed complete resolution of hydronephrosis (Fig. 1-c).

Case 2

A two-year-old girl was referred to our institute due to incidentally discovered hydronephrosis. She was investigated for abdominal pain, and abdominal ultrasound revealed SFU grade 4 right hydronephrosis without clear hydroureter (Fig. 2-a). Initially, vesicoureteric reflux was excluded based on a normal VCUG. A MAG3 renal scan revealed a hydronephrotic right kidney with reduced global cortical uptake, no response to Lasix, and split renal function of 32% on the right side. The patient was admitted electively, and right RGP showed right mid-ureteral stricture with a length of 1 cm (Fig. 2-b). Subsequently, the patient underwent laparoscopic excision of the stricture segment and ureteroureterostomy (Fig. 2-c, d). A pathological report indicated predominant sever chronic inflammation with foreign body giant cell infiltration of the ureteral wall with

* Correspondence: drhamdan@ksu.edu.sa
Division of Urology, Department of Surgery, College of Medicine and King Saud University Medical City, King Saud University, PO Box 7805, Riyadh 11472, Kingdom of Saudi Arabia

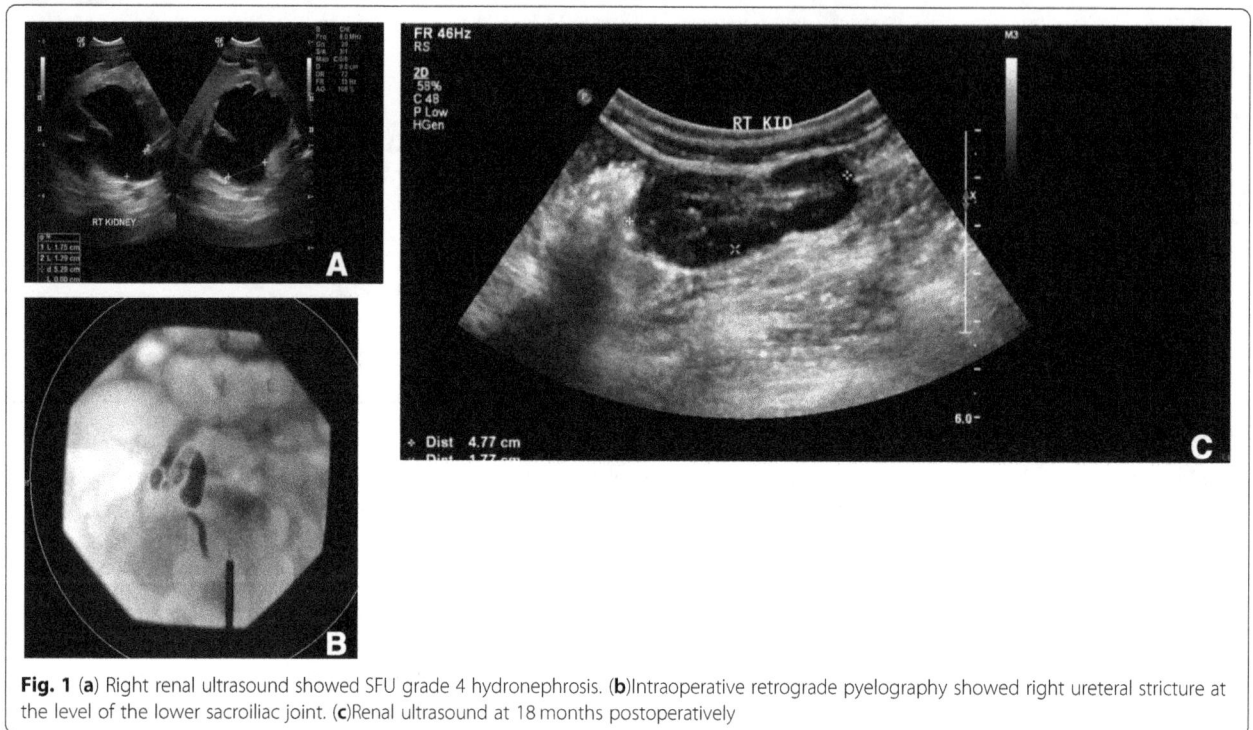

Fig. 1 (**a**) Right renal ultrasound showed SFU grade 4 hydronephrosis. (**b**)Intraoperative retrograde pyelography showed right ureteral stricture at the level of the lower sacroiliac joint. (**c**)Renal ultrasound at 18 months postoperatively

severely stenosed lumen. Right RGP was performed at the time of stent removal and showed smooth passage of contrast media up to the pelvicalyceal system (Fig. 2-e). An ultrasound examination performed 30 months postoperatively revealed SFU grade 1 hydronephrosis.

Discussion and conclusions

Mid-ureteral stricture is not a common cause of congenital hydronephrosis and is much less frequent than proximal or distal stricture [3]. Campbell published an autopsy series of 12 thousnads children. He found congenital ureteral obstruction in 1:150 autposies. Only 4% of them had a mid-ureteral obstruction. This outlines the rarity of CMS as a cause of congenital hydronephrosis [4].

Many theories have attempted to attribute stricture formation during embryogenesis to various causes, including a localized area of developmental arrest caused by extrinsic compression by foetal vessels during intrauterine life, a congenital ureteral valve, intrauterine ureteritis, and incomplete recanalization of the ureter [1, 5–8]. However, the exact explanation remains unclear. Mid-ureteral stricture may appear as a definite stricture or as a true valve without lumen stenosis [9]. The cases described here involved definite lumen stenosis, and no valves were detected.

CMS may be associated with other congenital renal anomalies, including crossed renal ectopia [2], multicystic dysplastic contralateral kidney [8, 10], solitary kidney [11], contralateral blind ending ureter [11, 12], and

ectopic ureter of a duplex system [13]. However, our current cases exhibited no congenital renal anomalies other than ureteral stricture. CMS is mostly diagnosed as a unilateral disorder; however, cases with bilateral anomalies have been reported in the literature [14]. Our cases involved CMS on one side with an apparently normal contralateral side.

CMS is typically not diagnosed preoperatively, and definite diagnoses have been reached via retrograde assessment of the ureter [3, 14]. Burgnara et al. reported one case of CMS diagnosed using foetal MRI in which prenatal ultrasound showed progressive left hydronephrosis with suspected proximal left ureteral dilatation; this diagnosis was confirmed postnatally by intraoperative RGP [15]. RGP remains controversial as a routine preoperative imaging procedure in cases of congenital hydronephrosis. Routine preoperative RGP is recommended in cases involving a diagnosis of an unexpected ureteral lesion, such as mid-ureteral stricture, ureteral polyp and retrocaval ureter. In addition to confirming this diagnosis, RGP will allow for the proposed surgical intervention to be performed without requiring extension of the incision or anastomosis with inappropriate exposure [8]. For this reason, Hawang et al. recommended routine RGP prior to repair, during the same anaesthesia session, unless the ureter distal to the point of obstruction has been well visualized by other means [3]. Conversely, Rushton et al. did not recommend routine RGP based on findings from 108 pyeloplasties performed between 1986

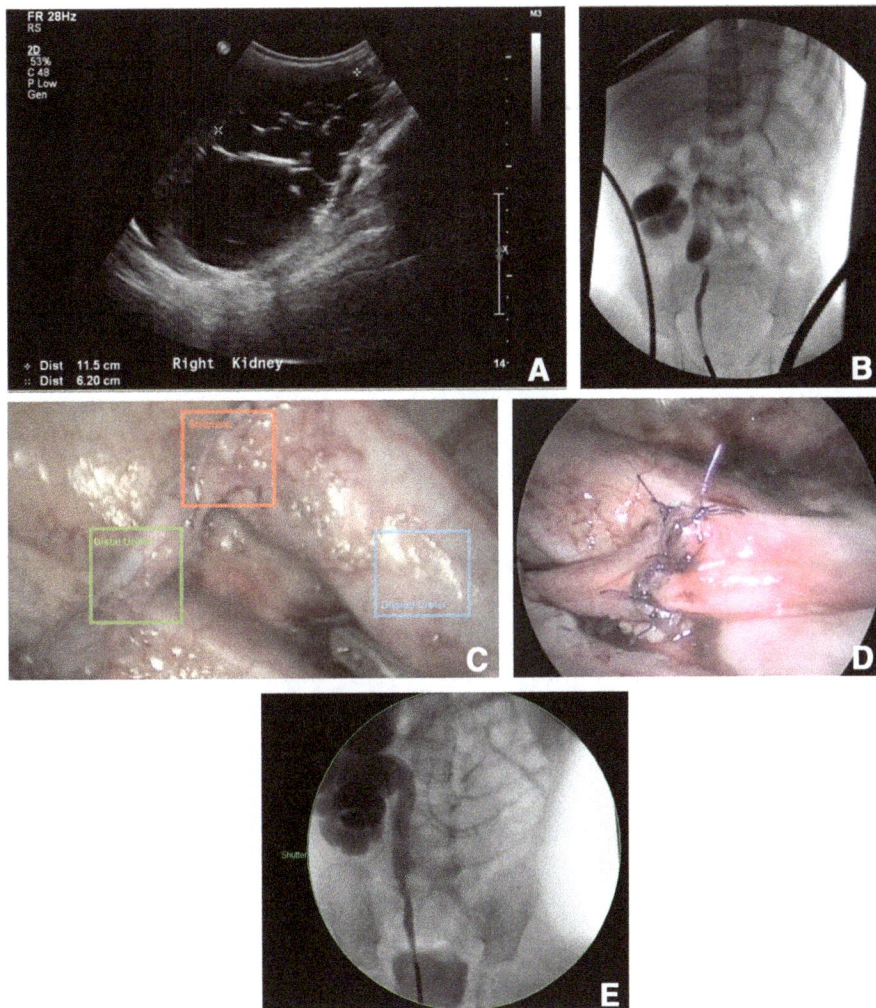

Fig. 2 (**a**) Preoperative ultrasound showed SFU grade 4 hydronephrosis. (**b**) Retrograde pyelogram demonstrated right ureteral stricture at the level of the right mid-sacroiliac joint with proximal mega-ureter. (**c**) Laparoscopic view of the mid-ureteral stricture. (**d**) Image obtained at the end of the laparoscopic ureteroureterostomy. (**e**) Retrograde pyelogram showed a patent ureteral lumen after double-J stent removal

and 1992, and they also found that RGP was not necessary for successful repair [16]. Both of the patients described in the present report were initially diagnosed using RGP. RGP was helpful for not only assessing stricture size and length but also ensuring appropriate decision making. We recommend routine preoperative RGP to avoid operator errors during ultrasound and the exclusion of unexpected ureteral lesions.

In our institution, postoperative renogram is only indicated if deterioration of hydronephrosis is observed in any of postoperative ultrasound scans or there is a poor renal function preoperatively. Both cases had improved hydronephrosis in consecutive postoperative renal ultrasound scans; thus, postoperative renal scan was no indicated. Moreover, the preoperative DRF of our included renal units was acceptable.

The management of CMS involves resection of the stricture and re-anastomosis of the ureter, with no role for conservative management [3]. Our definitive management, which was the same as that described in the literature, included resection of the stenotic area and re-anastomosis of the ureter. In our second case, this procedure was performed via transperitoneal laparoscopy.

In our cases, chronic inflammatory cells were predominant in the excised stricture segments. Hawang et al. reported the presence of inflammatory cells in the stenotic area, although these cells did not appear to be significant. In their study, they found asymmetry in the thickness of the muscularis mucosa with non-significan acute or chronic inflammation of the stenosed segment in some cases [3]. In our second case, sever chronic inflmmation was clearly observed and there was a focal inflammation in case 1. This may refelct the role of inflammation in some cases of CMS.

Postoperative long-term follow-up revealed the regression of hydronephrosis. In most of the relevant literature, improvement in hydronephrosis and promising renal function have been reported during short-term follow-up [2, 10, 16].

CMS is a rare cause of congenital hydronephrosis that should be considered whenever proximal mega-ureter is an associated finding. Despite advanced radiological modalities, RGP remains the mainstay approach for diagnosing ureteral anomalies.

Abbreviation

CMS: Congenital mid-ureteral stricture; MAG-3: Mercaptoacetyltriglycine; RGP: Retrograde pyelography; SFU: Society for Fetal Urology; VCUG: Voiding cysto-urethrogram

Acknowledgements

Not applicable

Funding

None

Authors' contributions

HH design the study, performed the treatment, wrote the manuscript and approve the final manuscript. AFN perform literature search, acquisition of the data, manuscript review and revising the manuscript. All authors read and approved the final manuscript.

Authors' information

HH: Associate Professor and Consultant Paediatric Urologist, Saudi Board of Urology and Arab Board of Urology; Fellowship in Paediatric Urology (Montreal, Canada), Fellowship in Laparoscopic Paediatric Urology (Paris, France) Deputy Chairman for Academic Affairs, Department of Surgery.

Consent for publication

Written informed consent for publication of clinical details and clinical images was obtained from the parents of both patients.

Competing interests

The authors declares that there are no competing interests.

References

1. Allen TD. Congenital ureteral strictures. J Urol. 1970;104:196–204.
2. Smith BG, Metwalli AR, Leach J, Cheng EY, Kropp BP. Congenital midureteral stricture in children diagnosed with antenatal hydronephrosis. Urology. 2004;64:1014–9.
3. Hwang AH, McAleer IM, Shapiro E, Miller OF, Krous HF, Kaplan GW. Congenital mid ureteral strictures. J Urol. 2005;174:1999–2002.
4. Campbell M. Clinical consideration of the anatomy, physiology, embryology, and anomalies of urogenital tract. Pediatric Urology New York: MacMillan Co. 1937;1:188.
5. Maizels M, Stephens F. Valves of the ureter as a cause of primary obstruction of the ureter: anatomic. embryologic and clinical aspects J Urol. 1980;123:742–7.
6. Albertson KW, Talner LB. Valves of the ureter. Radiology. 1972;103:91–4.
7. Sant GR, Barbalias GA, Klauber GT. Congenital ureteral valves--an abnormality of ureteral embryogenesis? J Urol. 1985;133:427–31.
8. Ruano-Gil D, Coca-Payeras A, Tejedo-Mateu A. Obstruction and normal recanalization of the ureter in the human embryo. Its relation to congenital ureteric obstruction. Eur Urol. 1975;1:287–93.
9. Cauchi JA, Chandran H. Congenital ureteric strictures: an uncommon cause of antenatally detected hydronephrosis. Pediatr Surg Int. 2005;21:566–8.
10. Kosto B. Congenital mid-ureteral stricture in a solitary kidney. J Urol. 1971; 106:529–31.
11. Ayyat FM, Adams G. Congenital midureteral strictures. Urology. 1985;26:170–2.
12. Hirai K, Ueda H, Segawa N, Yamamoto K, Kanehara H, Suzuki T, et al. Congenital midureteral stricture with ectopic ureter: a case report. Acta Urol Jpn. 1994;40:71–4.
13. Domenichelli V, De Biagi L, Italiano F, Carfagnini F, Lavacchini A, Federici S. Congenital bilateral mid-ureteral stricture: a unique case. J Pediatr Urol. 2008;4:401–3.
14. Rushton HG, Salem Y, Belman AB, Majd M. Pediatric pyeloplasty: is routine retrograde pyelography necessary? J Urol. 1994;152:604–6.
15. Burgnara M, Cecchetto M, Manfredi R, Zuffante M, Fanco V, Pietrobelli A, et al. Prenatal diagnosis of a rare form of congenital mid-ureteral stricture: a case report and literature revisited. BMC Urol. 2007;7:8.
16. Prieto JC, Castellan M, Gosalbez R, Labbie A, Perez-Brayfield M. Severe congenital midureteral dilatation. J Pediatr Surg. 2007;42:257–8.

34

Systemic analysis of urinary stones from the Northern, Eastern, Central, Southern and Southwest China

Rui-hong Ma[1]*![ID], Xiao-bing Luo[1], Qin Li[2] and Hai-qiang Zhong[1]

Abstract

Background: To provide some basis for the prevention of urinary stones in general population, we did a systemic analysis of urinary stones from Northern, Eastern, Central, Southern and Southwest China by a multi-center study.

Methods: A total of 11,157 urinary stones from Northern, Eastern, Central, Southern and Southwest China were obtained and analyzed by Fourier transform infrared spectroscopy. Combined with scanning electron microscopy and X-ray energy spectrometer, urinary stones were classified into different types. Furthermore, the correlation between stone types and clinical characteristics, as well as their regional distribution were elucidated.

Results: Calcium oxalate stones were the most common type in each region, followed by calcium oxalate-calcium phosphate mixed stones, uric acid stones and calcium phosphate stones. The distribution of calcium oxalate stones were highest prevalence in Southwest China (67.9%, $P < 0.05$), followed by Eastern and Northern China. Anhydrous uric acid stones, with a constituent ratio of 19.3% in Southern China, and 13.7% in Central China, were significantly higher than that in other regions ($P < 0.05$). Elements analysis indicated varieties among stone types as well as distribution regions. Moreover, the clinical characteristics were highly correlated with stone types and anatomical locations but not their distribution regions.

Conclusions: The material and elements composition of urinary stones among different regions showed some varieties. Calcium oxalate stone has the highest constituent ratio in Southwest China, while anhydrous uric acid stone has the highest constituent ratio in Southern China. Moreover, the clinical characteristics were highly correlated with stone types and anatomical locations but not their distribution regions.

Keywords: Urinary stones, Fourier transform infrared spectroscopy, Scanning electron microscopy, X-ray energy spectrometer, Calcium oxalate stones, Uric acid stones, Regional distribution

Background

Urinary stone disease, also known as urolithiasis, is one of the leading afflictions worldwide. The incidence differs with geographic distribution. In general, as described in detail previously [1, 2], the average prevalence is higher in western countries (5–9% in Europe, and 13% in North America) than the eastern (1–5% in Asia). While in Saudi Arabia, nearly 20% people suffer from it. In China, the disease approximately affects 4% of population and increases steadily during the recent 20 years, due to high calories intake from dietary and lack of exercise in lifestyle [3–5]. Therefore, effective prevention strategy and precise treatment are needed to alleviate the burden caused by high prevalence of urolithiasis.

Urolithiasis cause undoubtedly considerable burden on public health worldwide not only by its high prevalence but also for the recurrence rate. A report in Germany indicated that about 40% of patients suffered from recurrent urolithiasis once or more, and even over 10%

* Correspondence: olive5327@163.com
[1]The Department of Clinical Laboratory, The Sixth People's Hospital of Nansha, Xingye Road No. 7, Dagang Town, Nansha, Guangzhou 511470, People's Republic of China
Full list of author information is available at the end of the article

underwent five or more stone episodes [6]. Therefore, it is important to clearly define the etiology and establish an effective prevention program on urinary stones [7]. As the composition of urinary stone may provide some clue for the formation process, stone analysis is important in determining the possible etiology of urinary stones. Moreover, there exists a wide geographic variation in proportion for different stone types. The phenomenon is demonstrated well in the United States but still limited in China [8, 9]. Therefore, in the present study, we did a systemic analysis of urinary stones from Northern, Eastern, Central, Southern and Southwest China by a multi-center study to describe the commons and differences of stone composition, major and trace elements as well as clinical characteristics.

Methods

Ethics statement

The sample collection procedures were explained to all patients. Written informed consent was obtained from all patients. The principles outlined in the Declaration of Helsinki of 1975 (revised in 1983 and 1989) were followed throughout the study period. The study was approved by both the Ethics Committee of The Sixth People's Hospital of Nansha, Guangzhou (reference number is No: 20130821057P) and the Ethics Committee of The Kingmed Diagnostics Center of Guangzhou (KM20130149).

Subjects and specimens

Urinary stones from 11,157 urolithiasis patients were collected from department of the urinary surgery in The Sixth People's Hospital of Nansha, Guangzhou, and the Kingmed Diagnostics Center of Guangzhou during September 2013 to September 2017. The patients consisted of 7437 males, ranged from 18 to 95 years old, the mean age was 49.61 ± 14.40 (Mean ± S.D) years, and 3720 females, ranged from 20 to 88 years old, the mean age was 49.31 ± 13.23 (Mean ± S.D) years. The age of the two groups had no statistically significant difference.

China's regional division

Northern China includes: Beijing, Tianjin, Hebei, Shanxi, Inner Mongolia provinces; Eastern China includes: Shanghai, Shandong, Jiangsu, Anhui, Jiangxi, Zhejiang, Fujian provinces; Central China includes: Hubei, Hunan, Henan; Southern China includes: Guangdong, Guangxi, Hainan provinces; Southwest China includes: Chongqing, Sichuan, Guizhou, Yunnan, Tibet provinces.

The recruitment of the urinary lithiasis patients

Of the above patients, 844 from Northern China, including 646 males, with average age of 45.58 ± 13.45, and 198 females, with average age of 43.16 ± 14.87; 2149 from Eastern China, including 1277 males, with average age of 47.07 ± 13.19, and 872 females, with average age of 46.95 ± 12.56; 713 from Central China, including 463 males, with average age of 49.65 ± 14.36, and 250 females, with average age of 48.98 ± 13.11; 6423 from Southern China, including 4339 males, with the average of 50.50 ± 14.75, and 2084 females, with the average age of 50.31 ± 13.38; 1028 from Southwest China, including 712 males, with the average of 46.85 ± 14.00, and 316 females, with the average age of 47.92 ± 13.09. The proportion of males and females from each region is slightly different, with a higher proportion of males in Northern China, and a lower in Eastern China. The age has some differences among different regions, with older age in Southern China and Central China, and younger age in Northern China.

Systemic classification of urinary stones

A total of 11,157 urinary stones were classified into different types with systemic classification combing using FTIR spectroscopy, SEM and X-ray energy spectrometer, the procedure has been detailed in our previous work [7].

Comparison of stone composition and clinical characteristics in patients with different regions

Urinary lithiasis patients were divided into five groups according to the regions, such as Northern China, Eastern China, Central China, Southern China and Southwest China, and urinary stones were divided into five groups according to the composition, such as calcium oxalate stones, calcium phosphate stones, uric acid stones, calcium oxalate-calcium phosphate mixed stones and other kinds of stone group. Others consisted of magnesium ammonium phosphate, cystine, brushite, urate stones and some subtypes of mixed stones that were minority. Stone composition and clinical characteristics in different regions were compared and analyzed.

Statistic methods

Age was analyzed using One-Way ANOVA and presented as mean ± SD, while the ratio of male and female, and the ratio with different types of stones as well as from different anatomical locations or regions were analyzed using a chi square test. LSD and the partitions of the chi square methods were used for multiple comparisons using IBM SPSS Statistics 24 software. $P < 0.05$ was regarded as statistically significant.

Results

Urinary stone composition were distinct in different regions of China

Calcium oxalate (whewellite and weddellite) stones were the most common in each region, followed by calcium oxalate-calcium phosphate mixed, anhydrous uric acid and calcium phosphate stones. The distribution of calcium oxalate stones were highest prevalence in Southwest China (67.9%, $P < 0.05$), followed by Eastern and Northern China. Anhydrous uric acid stones, with a constituent ratio of 19.3% in Southern China, and 13.7% in Central China, were significantly higher than that in Northern, Eastern and Southwest China ($P < 0.05$). The constituent ratio of calcium phosphate stones (about 5%) among different regions had no statistical differences ($P > 0.05$). The stone type constitution in the five regions of China was shown in Table 1.

Element composition and distribution in each type of urinary stone

Besides the main elements (Italic), each type of stone still contains a small amount of metal and non-metallic elements, which had some varieties among stone types as well as regions. For calcium oxalate stones, besides the main elements carbon, oxygen, calcium, they still contain some sodium, kalium, magnesium, chlorine, aluminum, phosphorus, niobium, hafnium, sulphur, etc. For calcium phosphate stones, in addition to carbon, oxygen, calcium, phosphorus, they still contain some sodium, kalium, magnesium, chlorine, aluminium, niobium, fluorine, zinc, technetium, hafnium, chrome, etc.; and for those anhydrous uric acid stones, in addition to carbon, oxygen, nitrogen, they still had some sodium, calcium, aluminium, chlorine. Urinary stones from Southern China usually contained some zinc, and those from Southwest China usually contained some silicon, which seems more complex and diverse compared with other regions (Table 2). Mapping analysis of element distribution in general stones with X-ray energy spectrometer showed that for those calcium oxalate stones with micro dishes of calcium phosphate and calcium oxalate-calcium phosphate mixed stones, calcium oxalate crystals were always distributed in the outer layer while calcium phosphate crystals were in the core (Fig. 1a, b). Moreover, for those calcium phosphate stones, usually with a small amount of ammonium magnesium phosphate crystals scattered in the profile (Fig. 1c). Uric acid stones, mixed with micro or macro dishes of calcium oxalate crystals, displayed inconsistent crystal distribution

characteristics. In some of the uric acid stones, uric acid crystals were shown in the outer layer and calcium oxalate crystals were in the core. Calcium oxalate crystals in the outer layer while uric acid crystals in the center were also found in some kind of uric acid stones. Besides, uric acid crystals mixed with calcium oxalate crystals in circular layers were observed in uric acid stones (Fig. 2). Mapping analysis of element distribution in micro field with magnification of 3000 times showed that there was only calcium distribution in calcium oxalate crystals, and both calcium and phosphorus distribution in calcium phosphate crystals and calcium oxalate-calcium phosphate mixed crystals, with a consistent distribution in calcium phosphate crystals and inconsistent distribution in calcium oxalate-calcium phosphate mixed crystals. Calcium was distributed in both calcium oxalate and calcium phosphate crystals; phosphorus was distributed in calcium phosphate crystals (Fig. 3). Moreover, there was only nitrogen distribution in uric acid crystals, and both nitrogen and calcium distribution in uric acid-calcium oxalate mixed crystals (Fig. 4).

The clinical characteristics of each type of urinary stone

Urinary stones were divided as upper urinary stones (kidney and ureteral stones) and lower urinary stones (bladder and urethral stones) according to the anatomical location. In our current studies, we did correlation analysis on 9073 urinary stones and clinical characteristics of these patients. Interestingly, the clinical characteristics were highly correlated with stone types and anatomical locations but not their regions. As shown in Table 3, 7448 cases were upper urinary stones while 1625 were lower urinary stones, and the ratio were 4.6:1. Among the patients with upper urinary stones, 4523 were males, accounting for 60.7%, while those with lower urinary stones, 1504 were males, accounting for 92.6%, which had statistically significant difference ($P < 0.05$). It was indicated in the present study that calcium oxalate stone was the main stone type of upper urinary stones, constituting 60.6%, while uric acid stone was that of lower urinary stones, constituting 43.0% ($P < 0.05$). Patients with calcium oxalate stones were mainly males between the ages of 30 and 60, accounting for 49.4%, while those with calcium phosphate stones were mainly

Table 1 Distribution of stone types in five regions of China

Stone type/regions	Calcium oxalate	Calcium phosphate	Uric acid	Calcium oxalate-calcium phosphate mixed	Other types	Total
Northern	485 (57.5%)	42 (5.0%)	52 (6.2%)	183 (21.7%)	82 (9.7%)	844 (100%)
Eastern	1360 (63.3%)	121 (5.6%)	123 (5.7%)	490 (22.8%)	55 (2.6%)	2149 (100%)
Central	377 (52.9%)	36 (5.0%)	98 (13.7%)	177 (24.8%)	25 (3.5%)	713 (100%)
Southern	3317 (51.6%)	359 (5.6%)	1242 (19.3%)	1221 (19.0%)	284 (4.4%)	6423 (100%)
Southwest	698 (67.9%)	48 (4.7%)	60 (5.8%)	188 (18.3%)	34 (3.3%)	1028 (100%)
Total	6237 (55.9%)	606 (5.4%)	1575 (14.1%)	2259 (20.2%)	480 (4.3%)	11,157 (100%)

Table 2 Element composition in each type of urinary stone with different regions

Stone type/ region	Calcium Oxalate	Calcium Phosphate	Uric Acid	Calcium Oxalate-Calcium Phosphate Mixed
Northern	*C, O, Ca,* Na,Cl,Mg,Al,P,Nb,Tc	*C, O, Ca, P,* Na,Mg,F,Cl,Nb,Tc,Hf,Cr	*C, O, N,* Ca	*C, O, Ca, P,* Na,Mg,K,F,Cl,Al,Nb
Eastern	*C, O, Ca,*Na,Cl,Mg,Al,P,K,Nb,Tc,Br	*C, O, Ca, P,* Na,Mg,K,Al,Cl,Nb,Tc,Hf	*C, O, N,*Na,Al,Cl,Ca	*C, O, Ca, P,* Na,Mg,K,F,Cl,Al,Nb,Tc,Hf,Fe
Central	*C, O, Ca,*Na,Al, Mg,P	*C, O, Ca, P,* Na,Mg,Nb	*C, O, N,*Ca	*C, O, Ca, P,* Na,Mg,F,Cl,Nb,Tc
Southern	*C, O, Ca,*Na,Cl,Mg,Al,P,K,F,Si,Nb,Tc,Hf,Zn	*C, O, Ca, P,* Na,Mg,Nb, Tc,Hf, Zn,F	*C, O, N,*Al,Ca	*C, O, Ca, P,* Na,Mg,F,Cl,Al,Nb,Tc,Hf,Zn
Southwest	*C, O, Ca,* Na,Cl,Mg,Al,P,K,Nb,Tc,Zn,S,Fe,Si	*C, O, Ca, P,* Na,Mg,K,F,Cl, Nb, Tc,Si	*C, O, N,*Al,Cl,Ca,Si	*C, O, Ca, P,* Na,Mg,F,Cl,Al,Nb, Tc,Si

The italics are the main elements of corresponding stone types

females between the ages of 30 and 60, accounting for 42.1%, and those with uric acid stones were mainly elder males over the age of 60, accounting for 45.8%, the difference was statistically significant ($P < 0.05$). Calcium phosphate stones and calcium oxalate-calcium phosphate mixed stones were mainly from upper urinary tract. Patients with calcium oxalate-calcium phosphate mixed stones were males or females, the ratio tend to 1, while those with magnesium ammonium phosphate and urate stones were mainly females, and those with brushite and cystine stones were mainly males (not list in the table).

Discussion

Urolithiasis, a common urological disease with multiple etiologies, has been a public burden to the world. In the last few decades, urolithiasis has been steadily increased [6, 10]. The present data indicated that the highest incidence of urinary stones occurred in 40–49 years old males and 50–59 years old females respectively. Urinary stones can be classified as metabolic stones (calcium oxalate and some uric acid or urate) and infectious stones (struvite, apatite or a mixture of the two), males are more likely to have metabolic stones, while females, with a high probability of urinary tract infections than men, are more prone to infectious stones [11]. The present data showed that patients with calcium oxalate stones and uric acid stones were mainly males, while those with calcium phosphate stones and magnesium ammonium phosphate (struvite) stones were mainly females.

The present data showed calcium oxalate stone was the most frequent stone type in all age groups, with high frequency between the ages of 30 and 60 years, and relatively low frequency in the younger and elderly. As previously detailed [12], the intake of oxalate and calcium in the diet has an important effect on urinary oxalate excretion, which also play a major role in the formation of calcium oxalate stone. Increased intake of dietary oxalate lead to an increase of urinary oxalate excretion, and decreasing dietary oxalate lowers urinary oxalate excretion [13]. Dietary calcium has a bidirectional effect on urinary oxalate excretion, Borghi's study showed the

low-calcium (10 mmol/day) group presented a higher relapse of calcium oxalate stones than the normal-calcium (30 mmol/day) group [14]. The high percentage of calcium oxalate stone in Southwest China may be originated from water quality, soil and the local dietary structure. It was supposed that the major contributing factor maybe the increase of Ca^{2+}/Mg^{2+} ratio (in meq) in drinking water [15]. Additionally, the high calcium-content in local plants grown on karst soils along with the high ingestion of oxalate food may lead to the high incidence of calcium oxalate stones [15]. In China, karst soils mainly distributes in Southwest of China (Chongqing, Sichuan, Guizhou, Yunnan) [16], with a consistent distribution with calcium oxalate stones, which presents the highest constituent ratio in the Southwest among all areas of China. Meanwhile, calcium oxalate- calcium phosphate mixed stones account for a large proportion. In our opinion, it is difficult to manage urinary stones as stone recurrence is common because residual stone fragment contain bacteria and become the core of recurrent stone [11]. Furthermore, a previous research showed urinary tract infection was closely related to the existence of amorphous carbonated calcium phosphate (or whitlockite) and carbonated apatite [17]. Other research indicated that for recurrent stones, the admixed $CaOx/CaPO_4$ stones were converted from pure $CaPO_4$ more commonly than from pure CaOx stone [18]. Therefore, we conclude that calcium oxalate-calcium phosphate mixed or calcium oxalate stones with $CaPO_4$ in the core, the infectious factors maybe first involved in the stone process, and a considerable proportion of which may be recurrent stones.

Uric acid stones has a prevalence of about 10% among all stones [19], but this percentage become extremely high in those patients with gout [20]. Consistent with other reports [21], we found that uric acid stones increased with older age, elder males over the age of 60 accounted for 45.8% of total uric acid stones in the present study. UA urolithiasis is a complex disease that is affected by many factors. Diseases relevant with aging, such as obesity, insulin resistance and diabetes, are also associated with low urinary pH and UA stone formation [22–24]. Furthermore, as previously described [25], persistent acidic urine (pH ≤ 5.5) is considered to be the

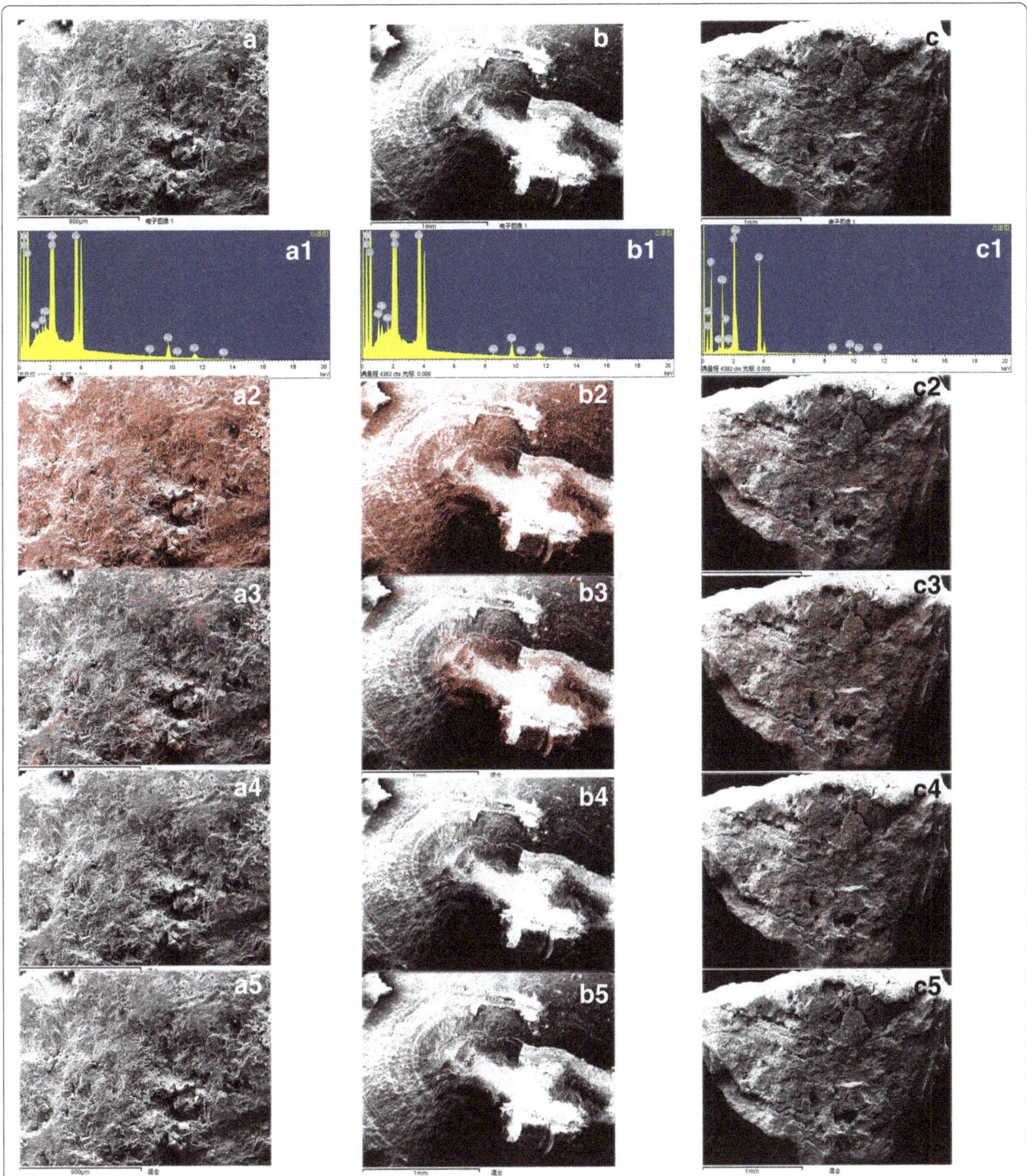

Fig. 1 Element distribution in general stones (the red dot represented element distribution). **a** calcium oxalate stones with micro dishes of calcium phosphate: calcium oxalate crystals were distributed in the outer layer and profile, with micro dishes of calcium phosphate crystals in the core. A1.The energy spectrum, A2. Calcium distribution, A3. Phosphorus distribution, A4. Magnesium distribution, A5. Natrium distribution; **b** calcium oxalate-calcium phosphate mixed stones: calcium oxalate crystals were distributed in the outer layer, calcium phosphate crystals were in the core. B1. The energy spectrum, B2. Calcium distribution, B3. Phosphorus distribution, B4. Aluminum distribution, B5. Natrium distribution; **c** Calcium phosphate stones: a small amount of ammonium magnesium phosphate crystals were scattered in the profile. C1. The energy spectrum, C2. Calcium distribution, C3. Phosphorus distribution, C4. Magnesium distribution, C5. Aluminum distribution

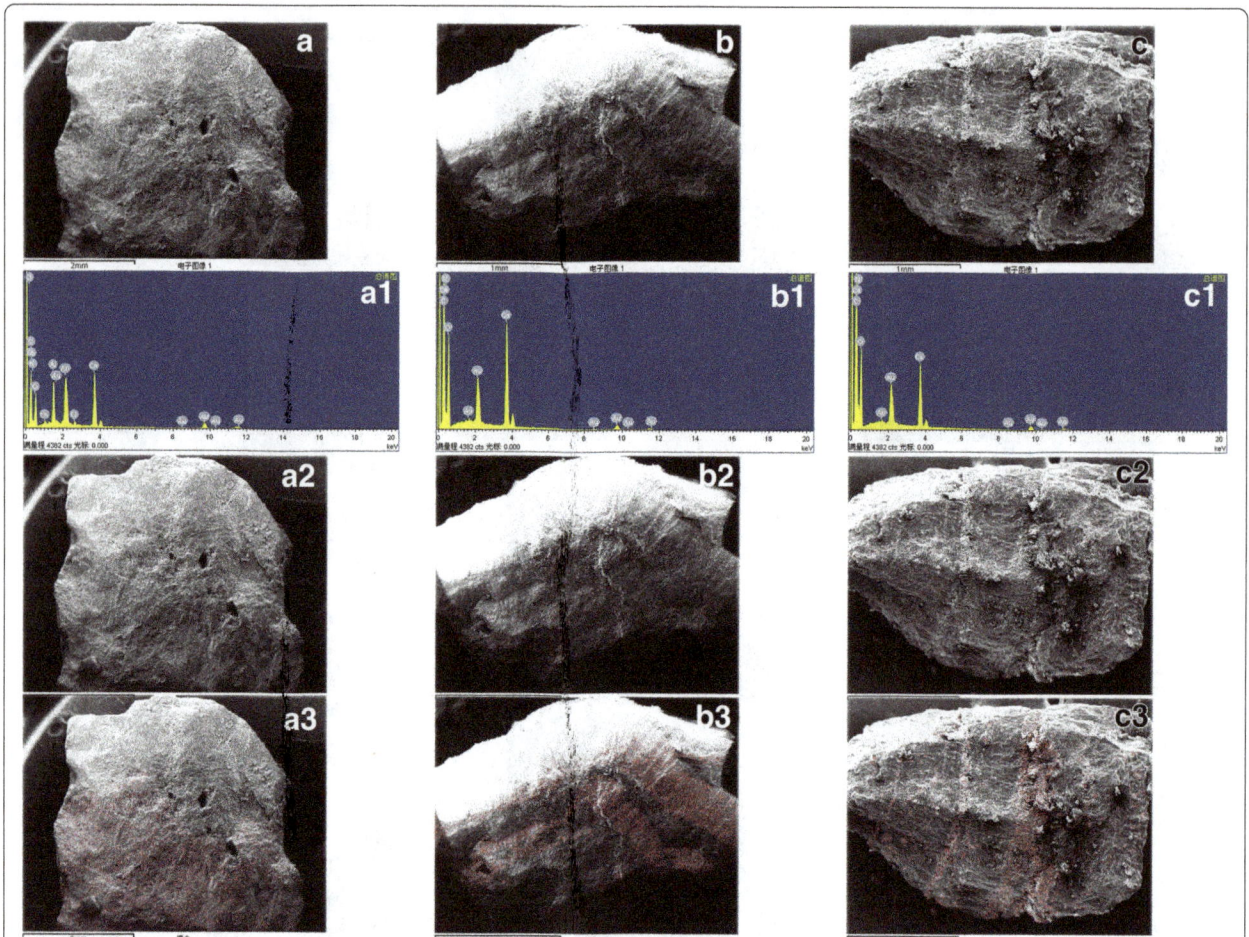

Fig. 2 Element distribution in general stones: uric acid stones mixed with some calcium oxalate crystals (the red dot represented element distribution). **a** Uric acid- calcium oxalate mixed stones: uric acid crystals were distributed in the outer layer, and calcium oxalate crystals in the core. A1. The energy spectrum, A2. Nitrogen distribution, A3. Calcium distribution; **b** Calcium oxalate - uric acid mixed stones: calcium oxalate crystals were distributed in the outer layer, and uric acid crystals in the core. B1. The energy spectrum, B2. Nitrogen distribution, B3. Calcium distribution; **c** Uric acid stones mixed with micro dishes of calcium oxalate crystals: uric acid crystals were distributed in circular layer, and calcium oxalate crystals were scattered between the layers: C1. The energy spectrum, C2. Nitrogen distribution, C3. Calcium distribution

most important risk factor for the formation of UA stones. Additionally, environmental factors may have a prominent influence on the composition of urinary stones. As reported [26], climate and diet play a crucial role in the formation of UA stones. Hot and dry climate increases fluid losses with reduced urinary volume and decreased urinary pH. Consistent with these, our studies showed the incidence of UA stone in Southern China was the highest, followed by Central, Northern, Eastern and Southwest in China. For those uric acid-calcium oxalate mixed stones, some research indicated that patients with this kind of mixed stones presented with metabolic abnormalities that promote both CaOx and UA stone formation [27, 28]. We supposed that the process of uric acid crystals deposition and that of calcium oxalate crystals deposition may promote each other, whichever occurred first, the formation process

probably accelerate when the other emerged. Therefore, uric acid and calcium oxalate crystals may be distributed in the core or outer layer or in circular layers.

There were other epidemiologic surveys in other countries. A study in the United States indicated that the prevalence of urinary stones in Southeast was almost twice of that in Northwest, which was ascribed to climatologic factors [29]. Moreover, another research based on five U.S. metropolitan areas further confirmed the strongest association between high temperature and kidney stones [30]. Furthermore, a multi-center analysis in Germany also showed significant regional differences in urinary stone distribution: a higher rate of uric acid stones in Southern Germany was supposed to be associated with their diets based on more red meat, and the higher incidence of infectious stones in Eastern Germany maybe due to lower standard medical care and infections [19].

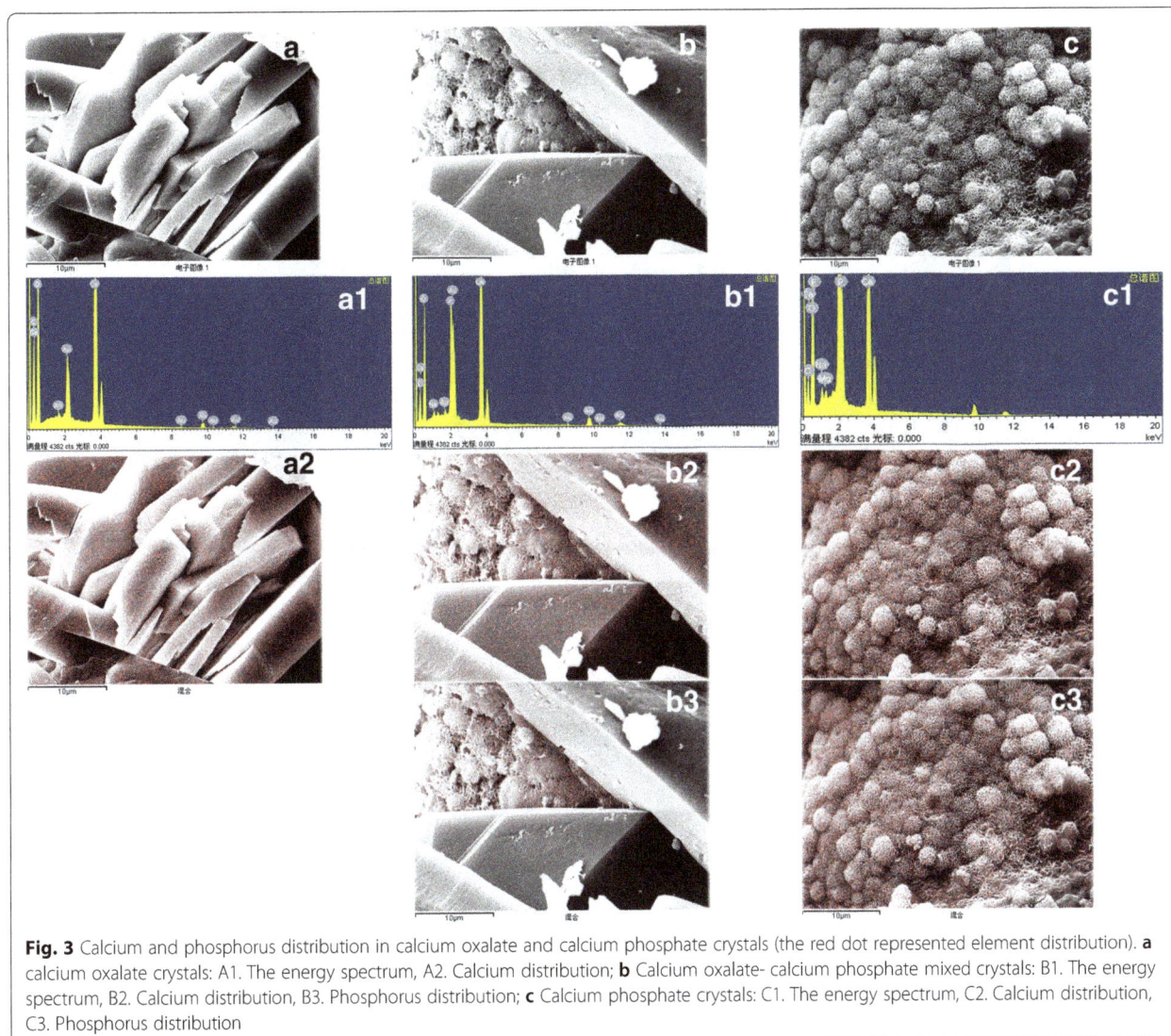

Fig. 3 Calcium and phosphorus distribution in calcium oxalate and calcium phosphate crystals (the red dot represented element distribution). **a** calcium oxalate crystals: A1. The energy spectrum, A2. Calcium distribution; **b** Calcium oxalate- calcium phosphate mixed crystals: B1. The energy spectrum, B2. Calcium distribution, B3. Phosphorus distribution; **c** Calcium phosphate crystals: C1. The energy spectrum, C2. Calcium distribution, C3. Phosphorus distribution

As reported, urinary stone form in multiphase steps, apart from the specific conditions like molar concentrations, pH, temperature, etc., different types of trace elements may also affect the crystallization process [31]. In the present study, X-ray energy spectrometer analysis indicated that besides the major elements of urinary stones, other minor elements, such as Na, Cl, Mg, Al, K, Fe, Zn, S, F, Nb, Tc, Hf, Cr and Si were also detected. According to the present study and the previous reports, we found they might play an important part in the urinary stone formation. What is the role of different elements? A study showed sodium concentration was marginally associated with increased risk of stone formation in elder participants (mean age of 61 years) with a history of kidney stone [32]. Nevertheless, the relationship between the sodium content and the risk of formation urinary stone is still under limited studies. Magnesium is also essential to stone formation. One

study suggested an oral of 500 mg magnesium oxide each day may inhibit the crystallization of CaO_X stones in normal volunteers [33], yet a research on rats implied that strict restriction of dietary magnesium may promote stone formation [34]. Potassium was also known as a lithogenesis inhibitor, a randomized trial demonstrated that potassium citrate can prevent the formation of new stones in idiopathic hypocitraturic calcium nephrolithiasis patients [35]. Aluminum is a non-essential element for human. One study showed that a positive correlation between aluminum level in the urine and stones, as well as between urine and hair, suggesting aluminum probably play a role in stone formation [36]. Another study indicated that Al^{3+} affected crystal growth of calcium phosphate at physiologic concentration, but evidence for the inhibitory role in calcium phosphate stone growth was insufficient [37]. Sulphur is an essential nonmetal element existing in all the cells of human body, and

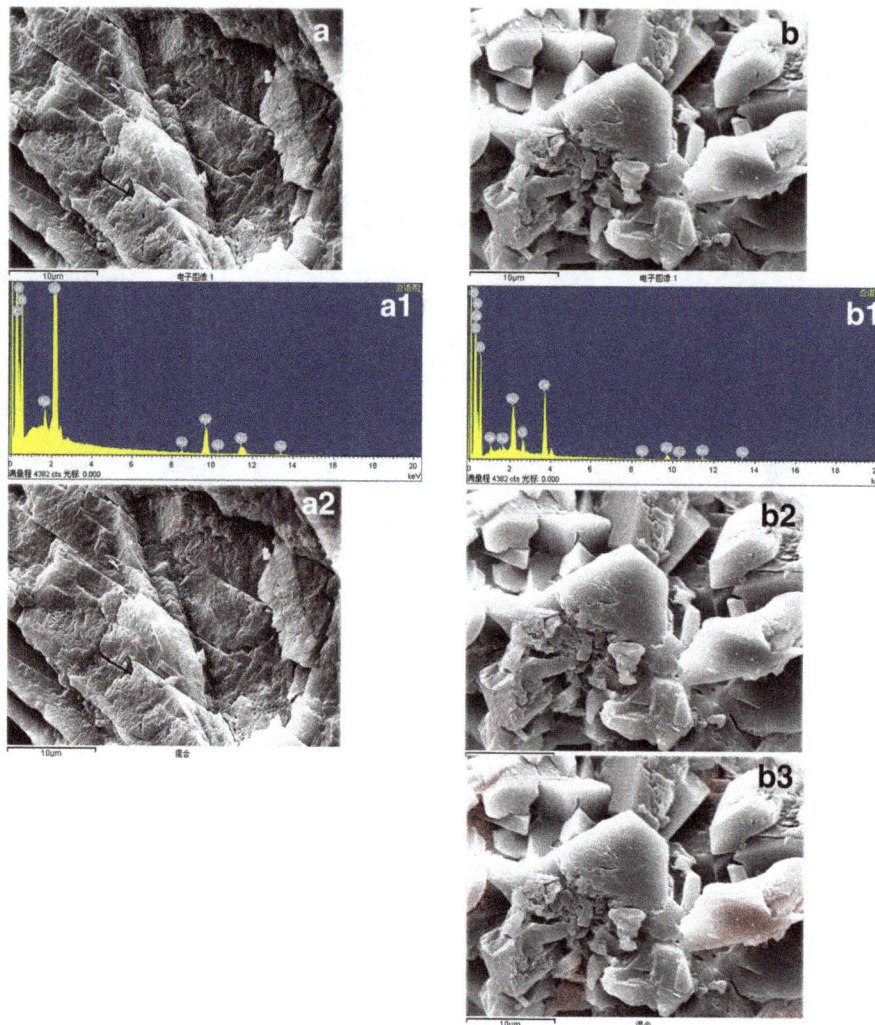

Fig. 4 Nitrogen and calcium distribution in uric acid and uric acid- calcium oxalate mixed crystals (the red dot represented element distribution). **a** Uric acid crystals: A1. The energy spectrum, A2. Nitrogen distribution; **b** Uric acid- calcium oxalate mixed crystals: B1. The energy spectrum, B2. Nitrogen distribution, B3. Calcium distribution

mainly obtained from sulfur-containing proteins in diet. The effects of sulphur on urinary stone formation are almost unknown, but yet a report indicated animal protein-induced hypercalciuria result in the presence of nonresorbable calcium sulfate in the tubular lumen, which may further lead to sulfate production and stone formation [38]. Moreover, the effects of zinc on urinary stone formation was controversial. One research suggested a positive correlation of dietary zinc intake and the risk of kidney stone [39], another showed zinc acts as an inhibitor on the formation of calcium oxalate stone [40]. Silicon may be an essential element for human. A previous research showed silicon plays an essential part in the metabolism of calcium and magnesium [41]. Furthermore, another research indicated ingestion of trisilicate may result in the formation stone entirely or partially composed of silica [42]. Nevertheless, how

silicon make an effect on urinary stone formation is still unclear. In the present study, sodium, magnesium, potassium presented a scattered distribution in the profile of urinary stones, while aluminum was more concentrated in the interior than the crust of the stones and usually accompanied with calcium phosphate crystals, which suggest that aluminum may play a role in the early phase of lithogenesis.

Conclusions

The systemic analysis of urinary stones from the Northern, Eastern, Central, Southern and Southwest China by a multi-center study indicated that the material and elements composition of urinary stones among different regions had some difference. Calcium oxalate stone has the highest constituent ratio in Southwest China, while anhydrous uric acid stones have a highest constituent

Table 3 Clinical characteristics of patients with each type of stone

Stone type		Calcium Oxalate		Calcium Phosphate		Uric Acid		Calcium oxalate-calcium phosphate mixed		Other rare type		Total
	No	4995		489		1398		1831		360		9073
	Rate (%)	55.05%		5.39%		15.41%		20.18%		3.97%		100%
	Age (years) & gender	Male	Female	Male	Female	Male	Female	Male	Female	Male	Female	
Upper urinary stones	< 20	48	18	0	6	0	0	12	6	0	6	96
	20~29	174	87	18	33	2	2	105	54	18	2	495
	30~39	546	204	18	71	46	8	213	120	21	15	1262
	40~49	909	432	24	60	132	40	258	225	48	29	2157
	50~59	753	522	51	62	168	80	183	189	42	48	2098
	60~69	396	273	24	29	95	78	72	75	15	33	1090
	>= 70	99	57	0	6	25	23	2	23	6	9	250
	Total	2925	1593	135	267	468	231	845	692	150	142	7448
Lower urinary stones	< 20	3	3	3	0	3	2	0	0	2	3	19
	20~29	3	3	0	1	10	1	42	12	0	0	72
	30~39	45	1	15	9	15	3	27	6	0	3	124
	40~49	87	2	9	1	33	3	36	3	9	3	186
	50~59	126	6	15	3	78	23	60	3	6	3	323
	60~69	108	3	15	1	205	3	54	2	12	3	406
	>= 70	87	0	12	3	315	5	48	1	21	3	495
	Total	459	18	69	18	659	40	267	27	50	18	1625
Total		3384	1611	204	285	1127	271	1112	719	200	160	9073

ratio in Southern China. It was confirmed that composition of urinary stones has wide geographic variation and the formation of which was associated with environmental factors (water quality and soil) as well as dietary structure, weather and climate. Moreover, the clinical characteristics were highly correlated with stone types and anatomical locations but not their regions. Furthermore, different type of urinary stones presented distinct elemental composition and distribution, and some minor element may play an important role in the formation of urinary stones. These findings would be meaningful to prevent stone occurrence and recurrence in general population from different areas of China in future.

Abbreviations
CaOx: Calcium oxalate; FTIR: Fourier transform infrared spectroscopy; SEM: Scanning electron microscopy; UA: Uric acid

Acknowledgments
We are grateful to Chun-yu Qi, Ming-quan Chen in the Urinary Surgery Department of our hospital and Yong Liu, Qi-jun Huang in the KingMed Dignostics Center of Guangzhou for kindly providing the specimens. We thank our colleagues in the Urinary Surgery Department and the operating room for their enthusiastic help, and the leaders of our hospital for their support.

Funding
This work was financed by grants from Medical and health science and technology project in Guangzhou (No. 20171A011354).

Authors' contributions
Conceived and designed the experiments or acquisition of data: RHM, XBL, QL and HQZ. Performed the experiments: RHM, XBL, HQZ. Analyzed the data: RHM, XBL, HQZ. Contributed reagents/materials/analysis tools: QL. Wrote the paper or involved in drafting the manuscript: RHM, XBL, HQZ. Critical revision of the manuscript: QL. All authors read and approved the final manuscript.

Ethics approval and consent to participate
The sample collection procedures were explained to all patients. Written informed consent was obtained from all patients. The principles outlined in the Declaration of Helsinki of 1975 (revised in 1983 and 1989) were followed throughout the study period. The study was approved by both the Ethics Committee of The Sixth People's Hospital of Nansha, Guangzhou (reference number is No: 20130821057P) and the Ethics Committee of The Kingmed Diagnostics Center of Guangzhou (KM20130149).

Competing interests
The authors have declared that no competing interests exist.

Author details
[1]The Department of Clinical Laboratory, The Sixth People's Hospital of Nansha, Xingye Road No. 7, Dagang Town, Nansha, Guangzhou 511470, People's Republic of China. [2]The Department of Pulmonary, Critical Care and Sleep, Yale School of Medicine, New Haven, USA.

References
1. Ramello A, Vitale C, Marangella M. Epidemiology of nephrolithiasis. J Nephrol. 2000;S(3):S45–50.

2. Alaya A, Nouri A, Belgith M, Saad H, Jouini R, Najjar MF. Changes in urinary stone composition in the Tunisian population: a retrospective study of 1,301 cases. Ann Lab Med. 2012;32(3):177–83.

3. Zeng Q, He Y. Age-specific prevalence of kidney stones in Chinese urban inhabitants. Urolithiasis. 2013;41:91–3.

4. Romero V, Akpinar H, Assimos DG. Kidney stones: a global picture of prevalence, incidence, and associated risk factors. Rev Urol. 2010;12:e86–96.

5. Ning X, Zhan C, Yang Y, Yang L, Tu J, Gu H, et al. Secular trends in prevalence of overweight and obesity among adults in rural Tianjin, China from 1991 to 2011: a population-based study. PLoS One. 2014;9:e116019.

6. Hesse A, Brandle E, Wilbert D, Kohrmann KU, Alken P. Study on the prevalence and incidence of urolithiasis in Germany comparing the years 1979 vs. 2000. Eur Urol. 2003;44:709–13.

7. Ma RH, Luo XB, Li Q, Zhong HQ. The systematic classification of urinary stones combine-using FTIR and SEM-EDAX. Int J Surg. 2017;41:150–61.

8. Lieske JC, Rule AD, Krambeck AE, Williams JC, Bergstralh EJ, Mehta RA, et al. Stone composition as a function of age and sex. Clin J Am Soc Nephrol. 2014;9:2141–6.

9. Scales CD Jr, Smith AC, Hanley JM, Saigal CS. Prevalence of kidney stones in the United States. Eur Urol. 2012;62:160–5.

10. Trinchieri A, Coppi F, Montanari E, Del Nero A, Zanetti G, Pisani E. Increase in the prevalence of symptomatic upper urinary tract stones during the last ten years. Eur Urol. 2000;37:23–5.

11. Rosenstein I, Osborn RS, Hopewell JP, Hamilton-Miller JM, Brumfitt W. Bacteriological and crystallographical analysis of urinary calculi: aid to patient management. J R Soc Med. 1984;77(6):478–82.

12. Holmes RP, Knight J, Assimos DG. Lowering urinary oxalate excretion to decrease calcium oxalate stone disease. Urolithiasis. 2016;44(1):27–32.

13. Lieske JC, Tremaine WJ, De Simone C, O'Connor HM, Li X, Bergstralh EJ, et al. Diet, but not oral probiotics, effectively reduces urinary oxalate excretion and calcium oxalate supersaturation. Kidney Int. 2010;78:1178–85.

14. Borghi L, Schianchi T, Meschi T, Guerra A, Allegri F, Maggiore U, et al. Comparison of two diets for the prevention of recurrent stones in idiopathic hypercalciuria. N Engl J Med. 2002;346:77–84.

15. Yang Y, Deng Y, Wang Y. Major geogenic factors controlling geographical clustering of urolithiasis in China. Sci Total Environ. 2016;571:1164–71.

16. Li D, Wen L, Jiang S, Song T, Wang K. Responses of soil nutrients and microbial communities to three restoration strategies in a karst area, Southwest China. J Environ Manag. 2018;207:456–64.

17. Carpentier X, Daudon M, Traxer O, Jungers P, Mazouyes A, Matzen G, et al. Relationships between carbonation rate of carbapatite and morphologic characteristics of calcium phosphate stones and etiology. Urology. 2009; 73(5):968–75.

18. Mandel N, Mandel I, Fryjoff K, Rejniak T, Mandel G. Conversion of calcium oxalate to calcium phosphate with recurrent stone episodes. J Urol. 2003; 169(6):2026–9.

19. Knoll T, Schubert AB, Fahlenkamp D, Leusmann DB, Wendt-Nordahl G, Schubert G. Urolithiasis through the ages: data on more than 200, 000 urinary stone analyses. J Urol. 2011;185(4):1304–11.

20. Marchini GS, Sarkissian C, Tian D, Gebreselassie S, Monga M. Gout, stone composition and urinary stone risk: a matched case comparative study. J Urol. 2013;189:1334.

21. Daudon M, Doré JC, Jungers P, Lacour B. Changes in stone composition according to age and gender of patients: A multivariate epidemiological approach. Urol Res. 2004;32:241–7.

22. Maalouf NM, Sakhaee K, Parks JH, Coe FL, Adams-Huet B, Pak CY. Association of urinary pH with body weight in nephrolithiasis. Kidney Int. 2004;65:1422–5.

23. Abate N, Chandalia M, Cabo-Chan AV Jr, Moe OW, Sakhaee K. The metabolic syndrome and uric acid nephrolithiasis: novel features of renal manifestation of insulin resistance. Kidney Int. 2004;65:386–92.

24. Daudon M, Traxer O, Conort P, Lacour B, Jungers P. Type 2 diabetes increases the risk for uric acid stones. J Am Soc Nephrol. 2006;17:2026–33.

25. Ordon M, Andonian S, Blew B, Schuler T, Chew B, Pace KT. CUA guideline: management of ureteral calculi. Can Urol Assoc J. 2015;9(11–12):E837–51.

26. Trinchieri A, Montanari E. Prevalence of renal uric acid stones in the adult. Urolithiasis. 2017;45(6):553–62.

27. Alvarez Arroyo MV, Traba ML, Rapado A. Hypocitraturia as a pathogenic risk factor in the mixed (calcium oxalate/uric acid) renal stones. Urol Int. 1992; 48(3):342–6.

28. Friedlander JI, Moreira DM, Hartman C, Elsamra SE, Smith AD, Okeke Z. Comparison of the metabolic profile of mixed calcium oxalate/uric acid stone formers to that of pure calcium oxalate and pure uric acid stone formers. Urology. 2014;84(2):289–94.

29. Soucie JM, Thun MJ, Coates RJ, McClellan W, Austin H. Demographic and geographic variability of kidney stones in the United States. Kidney Int. 1994;46(3):893–9.

30. Tasian GE, Pulido JE, Gasparrini A, Saigal CS, Horton BP, Landis JR, et al. Daily mean temperature and clinical kidney stone presentation in five U.S. metropolitan areas: a time-series analysis. Environ Health Perspect. 2014; 122(10):1081–7.

31. Wilson EV, Bushiri MJ, Vaidyan VK. Characterization and FTIR spectral studies of human urinary stones from southern India. Spectrochim Acta A Mol Biomol Spectrosc. 2010;77(2):442–5.

32. Curhan GC, Willett WC, Speizer FE, Stampfer MJ. Twenty-four-hour urine chemistries and the risk of kidney stones among women and men. Kidney Int. 2001;59:2290–8.

33. Kato Y, Yamaguchi S, Yachiku S, Nakazono S, Hori J, Wada N, et al. Changes in urinary parameters after oral administration of potassium-sodium citrate and magnesium oxide to prevent urolithiasis. Urology. 2004;63:7–11 discussion 11–12.

34. Kasaoka S, Kitano T, Hanai M, Futatsuka M, Esashi T. Effect of dietary magnesium level on nephrocalcinosis and growth in rats. J Nutr Sci Vitaminol (Tokyo). 1998;44:503–14.

35. Barcelo P, Wuhl O, Servitge E, Rousaud A, Pak CY. Randomized double-blind study of potassium citrate in idiopathic hypocitraturic calcium nephrolithiasis. J Urol. 1993;150:1761–4.

36. Słojewski M, Czerny B, Safranow K, Jakubowska K, Olszewska M, Pawlik A, et al. Microelements in stones, urine, and hair of stone formers: a new key to the puzzle of lithogenesis? Biol Trace Elem Res. 2010;137:301–16.

37. Meyer JL, Angino EE. The role of trace metals in calcium urolithiasis. Investig Urol. 1977;14:347–50.

38. Heilberg IP, Goldfarb DS. Optimum nutrition for kidney stone disease. Adv Chronic Kidney Dis. 2013;20:165–74.

39. Tang J, McFann K, Chonchol M. Dietary zinc intake and kidney stone formation: evaluation of NHANES III. Am J Nephrol. 2012;36:549–53.

40. Atakan IH, Kaplan M, Seren G, Aktoz T, Gül H, Inci O. Serum, urinary and stone zinc, iron, magnesium and copper levels in idiopathic calcium oxalate stone patients. Int Urol Nephrol. 2007;39:351–6.

41. Najda J, Gmiński J, Drózdz M, Danch A. The action of excessive, inorganic silicon (Si) on the mineral metabolism of calcium (ca) and magnesium (mg). Biol Trace Elem Res. 1993;37:107–14.

42. Haddad FS, Kouyoumdjian A. Silica stones in humans. Urol Int. 1986;41:70–6.

Permissions

The contributors of this book come from diverse backgrounds, making this book a truly international effort. This book will bring forth new frontiers with its revolutionizing research information and detailed analysis of the nascent developments around the world.

We would like to thank all the contributing authors for lending their expertise to make the book truly unique. They have played a crucial role in the development of this book. Without their invaluable contributions this book wouldn't have been possible. They have made vital efforts to compile up to date information on the varied aspects of this subject to make this book a valuable addition to the collection of many professionals and students.

This book was conceptualized with the vision of imparting up-to-date information and advanced data in this field. To ensure the same, a matchless editorial board was set up. Every individual on the board went through rigorous rounds of assessment to prove their worth. After which they invested a large part of their time researching and compiling the most relevant data for our readers.

The editorial board has been involved in producing this book since its inception. They have spent rigorous hours researching and exploring the diverse topics which have resulted in the successful publishing of this book. They have passed on their knowledge of decades through this book. To expedite this challenging task, the publisher supported the team at every step. A small team of assistant editors was also appointed to further simplify the editing procedure and attain best results for the readers.

Apart from the editorial board, the designing team has also invested a significant amount of their time in understanding the subject and creating the most relevant covers. They scrutinized every image to scout for the most suitable representation of the subject and create an appropriate cover for the book.

The publishing team has been an ardent support to the editorial, designing and production team. Their endless efforts to recruit the best for this project, has resulted in the accomplishment of this book. They are a veteran in the field of academics and their pool of knowledge is as vast as their experience in printing. Their expertise and guidance has proved useful at every step. Their uncompromising quality standards have made this book an exceptional effort. Their encouragement from time to time has been an inspiration for everyone.

The publisher and the editorial board hope that this book will prove to be a valuable piece of knowledge for researchers, students, practitioners and scholars across the globe.

List of Contributors

Jae Heon Kim, Seung Whan Doo, Won Jae Yang and Yun Seob Song
Department of Urology, Soonchunhyang University Hospital, Soonchunhyang University College of Medicine, Seoul, Korea

Soon Hyo Kwon
Department of Nephrology, Soonchunhyang University Hospital, Soonchunhyang University College of Medicine, Seoul, Korea

Eun Seop Song
Department of Obstetrics and Gynecology, Inha University School of Medicine, Incheon, Korea

Hong Jun Lee
Medical Research Institute, Chung-Ang University College of Medicine, Seoul, Korea

Ik Sung Lim
Department of Industrial Management and Engineering, Namseoul University College of Engineering, Cheonan, Korea

Hyun Hwang
North London Collegiate School, Jeju, Korea

Zlatibor Loncar, Vladimir Djukic and Branislav Olujic
Emergency Centre, Clinical Centre of Serbia, Faculty of Medicine, University of Belgrade, Pasterova 2, 11000 Belgrade, Serbia

Vladan Zivaljevic, Aleksandar Diklic, Nikola Slijepcevic and Ivan Paunovic
Centre for Endocrine Surgery, Clinical Centre of Serbia, Faculty of Medicine, University of Belgrade, Pasterova 2, 11000 Belgrade, Serbia

Tatjana Pekmezovic
Institute of Epidemiology, Faculty of Medicine, University of Belgrade, Visegradska 26A, Belgrade 11000, Serbia

Svetislav Tatic and Dusko Dundjerovic
Institute of Pathology, Faculty of Medicine, University of Belgrade, Dr Subotica 1, 11000 Belgrade, Serbia

Celeste De Monte, Simone Carradori and Arianna Granese
Department of Drug Chemistry and Technologies, Sapienza University of Rome, P.le A. Moro 5, Rome 00185, Italy

Giovanni Battista Di Pierro and Costantino Leonardo
Department of Obstetrics, Gynecology and Urology, Sapienza University of Rome, Viale del Policlinico 155, Rome 00161, Italy
Department of Urology, Ospedale Sant'Andrea, Sapienza

Cosimo De Nunzio
University of Rome, Via di Grottarossa 1035/1039, Rome 00189, Italy

Hasan S Sağlam, Şükrü Kumsar, Salih Budak, Hüseyin Aydemir and Öztuğ Adsan
Department of Urology, Faculty of Medicine, Sakarya University and Training and Research Hospital, 54100 Sakarya, Turkey

Osman Köse
Department of Urology, Faculty of Medicine, Sakarya University and Training and Research Hospital, 54100 Sakarya, Turkey
Beyaz Kent Sitesi, Beşköprü M. Girne C., 54100 Sakarya, Turkey

Tzu-Ping Lin, Yen-Hwa Chang, William JS Huang, Alex TL Lin and Kuang-Kuo Chen
Department of Urology, Taipei Veterans General Hospital, Taipei, Taiwan
Department of Urology, National Yang-Ming University School of Medicine, Taipei, Taiwan Shu-Tien Urological Science Research Center, Taipei, Taiwan

Ching-Hsin Chang
Department of Urology, Taipei Veterans General Hospital, Taipei, Taiwan
Department of Urology, Taipei Medical University Hospital, Taipei, Taiwan
Graduate Institute of Medical Sciences, College of Medicine, Taipei Medical University, Taipei, Taiwan

Daiki Ueno, Kazuhide Makiyama, Hiroyuki Yamanaka and Yoshinobu Kubota
Department of Urology, Yokohama City University School of Medicine, 3-9 Fukuura, Kanagawa-ku, Yokohama, Kanagawa 236-0004, Japan

Takashi Ijiri and Hideo Yokota
Image Processing Research Tea, RIKEN, Wako, Japan

Doreth T. A. M Teunissen, Marjolein M. Stegeman, Hans H. Bor and Toine A. L. M Lagro-Janssen
Department Primary and Community Care, Gender & Women's Health, Radboud University Medical Centre Nijmegen, Internal postal code 118, 6500 HB Nijmegen, The Netherlands

Meiling Chen and Yongzhong He
Urology Department, Fifth Affiliated Hospital, Guangzhou Medical University, 621 Gangwan Road, Huangpu District, Guangzhou, Guangdong 510700, China

Dehui Lai and Xun Li
Urology Department, Fifth Affiliated Hospital, Guangzhou Medical University, 621 Gangwan Road, Huangpu District, Guangzhou, Guangdong 510700, China
Translational Medical Center, Minimally Invasive Technology and Product, Guangzhou Medical University, Guangzhou, Guangdong, China

J. Koenig, S. Sevinc, C. Frohme, H. Heers, R. Hofmann and A. Hegele
Department of Urology and Pediatric Urology, University hospital Marburg, Philipps University, Marburg, Germany

Stephanie C Knüpfer, Martina D Liechti, Marc P Schneider, Elena Miramontes and Thomas M Kessler
Neuro-Urology, Spinal Cord Injury Center & Research, University of Zürich, Balgrist University Hospital, Forchstrasse 340, 8008 Zürich, Switzerland

Livio Mordasini, Dominik Abt and Daniel S Engeler
Department of Urology, Cantonal Hospital St. Gallen, St. Gallen, Switzerland

Jens Wöllner and Jürgen Pannek
Neuro-Urology, Swiss Paraplegic Center, Nottwil, Switzerland

Bernhard Kiss and Fiona C Burkhard
Department of Urology, University of Bern, Bern, Switzerland

Alfons G Kessels
Department of Clinical Epidemiology and Medical Technology Assessment, Maastricht University Medical Center, Maastricht, The Netherlands

Lucas M Bachmann
Medignition Inc., Research Consultants, Zug, Switzerland

Michele Rossi, Gianluca Maria Varano, Gianluigi Orgera and Florindo Laurino
Department of Radiology Interventional Radiology Unit, Ospedale Sant'Andrea, University "La Sapienza", Via di Grottarossa 1035/1039 00189, Rome, Italy

Alberto Rebonato
Department of Surgery, Radiology, and Odontostomatology Sciences, Santa Maria della Misericordia University Hospital, University of Perugia, Sant'Andrea delle Fratte, 06129 Perugia, Italy

Cosimo De Nunzio
Division of Urology, Ospedale Sant'Andrea, University "La Sapienza", Roma Via di, Grottarossa 1035/1039 00189, Rome, Italy

Lu Tian, Hongkun Zhang, Wei Jin and Ming Li
Department of Vascular Surgery, the First Affiliated Hospital of Medical College, Zhejiang University, Hangzhou 310003, China

Shanwen Chen
Department of Urology, the First Affiliated Hospital of Medical College, Zhejiang University, No. 79 Qing Chun Road, HangZhou 310003, China

Gaoyue Zhang
Department of Urology, the Second Affiliated Hospital of Zhejiang Chinese Medical University, Hangzhou 310005, China

Jae Heon Kim and Yun Seob Song
Department of Urology, Soonchunhyang University Hospital, 657 Hannam-Dong, Yongsan-Gu, Seoul 140-743, Korea

Sun Young Park and Mun Gyu Kim
Department of Anesthesiology and Pain Medicine, Soonchunhyang University Hospital, Seoul, Korea

Hoon Choi
Department of Urology, Korea University Hospital, Ansan, Korea

Dan Song and Sung Woo Cho
Department of Surgery, Soonchunhyang University Hospital, Seoul, Korea

Sigve Andersen, Tom Donnem and Roy M Bremnes
Institute of Clinical Medicine, The Arctic University of Norway, Tromso, Norway
Department Oncology, University Hospital of North Norway, Tromso 9038, Norway

Nora Ness
Institute of Medical Biology, The Arctic University of Norway, Tromso, Norway

Elin Richardsen and Lill-Tove Busund
Institute of Medical Biology, The Arctic University of Norway, Tromso, Norway
Department Pathology, University Hospital of North Norway, Tromso, Norway

Yngve Nordby
Institute of Clinical Medicine, The Arctic University of Norway, Tromso, Norway
Department of Urology, University Hospital of North Norway, Tromso, Norway

Øystein Størkersen
Department Pathology, St. Olavs Hospital, Trondheim University Hospital, Trondheim, Norway

Khalid Al-Shibli
Department Pathology, Nordland Hospital, Bodoe, Norway

Helena Bertilsson and Anders Angelsen
Department of Urology, St. Olavs Hospital, Trondheim University Hospital, Trondheim, Norway
Institute of Cancer research and Molecular Medicine, Norwegian University of Science and Technology, Trondheim, Norway

Mário Maciel de Lima Jr and Mário Maciel de Lima
Department of Urology, Coronel Mota Hospital, Rua Levindo Inácio de Oliveira, 1547, Paraviana, Boa Vista, RR CEP: 69307-272, Brazil

Fabiana Granja
Biodiversity Research Center, Federal University of Roraima (CBio/UFRR), Boa Vista, Brazil

Jae Heon Kim, Hwa Yeon Sun, Seung Whan Doo, Jong Hyun Yoon, Won Jae Yang and Yun Seob Song
Department of Urology, Soonchunhyang University College of Medicine, Seoul Hospital, 59, Daesagwan-ro, Yongsan-gu, Seoul 140-743, The Republic of Korea

Hoon Choi
Department of Urology, Korea University College of Medicine, Ansan Hospital, Ansan, Korea

Byung Wook Yoo
Department of Family Medicine, Soonchunhyang University School of Medicine, Seoul, Korea

Joyce Mary Kim
International Clinic Center, Soonchunhyang University Hospital, Seoul, Korea

Soon-Sun Kwon
Biomedical Research Institute, Seoul National University Bundang Hospital, Seongnam, South Korea

Eun Seop Song
Department of Obstetrics and Gynecology, Inha University School of Medicine, Incheon, Korea

Hong Jun Lee
Medical Research Institute, Chung-Ang University College of Medicine, Seoul, Korea

Ik Sung Lim
Department of Industrial Management and Engineering, Namseoul University College of Engineering, Cheonan, Korea

Shay Golan, Andrei Nadu and David Lifshitz
Institute of Urology, Rabin Medical Center, Petah Tikva, and Sackler Faculty of Medicine, Tel Aviv University, Tel Aviv, Israel

Toshikazu Tanaka, Shingo Hatakeyama, Hayato Yamamoto, Takuma Narita, Itsuto Hamano, Teppei Matsumoto, Osamu Soma, Yuki Tobisawa, Takahiro Yoneyama and Takuya Koie
Department of Urology, Hirosaki University Graduate School of Medicine, 5 Zaifu-chou, Hirosaki 036-8562, Japan

Tohru Yoneyama and Yasuhiro Hashimoto
Department of Advanced Transplant and Regenerative Medicine, Hirosaki University Graduate School of Medicine, Hirosaki, Japan

Chikara Ohyama
Department of Urology, Hirosaki University Graduate School of Medicine, 5 Zaifu-chou, Hirosaki 036-8562, Japan
Department of Advanced Transplant and Regenerative Medicine, Hirosaki University Graduate School of Medicine, Hirosaki, Japan

Yuriko Terayama and Tomihisa Funyu
Department of Urology, Oyokyo Kidney Research Institute, Hirosaki, Japan

Ippei Takahashi and Shigeyuki Nakaji
Department of Social Medicine, Hirosaki University School of Medicine, Hirosaki, Japan

Suzanne Ryan and Claire Boswell-Ruys
Neuroscience Research Australia [NeuRA] and the University of New South Wales, Sydney, Australia

Bonsan Bonne Lee
Neuroscience Research Australia [NeuRA] and the University of New South Wales, Sydney, Australia
Department of Spinal and Rehabilitation Medicine, Prince of Wales Hospital, Sydney, Australia

Swee-Ling Toh
Department of Spinal and Rehabilitation Medicine, Prince of Wales Hospital, Sydney, Australia
School of Public Health, University of Sydney, Sydney, Australia

Judy M. Simpson
School of Public Health, University of Sydney, Sydney, Australia

Kate Clezy
Department of Infectious Diseases, Prince of Wales Hospital, Sydney, Australia

Laetitia Bossa
Neuroscience Research Australia [NeuRA] and the University of New South Wales, Sydney, Australia
Centre for Marine Bio-Innovation, University of New South Wales, Sydney, Australia

Gerard Weber
Royal Rehabilitation Centre Sydney, Sydney, Australia

Jasbeer Kaur, Mark Tudehope and George Kotsiou
Royal North Shore Hospital, Sydney, Australia

Obaydullah Marial
Department of Spinal and Rehabilitation Medicine, Prince of Wales Hospital, Sydney, Australia
Royal Rehabilitation Centre Sydney, Sydney, Australia
Royal North Shore Hospital, Sydney, Australia

Stephen Goodall
Centre for Health Economics Research and Evaluation [CHERE], University of Technology Sydney, Sydney, Australia

Scott A. Rice
Centre for Marine Bio-Innovation, University of New South Wales, Sydney, Australia
The Singapore Centre for Life Sciences Engineering and the School of Biological Sciences, Nanyang Technological University, Singapore, Singapore

James Middleton
John Walsh Centre for Rehabilitation Research, Kolling Institute, Northern Sydney Local Health District, St Leonards, NSW 2065, Australia
Sydney Medical School Northern, University of Sydney, Sydney, Australia

Yanping Wang, Alicia Olivant Fisher, Deborah Stabley and Katia Sol-Church
Nemours Biomedical Research, Nemours /Alfred I. duPont Hospital for Children, Wilmington, DE 19803, USA

T. Ernesto Figueroa, Ahmad H. BaniHani and Jennifer A. Hagerty
Division of Urology, Nemours/Alfred I. duPont Hospital for Children, Wilmington, DE 19803, USA

Julia Spencer Barthold
Nemours Biomedical Research, Nemours /Alfred I. duPont Hospital for Children, Wilmington, DE 19803, USA
Division of Urology, Nemours/Alfred I. duPont Hospital for Children, Wilmington, DE 19803, USA

Jin Li, Rosetta M. Chiavacci, Kisha R. Harden, Debra J. Abrams and Cecilia E. Kim
Center for Applied Genomics, The Children's Hospital of Philadelphia, Philadelphia, PA 19104, USA

Thomas F. Kolon
Division of Urology, The Children's Hospital of Philadelphia, Philadelphia, PA 19104, USA

Hakon Hakonarson
Center for Applied Genomics, The Children's Hospital of Philadelphia, Philadelphia, PA 19104, USA
Division of Genetics, The Children's Hospital of Philadelphia, Philadelphia, PA 19104, USA
Department of Pediatrics, Perelman School of Medicine, University of Pennsylvania, Philadelphia, PA 19104, USA

Marcella Devoto
Division of Genetics, The Children's Hospital of Philadelphia, Philadelphia, PA 19104, USA
Department of Pediatrics, Perelman School of Medicine, University of Pennsylvania, Philadelphia, PA 19104, USA
Department of Biostatistics and Epidemiology, Perelman School of Medicine, University of Pennsylvania, Philadelphia, PA 19104, USA
Department of Molecular Medicine, Sapienza University, Rome, Italy

Ricardo Gonzalez
Division of Urology, Nemours/Alfred I. duPont Hospital for Children, Wilmington, DE 19803, USA
Auf der Bult Kinder- und Jugendkrankenhaus, Hannover, Germany

Paul H. Noh
Division of Urology, Nemours/Alfred I. duPont Hospital for Children, Wilmington, DE 19803, USA
Division of Pediatric Urology, Cincinnati Children's Hospital Medical Center, Cincinnati, OH, USA

Kazuhide Makiyama, Hiroji Uemura and Masahiro Yao
Department of Urology, Yokohama City University, Graduate School of Medicine, 3-9 Fukuura, Kanazawa-ku, Yokohama, Kanagawa 2360004, Japan

Kentaro Sakamaki
Departments of Biostatistics, Yokohama City University Graduate School of Medicine, Yokohama, Japan

Shinnosuke Kuroda, Hideyuki Terao and Junichi Matsuzaki
Department of Urology, Ohguchi Higashi General Hospital, Yokohama, Japan

Takashi Kawahara and Hiroki Ito
Department of Urology, Yokohama City University, Graduate School of Medicine, 3-9 Fukuura, Kanazawa-ku, Yokohama, Kanagawa 2360004, Japan

Department of Urology, Ohguchi Higashi General Hospital, Yokohama, Japan

Hiroshi Miyamoto
Departments of Pathology and Urology, Johns Hopkins University School of Medicine, Baltimore, USA

Daniel S. Engeler, Daniel Meyer, Dominik Abt and Hans-Peter Schmid
Department of Urology, Cantonal Hospital St. Gallen, St. Gallen, Switzerland

Stefanie Müller
Department of Neurology, Cantonal Hospital St. Gallen, St. Gallen, Switzerland

Shinobu Shimizu, Yachiyo Kuwatsuka and Masaaki Mizuno
Center for Advanced Medicine and Clinical Research, Nagoya University Hospital, 65 Tsurumai-cho, Showa-ku, Nagoya, Aichi 466-8560, Japan

Tokunori Yamamoto, Yasuhito Funahashi, Yoshihisa Matsukawa and Momokazu Gotoh
Department of Urology, Nagoya University Graduate School of Medicine, 65 Tsurumai-cho, Showa-ku, Nagoya, Aichi 466-8550, Japan

Yuzuru Kamei and Keisuke Takanari
Department of Plastic and Reconstructive Surgery, Nagoya University Graduate School of Medicine, 65 Tsurumai-cho, Showa-ku, Nagoya, Aichi 466-8550, Japan

Kazuhiro Toriyama
Department of Plastic and Reconstructive Surgery, Nagoya University Graduate School of Medicine, 65 Tsurumai-cho, Showa-ku, Nagoya, Aichi 466-8550, Japan
Department of Plastic and Reconstructive Surgery, Nagoya City University Hospital, 1-Kawasumi, Mizuho-cho, Mizuho-ku, Nagoya, Aichi 467-8602, Japan

Kazutaka Narimoto
Department of Integrative Cancer Therapy and Urology, Kanazawa University Graduate School of Medical Sciences, 13-1 Takara-machi, Kanazawa, Ishikawa 920-8640, Japan

Tomonori Yamanishi
Department of Urology, Continence Center, Dokkyo Medical University, 880 Kita-Kobayashi, Mibu-machi, Shimotsuga-gun, Tochigi 321-0293, Japan

Osamu Ishizuka
Department of Urology, Shinshu University School of Medicine, 3-1-1 Asahi, Matsumoto 390-8621, Japan

Shinobu Nakayama
Center for Advanced Medicine and Clinical Research, Nagoya University Hospital, 65 Tsurumai-cho, Showa-ku, Nagoya, Aichi 466-8560, Japan
Department of Clinical Research Management, Clinical Research Center, National Hospital Organization Nagoya Medical Center, 4-1-1, Sannomaru, Naka-ku, Nagoya Aichi 460-0001, Japan

Akihiro Hirakawa
Center for Advanced Medicine and Clinical Research, Nagoya University Hospital, 65 Tsurumai-cho, Showa-ku, Nagoya, Aichi 466-8560, Japan
Department of Biostatistics and Bioinformatics, Graduate School of Medicine, The University of Tokyo, 7-3-1 Hongo, Bunkyo-ku, Tokyo 113-0033, Japan

Stéphanie van der Lely, Martina Stefanovic, Melanie R. Schmidhalter, Martina D. Liechti, Thomas M. Kessler and Ulrich Mehnert
Neuro-Urology, Spinal Cord Injury Center & Research, University of Zürich, Balgrist University Hospital, Forchstrasse 340, 8008 Zürich, Switzerland

Marta Pittavino and Reinhard Furrer
Institute of Mathematics, University of Zürich, Winterthurerstrasse 190, 8057 Zürich, Switzerland

Martin Schubert
Neurophysiology, Spinal Cord Injury Center & Research, University of Zürich, Balgrist University Hospital, Forchstrasse 340, 8008 Zürich, Switzerland

Christopher Naugler
Department of Pathology and Laboratory Medicine, University of Calgary, Calgary, AB, Canada
Department of Family Medicine, University of Calgary, Calgary, AB, Canada

Thomas P. Griener and Wilson W. Chan
Department of Pathology and Laboratory Medicine, University of Calgary, Calgary, AB, Canada
Division of Microbiology, Department of Pathology and Laboratory Medicine, University of Calgary, Calgary, AB, Canada

Deirdre L. Church
Department of Pathology and Laboratory Medicine, University of Calgary, Calgary, AB, Canada

Division of Microbiology, Department of Pathology and Laboratory Medicine, University of Calgary, Calgary, AB, Canada
Department of Medicine, University of Calgary, Calgary, AB, Canada
1W-410, Diagnostic and Scientific Centre, 9-3535 Research Road NW, Calgary, AB T2L 2K8, Canada

Giorgio Bozzini, Mauro Seveso, Alberto Mandressi and Gianluigi Taverna
Departmentt of Urology, Humanitas Mater Domini, Via Gerenzano 2, I - 21053 Castellanza, Varese, Italy

Marco Provenzano
Humanitas University, Milan, Italy

Giorgio Guazzoni
Humanitas University, Milan, Italy
Department of Urology, Humanitas Research Hospital, Milan, Italy

Nicolò Buffi and Giovanni Lughezzani
Department of Urology, Humanitas Research Hospital, Milan, Italy

Junming Zheng, Jiangang Pan, Yi Qin and Xing Zhou
Department of Urology, The Second Affiliated Hospital of Guangzhou Medical University, 250 Changgang road, Guangzhou 510260, China

Jiale Huang
School of Mechanical and Automotive Engineering, South China University of Technology, Guangzhou, China

Yun Luo and Xin Gao
Department of Urology, Third Affiliated Hospital of Sun Yat-sen University, Guangzhou 510630, China

Feng Guo, Tianyou Li, Wei Liu, Gang Wang and Rongde Wu
Department of Pediatric Surgery, Shandong Provincial Hospital Affiliated to Shandong University, 324 Jingwu Road, Jinan 250021, Shandong Province, People's Republic of China

Rui Ma
Shandong Medical Imaging Research Institute, Medical School of Shandong University, Jinan, Shandong Province, People's Republic of China

Gaurav Aggarwal and Samiran Das Adhikary
Department of Urology, Apollo Hospital, Bhubaneshwar 751005, Odisha, India

Magdalena Stania, Daria Chmielewska, Krystyna Kwaśna, Agnieszka Smykla and Jakub Taradaj
Department of Physiotherapy Basics, Jerzy Kukuczka Academy of Physical Education, Mikołowska 72a, 40-065 Katowice, Poland

Grzegorz Juras
Department of Human Motor Behavior, Jerzy Kukuczka Academy of Physical Education, Mikołowska 72a, 40-065 Katowice, Poland

Frank C. Lin and Jonathan R. Walker
Division of Urology, Department of Surgery, University of Arizona, 1501 N. Campbell Ave, Tucson, AZ 85724, USA

Jamie S. Lin
Renal-Electrolyte and Hypertension Division, Department of Medicine, University of Pennsylvania, Perelman School of Medicine, 3400 Civic Blvd, Philadelphia, PA 19104, USA

Samuel Kim
Division of Cardiothoracic Surgery, Department of Surgery, University of Arizona, 1501 N. Campbell Ave, Tucson, AZ 85724, USA

Evaldo Favi
Transplant Unit, Renal Department, Royal London Hospital, Whitechapel Road, London E1 1BB, UK

Samuele Iesari
General Surgery, Department of Biotechnological and Applied Clinical Sciences, University of L'Aquila, Via Pompeo Spennati, 67100 L'Aquila, Italy

Alessandro Cina
Department of Bioimaging, Università Cattolica del "Sacro Cuore", Policlinico Universitario "Agostino Gemelli", Largo Agostino Gemelli 8, 00168 Rome, Italy

Franco Citterio
Renal Transplant Unit, Department of Surgery, Università Cattolica del "Sacro Cuore", Policlinico Universitario "Agostino Gemelli", Largo Agostino Gemelli 8, 00168 Rome, Italy

Hamdan Alhazmi and Abdullah Fouda Neel
Division of Urology, Department of Surgery, College of Medicine and King Saud University Medical City, King Saud University, Riyadh 11472, Kingdom of Saudi Arabia

Rui-hong Ma, Xiao-bing Luo and Hai-qiang Zhong
The Department of Clinical Laboratory, The Sixth People's Hospital of Nansha, Xingye Road No. 7, Dagang Town, Nansha, Guangzhou 511470 People's Republic of China

Qin Li
The Department of Pulmonary, Critical Care and Sleep, Yale School of Medicine, New Haven, USA

Index

A

Adipose-derived Regenerative Cells, 150-151, 154-156

Adrenalectomy, 8-11, 13, 119, 122

Adrenocortical Carcinoma, 7, 13

Alpha-blockers, 102, 172, 177

Anesthesia, 32, 53, 63, 71, 75, 79, 81-84, 153

Aneurysm, 70-74, 191

Anterior Vaginal Wall, 25-29

Aortic Calcification, 114-122

Asymptomatic Renal Stone, 52

Atherosclerosis, 70, 115, 122

Azoospermia, 135, 138

B

Beclomethasone Dipropionate, 171-172, 174, 177-178

Benign Prostate Enlargement, 31

Benign Prostatic Hyperplasia, 14, 19, 23-24, 37, 107-108, 163, 167, 178, 186-187

Biofilm, 124, 127

Biopsy, 8, 10, 32-33, 35, 93, 109-113, 172, 211

C

Calcium Oxalate Stones, 221-225

Chemotherapy, 8, 111, 188-189

Chronic Renal Failure, 1, 4-6, 110

Computed Tomography, 38, 42, 57, 71-73, 109, 113, 115-116, 121, 188-191, 207-208, 215

Cryptorchidism, 131-132, 135-137

Cystoscopy, 58, 63, 65-66, 79-84, 110, 140, 145, 193, 211

D

Diaphragmatic Ureteral Herniation, 206, 208

Dj Stenting, 192-193, 195

E

Electrical Stimulation, 145, 157-159

Electromyography, 196-198, 200, 204

Embolization, 70-71, 73-75, 77

Endovascular Treatment, 71, 78

F

Fistula, 26, 28-29, 215

Fourier Transform Infrared Spectroscopy, 221, 229

G

Genital Lesions, 96-97, 99

Genome, 122, 131-133, 135-138

H

Hemodialysis, 1, 5-6, 115, 122

Heterogeneity, 14, 65, 135, 169

Hydronephrosis, 54, 121, 126, 207, 209, 211, 217-220

Hypospadias, 132, 136

I

Inferior Vena Cava, 12, 75-77, 188-191

Intravesical Prostatic Protrusion, 179, 183-184, 186-187

L

Laser Diode Vaporization, 96-99

Lesion, 70, 77, 96-99, 110, 125, 188-189, 218

Lithotripsy, 52-53, 57

Lower Urinary Tract Symptoms, 14, 23, 37, 101, 107-108, 144, 149, 151, 157-158, 162-163, 167, 170, 178, 180, 186-187

M

Micturition, 48-49, 144-145, 147-149, 197

Mitotane, 7-13

N

Nephrectomy, 38-42, 71, 114-116, 188, 190-191, 207, 212, 215

Nephroureterectomy, 43, 109-113

Neurogenic Detrusor, 144, 148

Neurogenic Lower Urinary Tract Dysfunction, 64, 66, 144, 149, 162

Neuromodulation, 64-69, 144-145, 149

Nonbacterial Prostatitis, 171-173, 176, 178

Nutcracker Syndrome, 75, 78

P

Partial Nephrectomy, 38-42

Pelvic Floor Muscles, 196-197, 199-205

Pelvic Organ Prolapse, 25, 28-30

Penumbra, 70, 72-73

Perineural Infiltration, 85, 87, 89

Placebo, 22-23, 64-65, 84, 107, 123-125, 127, 130, 149, 152, 163, 172

Primary Care, 44-46, 51

Prognosis, 7, 12, 73, 92-93, 95, 113, 137, 179, 195, 212

Prophylaxis, 123-124, 145

Prostate Cancer, 21, 23, 85-86, 88-91, 93-95, 108, 152, 154, 156, 178

Prostatectomy, 37, 85-86, 92-95, 150-152, 154, 156, 163

R

Radical Prostatectomy, 85-86, 93-95, 150-152, 154, 156, 163

Radiotherapy, 8, 11, 13, 86, 89, 92, 94, 152, 187

Renal Artery Aneurysm, 70, 73-74

Retrograde Intrarenal Surgery, 52, 57

S

Sacral Neuromodulation, 64, 66, 68-69, 144-145, 149

Scanning Electron Microscopy, 221, 229

Sclerosis, 124-126, 130, 144-145, 149, 162, 197, 204

Serenoa Repens, 14, 16, 19-20, 23-24, 171-174, 176-178

Sphincter, 66-67, 144-146, 151, 153-156, 205

Sphincter Dyssynergia, 67, 144-146

Stent, 53-54, 56-57, 71, 73-80, 83, 111, 139-143, 192-194, 206-207, 209, 211, 218-219

Stent Migration, 75-78, 139, 142

Stent Removal, 79, 83, 193-194, 218-219

Stress Urinary Incontinence, 25, 29-30, 107, 150-152, 155-156, 196-198, 202-205

Supercritical Fluid, 14, 17-18, 23

Symptomatic Ureteral Stone, 52-54, 57

U

Ultrasonography, 27, 31, 33, 78, 102, 153-154, 187-188

Urea Clearance, 1-3, 5

Ureteral, 52-57, 79-80, 83-84, 111, 139-142, 195, 206-209, 211-212, 217-220, 223, 230

Ureteroscopy, 52, 57, 83, 109-113, 192-193, 207

Urethrocystoscopy, 58-63

Uric Acid Stones, 221-224, 226, 228, 230

Urinary Incontinence, 25, 28-30, 44, 46, 51, 69, 105, 107, 129, 144, 148, 150-152, 154-156, 162, 196-198, 202-205

Urinary Tract Symptoms, 14, 19, 23, 37, 101, 107-108, 144, 148-149, 151, 157-158, 162-163, 167, 170, 178, 180, 186-187

Urography, 109, 113, 139-140, 142, 193

Urolithiasis, 57, 79, 114-115, 119-122, 152, 221-222, 224, 230

Urothelial Carcinoma, 43, 109-110, 112-113

V

Vapoenucleation, 31-32, 34-37

www.ingramcontent.com/pod-product-compliance
Lightning Source LLC
Chambersburg PA
CBHW061259190326

41458CB00011B/3719